Current Clinical Psychiatry

Series Editor:

Jerrold F. Rosenbaum
Department of Psychiatry
Massachusetts General Hospital
Boston, MA, USA

Current Clinical Psychiatry offers concise, practical resources for clinical psychiatrists and other practitioners interested in mental health. Covering the full range of psychiatric disorders commonly presented in the clinical setting, the Current Clinical Psychiatry series encompasses such topics as cognitive behavioral therapy, anxiety disorders, psychotherapy, ratings and assessment scales, mental health in special populations, psychiatric uses of nonpsychiatric drugs, and others. Series editor Jerrold F. Rosenbaum, MD, is Chief of Psychiatry, Massachusetts General Hospital, and Stanley Cobb Professor of Psychiatry, Harvard Medical School.

More information about this series at http://www.springer.com/series/7634

Eric P. Hazen • Christopher J. McDougle
Editors

The Massachusetts General Hospital Guide to Medical Care in Patients with Autism Spectrum Disorder

Humana Press

Editors
Eric P. Hazen
Department of Psychiatry
Massachusetts General Hospital
Boston, MA
USA

Christopher J. McDougle
Department of Psychiatry
Massachusetts General Hospital
Boston, MA
USA

ISSN 2626-241X ISSN 2626-2398 (electronic)
Current Clinical Psychiatry
ISBN 978-3-319-94456-2 ISBN 978-3-319-94458-6 (eBook)
https://doi.org/10.1007/978-3-319-94458-6

Library of Congress Control Number: 2018959218

This Humana Press imprint is published by the registered company Springer Nature Switzerland AG
The registered company address is: Gewerbestrasse 11, 6330 Cham, Switzerland

Foreword

The Massachusetts General Hospital (MGH) is a nonprofit, Harvard Medical School-affiliated, academic medical center serving the entire New England area and beyond and is a founding member of Partners Health Care. Consisting of primary care and specialty physicians, a medical center in downtown Boston, suburban and regional partnering hospitals, specialty facilities, and community health centers, the MGH employs more than 25,000 individuals. In addition to approximately 1,000 inpatient beds, the MGH also provides quality health care at many outpatient sites. A key component of the MGH Mission Statement is to improve the health and well-being of the diverse communities we serve.

In 2013 the leadership group at the MGH made a hospital system-wide commitment to providing high-quality and accessible medical care for children, adolescents, and adults with autism spectrum disorder (ASD) and other developmental disorders. Expanding upon previous efforts that included the remediation of architectural barriers, installation of accessible medical equipment, and adoption of policies and procedures to improve access to health care for individuals with disabilities, a program called the Autism Care Collaborative (ACC) Project was launched. Dedicating personnel, including several executive leaders, and other resources to the ACC, committees were formed focusing on improving inpatient medical care, administrative processes, information technology/communication, and employee education. These work groups included individuals from numerous disciplines and departments throughout the hospital, as well as parent volunteers from the Lurie Center for Autism.

To date, the ACC Project has made significant progress towards achieving its initial goals. Two medical inpatient units in the care of adults with ASD and other developmental disorders with comorbid medical illness have been created and engage physicians, nurses, and other care team members with a passion for and interest and experience in providing medical care for these individuals. In parallel, improvements in the care of children and adolescents with ASD were made on the general pediatric units. Video teaching tools, including recommendations about how to interact with patients with ASD and their family members in a supportive manner, have been developed to educate all professional staff and employees of MGH. In addition, the ACC Project has developed a tool called the Autism Care Questionnaire (ACQ). The ACQ is designed to give medical staff a quick way to learn about patients' unique communication methods, sensory differences, and other potential stressors or safety concerns. Parents of outpatients with ASD and other developmental disorders are encouraged to complete this tool online at home or in the MGH outpatient clinics or hospital. The completed form is then added to the patient's electronic medical record. When a patient with ASD or other developmental disorder is admitted to the hospital, the ACQ can be quickly accessed and used to inform the treatment plan so that all staff can optimally interact with and provide care for the patient.

The ACC Project has also created a new position within the hospital called the Autism Patient Navigator. This position is currently filled by an experienced occupational therapist whose role is to act as a liaison to the patient and family and facilitate and coordinate the care provided during an inpatient admission for medical care, outpatient procedure, or diagnostic testing. The Navigator also serves as a catalyst to help individual departments in the hospital develop systems of care designed to better serve individuals with ASD and other developmental disorders and their family members.

When the ACC Project began its work, it became evident that many physicians, nurses, and other care providers throughout the hospital system knew very little about the diagnosis and treatment of comorbid medical illness in children, adolescents, and adults with ASD and other developmental disorders. We are confident that *The Massachusetts General Hospital Guide to Medical Care in Patients with Autism Spectrum Disorder*, edited by Eric P. Hazen, MD, and Christopher J. McDougle, MD, will address this knowledge gap for care providers at hospitals and outpatient sites not only throughout the MGH system but across the country and beyond, as well. In addition, we are hopeful that the knowledge gained through the ACC Project will prove helpful to other institutions across the nation that want to implement a similar program.

We would like to thank the Ruderman Family Foundation, the Working for Inclusive and Transformative Healthcare (WITH) Foundation, the Nancy Lurie Marks Family Foundation, and Matt and Eve Megargel for their generous support of the ACC Project.

Debra Burke, RN, DNP, MBA, NEA-BC
Senior Vice President for Patient Care and Chief Nurse
Jeanette Ives and Paul Erickson Endowed Chair in Nursing
Massachusetts General Hospital
Boston, MA, USA

Peter Greenspan, MD
Medical Director, MassGeneral Hospital for Children, Vice Chair
Department of Pediatrics, Massachusetts General Hospital, Assistant
Professor of Pediatrics, Harvard Medical School
Boston, MA, USA

Ronald E. Kleinman, MD
Physician-in-Chief, MassGeneral Hospital for Children, Chair
Department of Pediatrics, Massachusetts General Hospital
Charles Wilder Professor of Pediatrics, Harvard Medical School
Boston, MA, USA

Jerrold F. Rosenbaum, MD
Psychiatrist-in-Chief, Chair, Department of Psychiatry
Massachusetts General Hospital
Stanley Cobb Professor of Psychiatry, Harvard Medical School
Boston, MA, USA

Katrina Armstrong, MD, MSCE
Physician-in-Chief, Chair, Department of Medicine
Massachusetts General Hospital, Jackson Professor of Medicine
Harvard Medical School
Boston, MA, USA

Keith Lillemoe, MD
Surgeon-in-Chief, Chair, Department of Surgery
Massachusetts General Hospital, W. Gerald Austen Professor of Surgery
Harvard Medical School
Boston, MA, USA

Joan Sapir, EdM, MBA
Senior Vice President, Massachusetts General Hospital
Mass General Physicians Organization
Boston, MA, USA

W. Gerald Austen, MD
Surgeon-in-Chief Emeritus, Massachusetts General Hospital
Edward D. Churchill Distinguished Professor of Surgery
Harvard Medical School
Boston, MA, USA

Peter L. Slavin, MD
President, Massachusetts General Hospital
Professor of Health Care Policy, Harvard Medical School
Boston, MA, USA

Contents

Contributors

Robert E. Accordino, MD, MSc Child and Adolescent Psychiatry, Massachusetts General Hospital, Boston, MA, USA

Joseph H. Bahn, DPM Kaiser Permanente Northern California, Sacramento, CA, USA

Phil Bartel University of Pittsburgh School of Medicine, Pittsburgh, PA, USA

Nicole M. Benson, MD Child and Adolescent Psychiatry, Massachusetts General Hospital, Boston, MA, USA

Kathryn S. Brigham, MD Department of Pediatrics, Division of Adolescent and Young Adult Medicine, Massachusetts General Hospital, Boston, MA, USA

Jocelyn Carter, MD Department of Medicine, Massachusetts General Hospital, Boston, MA, USA

Anne-Frederique Chouinard, DMD, MSc Department of Oral Maxillofacial Surgery, Massachusetts General Hospital, Boston, MA, USA

John M. Dobrowski, MD Department of Otolaryngology, Massachusetts Eye and Ear Infirmary, Massachusetts General Hospital, Boston, MA, USA

Molly A. Dobrowski, RN St. Louis University School of Nursing, and Amego, Inc., Boston, MA, USA

Anna Cristina Garza-Mayers, MD, PhD Harvard Combined Program in Dermatology, Massachusetts General Hospital, Boston, MA, USA

Aubrey L. Gilbert, MD Department of Ophthalmology, Boston Children's Hospital, Massachusetts Eye and Ear Infirmary, Boston, MA, USA

Eric P. Hazen, MD Department of Psychiatry, Massachusetts General Hospital, Boston, MA, USA

Jason G. Ho, MD Department of Cardiology, University of Florida College of Medicine, Jacksonville, FL, USA

Yamini Jagannath Howe, MD Developmental-Behavioral Pediatrics, Massachusetts General Hospital, Lurie Center for Autism, Lexington, MA, USA

Christiana Iyasere, MD, MBA Department of Medicine, Massachusetts General Hospital, Boston, MA, USA

Sarah M. Kadzielski, MD Pediatric Gastroenterology and Nutrition, Massachusetts General Hospital, Boston, MA, USA

Lurie Center for Autism, Lexington, MA, USA

Ann Kao, MD, MPH Department of Pediatrics and Internal Medicine, Massachusetts General Hospital, Boston, MA, USA

Melanie Kazlas, MD Department of Ophthalmology, Boston Children's Hospital, Massachusetts Eye and Ear Infirmary, Boston, MA, USA

Donald Keamy Jr., MD, MPH Department of Otolaryngology, Massachusetts Eye and Ear Infirmary, Massachusetts General Hospital, Boston, MA, USA

Stuart E. Kigner, DPM Department of Orthopaedic Surgery, Massachusetts General Hospital, Boston, MA, USA

T. Bernard Kinane, MD Department of Pediatrics, Massachusetts General Hospital, Boston, MA, USA

Shelly King, MSN, RN, CPNP Pediatric Urology, Riley Hospital for Children, Indiana University School of Medicine, Indianapolis, IN, USA

Daniela Kroshinsky, MD, MPH Department of Dermatology, Massachusetts General Hospital, Boston, MA, USA

Archibald J. Loch, DPM Mercyhealth Hospital and Medical Center-Walworth, Lake Geneva, WI, USA

Jennifer A. Magee, DMD, MPH Department of Oral Maxillofacial Surgery, Massachusetts General Hospital, Danvers, MA, USA

Jessica McCannon, MD Department of Pediatrics, Massachusetts General Hospital, Boston, MA, USA

Christopher J. McDougle, MD Department of Psychiatry, Massachusetts General Hospital, Boston, MA, USA

Lurie Center for Autism, Lexington, MA, USA

Susanna Mierau, MD, PhD Department of Physiology, Development and Neuroscience, University of Cambridge, Cambridge, UK

Jennifer Mullett, RN, BC Lurie Center for Autism, Lexington, MA, USA

Ann Neumeyer, MD Department of Neurology, Massachusetts General Hospital, Boston, MA, USA

Lurie Center for Autism, Lexington, MA, USA

Jonathan Paolino, MD Department of Pediatrics, Massachusetts General Hospital, Boston, MA, USA

Jill Pineda, PhD Neuropsychology Department, Kennedy Krieger Institute, Baltimore, MD, USA

Anne Althausen Plante, MD Department of Obstetrics and Gynecology, Massachusetts General Hospital, Boston, MA, USA

Gleeson Rebello, MD Department of Orthopedic Surgery, Massachusetts General Hospital, Boston, MA, USA

Hillary Risk, MSN, RN, FNP Pediatric Urology, Riley Hospital for Children, Indiana University School of Medicine, Indianapolis, IN, USA

Ana Maria Rosales, MD Department of Pediatrics, Massachusetts General Hospital, Boston, MA, USA

Amita Sharma, MD Department of Pediatrics, Massachusetts General Hospital, Boston, MA, USA

Taylor Wang, MSN, RN, CPNP Pediatric Urology, Riley Hospital for Children, Indiana University School of Medicine, Indianapolis, IN, USA

Melissa Young, MSN, RN, CPNP Pediatric Urology, Riley Hospital for Children, Indiana University School of Medicine, Indianapolis, IN, USA

Part I

General Principles

Introduction

1

Eric P. Hazen and Christopher J. McDougle

An understanding of autism spectrum disorder (ASD) and its potential impact on a patient's medical care is essential for health-care providers in the twenty-first century. The prevalence of ASD has risen significantly over recent decades and continues to rise. The most recent estimate by the Centers for Disease Control and Prevention is that 1 out of every 68 children in the United States has ASD [3]. This represents a significant increase from the survey conducted just 10 years prior, which placed the prevalence at 1 out of 110 children [2]. The number of children diagnosed with ASD increased 600% between the 1960s and the 1980s, and it has increased another 600% over the last 20 years [24]. The reasons for this rise are unclear and the source of some debate. Changes in the diagnostic criteria and improvements in the early detection of children with ASD likely explain most of the increased prevalence [12]. Whether the rates of ASD are not merely an artifact of increased detection and diagnostic patterns but represent a true rise in the incidence of the condition, in part, has not been entirely explained. Regardless, there are millions of children and adults affected by ASD in the United States.

The prevalence of ASD alone indicates that individuals with ASD would make up a significant proportion of patients in any medical setting. However, individuals with ASD also have higher rates of medical comorbidity than the general population, including higher rates of epilepsy, gastrointestinal disorders, allergies, nutritional deficiencies, obesity, sleep problems, and certain kinds of immunologic disorders [9]. One of the few large-scale studies of medical comorbidity in an adult population showed that nearly all of the medical conditions examined, including immune conditions, gastrointestinal and sleep disorders, seizures, obesity, dyslipidemia, hypertension, diabetes, stroke, and Parkinson's disease, were more common in adults with ASD compared to a non-ASD control group [7].

For some individuals, the risk of developing particular medical conditions is clearly tied to the same underlying genetic disorder that puts them at risk for ASD. For example, approximately 60% of male patients with fragile X syndrome, which is secondary to a defect of the FMR1 gene on the X chromosome, meet the criteria for ASD [19]. This mutation also puts those with this condition at risk for health conditions that include seizures, strabismus, flat feet, frequent ear infections, and hypermobile joints.

E. P. Hazen (✉) · C. J. McDougle
Department of Psychiatry, Massachusetts General Hospital, Boston, MA, USA

Lurie Center for Autism, Lexington, MA, USA
e-mail: eric.hazen@mgh.harvard.edu; CMCDOUGLE@mgh.harvard.edu

E. P. Hazen, C. J. McDougle (eds.), *The Massachusetts General Hospital Guide to Medical Care in Patients with Autism Spectrum Disorder*, Current Clinical Psychiatry,
https://doi.org/10.1007/978-3-319-94458-6_1

In some cases, medical comorbidities in ASD appear clearly linked to behavioral patterns related to the disorder. For instance, the restricted diets of many of ASD patients often lead to nutritional deficiencies, while sensory sensitivities may make dental hygiene a challenge for some individuals, resulting in dental caries or periodontal disease.

In other cases, the relationship between ASD and associated medical comorbidities is less clear. Some conditions may be due to common underlying genetic or physiologic abnormalities that have not yet been identified. For instance, some have postulated that the increased rate of familial autoimmunity in children with ASD may be due to immune dysregulation that also plays a role in the development of ASD in a subset of patients [23]. Some investigators have proposed the "leaky gut" hypothesis, in which abnormalities in intestinal absorption allow neurotoxic chemicals to pass into the bloodstream and cross the blood-brain barrier, which in turn may play a role in the development of ASD [13]. This hypothesis is controversial, but the frequency of gastrointestinal disorders in the ASD population is very high and the reason for this is not well-understood.

Given the rates of medical comorbidities in ASD patients, it is not surprising that this group has a high degree of health-care utilization. Most of the available data in this area comes from pediatric patients. It has been shown that children with ASD have a higher frequency of both outpatient medical visits and inpatient medical hospitalizations [6] and that the length of stay for medical admissions is approximately 50% greater for patients with ASD compared to typically developing patients [18]. One recent study showed that adolescents with ASD use the emergency department four times as often as adolescents without ASD and that there has been a trend toward increasing use over recent years [17]. Overall medical expenditures are four to six times higher for pediatric patients with ASD [26].

Despite these high rates of health-care utilization and the high levels of expenditure on patients with ASD, there is clear evidence that our health-care system is failing these patients. Families of children with ASD and a special health-care need are more likely to report unmet health-care needs, difficulty accessing care, difficulty receiving subspecialist referrals, financial hardship for the family related to medical expenses, and having a family member reducing or stopping employment due to the child's condition [5, 14]. Patients with ASD have also been shown to be less likely to receive important preventive care services such as flu shots, for example [8].

Patient and family satisfaction with care also tends to be low. Families of patients with ASD are much more likely to report dissatisfaction with their doctors, perceived suboptimal clinical care, and longer delays in receiving care [4, 16, 28]. Patients with ASD who belong to racial or ethnic minority groups may suffer from even greater disparities in the quality of their care. The health care of Black and Latino children with ASD has been shown to be lower on quality indicators compared to that of White children [21], and families of Black and Latino families of children with ASD are less likely to report that their health-care provider spent enough time with them and that the provider was sensitive to their family's values [20].

One of the contributors to the poor quality of care and difficulties accessing care experienced by patients with ASD appears to be shortcomings in our medical education system. In survey studies, practicing primary care pediatricians have indicated low perceived competency in the care of patients with ASD as well as a desire for more education about the needs of children with ASD, and they further indicated that they perceived these factors as barriers to care for patients [10].

Recent survey studies show similar perceived knowledge and training gaps in current pediatric residents, suggesting that the medical education has not adapted sufficiently to meet the needs of patients with ASD [1]. While these educational shortcomings have been better studied among pediatric providers, there is no reason to believe that they are isolated to this group and in fact pediatricians may receive more training about ASD than most other medical specialties [22]. A recent large-scale survey study of adult primary care providers demonstrated that most of the providers did not believe they had the skills and tools needed to care for patients with ASD, and a high proportion of the surveyed providers were not even aware that they had patients with ASD in their panel [29]. Similar deficiencies of knowledge and comfort level have been reported in emergency service personnel as well [27].

Education for medical providers is particularly important because the features of the disorder make it challenging for those with ASD to interface with the medical system. Individuals with ASD commonly have difficulty with departures from familiar routines, anxiety around strangers, and impairments in communication, including difficulty expressing pain. Sensitivity to sensory stimuli is also very common in ASD [11]. Medical settings generally present patients with a flood of unfamiliar sensory stimuli that may provoke anxiety or agitation in some patients. Sensory inputs that seem routine to medical staff, such as the feel of an identification bracelet or the sound of hospital monitors, may be overwhelming for some patients with ASD [15]. Common medical procedures, such as blood pressure monitoring or a physical examination, can be extremely stressful for patients with ASD due to the troubling sensory input, the close physical proximity to the medical provider, or a lack of understanding about what is happening. The distress related to medical encounters does not only affect patients with ASD and their families, but it also has the potential to lead to emotional distress for providers, risk of physical assault to providers, hindered workflow due to additional time required for medical procedures, and decreased quality of the care that is delivered [25].

At Massachusetts General Hospital, a group of motivated providers, administrators, and patient families began an initiative to improve the quality of care and patient experience for individuals with ASD. This initiative, begun in 2013, is described in detail in Chapter 5, "Quality Improvement." Key features of the initiative included the development of resources and materials for patients and families, improvements in communication with patients and families about their individual needs, development of clinical care algorithms to facilitate efficient patient flow and reduce wait times for admissions and discharges, and a broad-based education program that included all staff that might interface with a patient with ASD, including nonclinical staff such as food service workers and facility maintenance staff. As part of this initiative, a new position was created, the Autism Patient Navigator, who is a clinical professional whose duty is to guide patients with ASD and their families through the hospitalization process as well as to provide support and education for providers. The initiative has been a great success in improving the patients' health-care experiences and the comfort and skill of hospital staff in caring for patients with ASD. *The Massachusetts General Hospital Guide to Medical Care in Patients with Autism Spectrum Disorder* is intended as a means of extending this educational effort beyond the grounds of our hospital to the community of potential medical providers for children, adolescents, and adults with ASD.

In discussing this book with some medical colleagues, we most often were met with enthusiasm and support, but we also commonly heard the following sentiment, variously expressed: "I don't understand why this is needed. I approach the treatment of my patients with ASD the same as I would any other patient." Often, such statements carried an edge of indignation, as though to treat patients with ASD any differently than other patients would be a form of discrimination against them. We believe, however, that this belief is misguided in that it does not account for the mounting evidence that individuals with ASD have difficulty accessing and interacting with our health-care system as it is currently structured. Nor does it account for the fact that certain illnesses might be more likely in individuals with ASD than the general population and that the presentation of those illnesses may be quite different in the patient with ASD, who may, for example, express pain or discomfort through changes in behavior rather than words. As we will describe, approaches to office visits, inpatient hospitalization, diagnostic evaluation, medical procedures, and treatment approaches can all be modified to make them safer, more effective, and better tolerated for patients with ASD.

Just as we have made great strides over recent decades in adapting buildings and sidewalks to accommodate the needs of individuals with physical disabilities, assuring that ramps and elevators allow those who cannot navigate stairs or step over curbs to move freely, our medical system and individual medical providers must learn to accommodate the needs of the growing segment of our population with ASD. We present this book as a step in that direction.

References

1. Broder-Fingert S, Ferrone CF, Giauque A, Connors SL. Residents' knowledge and comfort with caring for children with autism spectrum disorder. Clin Pediatr (Phila). 2014;53(14):1390–2. https://doi.org/10.1177/0009922814526982. Epub 2014 Mar 18. PubMed PMID: 24647693.
2. Centers for Disease Control and Prevention. Prevalence of autism spectrum disorders – autism and developmental disabilities monitoring network, United States, 2006. MMWR Surveill Summ. 2009;58(10):1–20.
3. Christensen DL, Baio J, Van Naarden Braun K, Bilder D, Charles J, Constantino JN, Daniels J, Durkin MS, Fitzgerald RT, Kurzius-Spencer M, Lee LC, Pettygrove S, Robinson C, Schulz E, Wells C, Wingate MS, Zahorodny W, Yeargin-Allsopp M, Centers for Disease Control and Prevention (CDC). Prevalence and characteristics of autism Spectrum disorder among children aged 8 years – autism and developmental disabilities monitoring network, 11 sites, United States, 2012. MMWR Surveill Summ. 2016;65(3):1–23. https://doi.org/10.15585/mmwr.ss6503a1.
4. Carbone PS, Murphy NA, Norlin C, Azor V, Sheng X, Young PC. Parent and pediatrician perspectives regarding the primary care of children with autism spectrum disorders. J Autism Dev Disord. 2013;43(4):964–72. https://doi.org/10.1007/s10803-012-1640-7. PubMed PMID: 22948548.
5. Chiri G, Warfield ME. Unmet need and problems accessing core health care services for children with autism spectrum disorder. Matern Child Health J. 2012;16(5):1081–91. https://doi.org/10.1007/s10995-011-0833-6. PubMed PMID: 21667201.
6. Croen LA, Najjar DV, Ray GT, Lotspeich L, Bernal P. A comparison of health care utilization and costs of children with and without autism spectrum disorders in a large group-model health plan. Pediatrics. 2006;118(4):e1203–11. PubMed PMID: 17015508.
7. Croen LA, Zerbo O, Qian Y, Massolo ML, Rich S, Sidney S, Kripke C. The health status of adults on the autism spectrum. Autism. 2015;19(7):814–23. https://doi.org/10.1177/1362361315577517. Epub 2015 Apr 24. PubMed PMID: 25911091.
8. Cummings JR, Lynch FL, Rust KC, Coleman KJ, Madden JM, Owen-Smith AA, Yau VM, Qian Y, Pearson KA, Crawford PM, Massolo ML, Quinn VP, Croen LA. Health services utilization among children with and without autism Spectrum disorders. J Autism Dev Disord. 2016;46(3):910–20. https://doi.org/10.1007/s10803-015-2634-z. PubMed PMID: 26547921; PubMed Central PMCID: PMC4747787.
9. Gurney JG, McPheeters ML, Davis MM. Parental report of health conditions and health care use among children with and without autism: National Survey of Children's Health. Arch Pediatr Adolesc Med. 2006;160(8):825–30. PubMed PMID: 16894082.
10. Golnik A, Ireland M, Borowsky IW. Medical homes for children with autism: a physician survey. Pediatrics. 2009;123(3):966–71. https://doi.org/10.1542/peds.2008-1321. PubMed PMID: 19255027.
11. Hazen EP, Stornelli JL, O'Rourke JA, Koesterer K, McDougle CJ. Sensory symptoms in autism spectrum disorders. Harv Rev Psychiatry. 2014;22(2):112–24. https://doi.org/10.1097/01.HRP.0000445143.08773.58. Review. PubMed PMID: 24614766.
12. Hansen SN, Schedel DE, Parner ET. Explaining the increase in prevalence of autism spectrum disorders: the proportion attributable to changes in reporting practices. JAMA Pediatr. 2015;169(1):56–62.
13. Hsaio EY. Gastrointestinal issues in autism spectrum disorder. Harv Rev Psychiatry. 2014;22(2):104–11.
14. Kogan MD, Strickland BB, Blumberg SJ, Singh GK, Perrin JM, van Dyck PC. A national profile of the health care experiences and family impact of autism spectrum disorder among children in the United States, 2005–2006. Pediatrics. 2008;122(6):e1149–58. https://doi.org/10.1542/peds.2008-1057.
15. Kopecky K, Broder-Fingert S, Iannuzzi D, Connors S. The needs of hospitalized patients with autism spectrum disorders: a parent survey. Clin Pediatr (Phila). 2013;52(7):652–60. https://doi.org/10.1177/0009922813485974. Epub 2013 Apr 25. PubMed PMID: 23624619.
16. Liptak GS, Orlando M, Yingling JT, Theurer-Kaufman KL, Malay DP, Tompkins LA, Flynn JR. Satisfaction with primary health care received by families of children with developmental disabilities. J Pediatr Health Care. 2006;20(4):245–52. PubMed PMID: 16831632.
17. Liu G, Pearl AM, Kong L, Leslie DL, Murray MJ. A profile on emergency department utilization in adolescents and young adults with autism spectrum disorders. J Autism Dev Disord. 2017;47(2):347–58. https://doi.org/10.1007/s10803-016-2953-8. Erratum in: J Autism Dev Disord. 2017 Mar 23:.PubMed PMID: 27844247.

18. Lokhandwala T, Khanna R, West-Strum D. Hospitalization burden among individuals with autism. J Autism Dev Disord. 2012;42(1):95–104. https://doi.org/10.1007/s10803-011-1217-x.
19. Lozano R, Rosero CA, Hagerman RJ. Fragile X spectrum disorders. Intractable Rare Dis Res. 2014;3(4):134–46. https://doi.org/10.5582/irdr.2014.01022. Review. PubMed PMID: 25606363; PubMed Central PMCID: PMC4298643.
20. Magaña S, Parish SL, Son E. Have racial and ethnic disparities in the quality of health care relationships changed for children with developmental disabilities and ASD? Am J Intellect Dev Disabil. 2015;120(6):504–13. https://doi.org/10.1352/1944-7558-120.6.504. PubMed PMID: 26505871.
21. Magaña S, Parish SL, Rose RA, Timberlake M, Swaine JG. Racial and ethnic disparities in quality of health care among children with autism and other developmental disabilities. Intellect Dev Disabil. 2012;50(4):287–99. https://doi.org/10.1352/1934-9556-50.4.287. PubMed PMID: 22861130.
22. McDougle CJ. Sounding a wake-up call: improving the lives of adults with autism. J Am Acad Child Adolesc Psychiatry. 2013;52(6):566–8.
23. McDougle CJ, Landino SM, Vahabzadeh A, O'Rourke J, Zurcher NR, Finger BC, Palumbo ML, Helt J, Mullett JE, Hooker JM, Carlezon WA Jr. Toward an immune-mediated subtype of autism spectrum disorder. Brain Res. 2015;1617:92.
24. Rice CE, Rosanoff M, Dawson G, Durkin MS, Croen LA, Singer A, Yeargin-Allsopp M. Evaluating changes in the prevalence of the autism spectrum disorders (ASDs). Public Health Rev. 2012;34(2):1–22.
25. Sakai C, Miller K, Brussa AK, MacPherson C, Augustyn M. Challenges of autism in the inpatient setting. J Dev Behav Pediatr. 2014;35(1):82–4. https://doi.org/10.1097/DBP.0000000000000024. PubMed PMID: 24399104.
26. Shimabukuro TT, Grosse SD, Rice C. Medical expenditures for children with an autism spectrum disorder in a privately insured population. J Autism Dev Disord. 2008;38(3):546–52. Epub 2007 Aug 10
27. Wachob D, Pesci LJ. Brief report: knowledge and confidence of emergency medical service personnel involving treatment of an individual with autism spectrum disorder. J Autism Dev Disord. 2017;47(3):887–91. https://doi.org/10.1007/s10803-016-2957-4. PubMed PMID: 27909851.
28. Zablotsky B, Kalb LG, Freedman B, Vasa R, Stuart EA. Health care experiences and perceived financial impact among families of children with an autism spectrum disorder. PsychiatrServ. 2014;65(3):395–8. https://doi.org/10.1176/appi.ps.201200552. PubMed PMID: 24584528; PubMed Central PMCID: PMC4384426
29. Zerbo O, Massolo ML, Qian Y, Croen LA. A study of physician knowledge and experience with autism in adults in a large integrated healthcare system. J Autism Dev Disord. 2015;45(12):4002–14. https://doi.org/10.1007/s10803-015-2579-2. PubMed PMID: 26334872.

2 Office-Based Medical Care

Yamini Jagannath Howe, Phil Bartel, and Robert E. Accordino

Introduction

Autism spectrum disorder (ASD) is a neurodevelopmental condition characterized by social communication impairments and restricted and repetitive patterns of interests and behaviors [1]. The reported incidence of ASD has been increasing, with 1 in 59 children aged 8 years estimated to be affected in the USA [2]. Symptoms of ASD first manifest in early childhood and are highly variable from person to person, leading to functional impairments throughout a person's life span [3, 4]. It is therefore imperative that all healthcare providers, both in pediatrics and adult medicine, recognize the unique challenges that individuals with ASD face.

The hallmark social and communication impairments and related emotional and behavioral regulation difficulties seen in ASD make interacting with others – including healthcare professionals – particularly challenging. For example, individuals with ASD may be unable to express pain reliably, leading to a delay in the recognition and treatment of medical conditions by their healthcare providers [5]. Individuals with ASD may experience anxiety with social interactions as well as difficulties with the sensory environment of the healthcare setting, understanding instructions given, and communicating with their healthcare provider [6, 7]. As compared with other individuals with special healthcare needs, individuals with ASD are more likely to have unmet medical needs and problems accessing care and to experience lower quality of healthcare, perhaps as a result of these impairments [8–10].

Medical providers themselves may also feel unequipped or unprepared to provide care for people with ASD. Healthcare providers cite worries about behavior, communication limitations, and lack of knowledge about the individual's specific needs as barriers to delivering effective healthcare [6, 11]. The busy nature of most ambulatory, office-based medical practices, with long wait times and short appointment times, makes it difficult to address individual patients' needs. With planning, preparation, and practice, however, patients with ASD can learn to accommodate to an outpatient medical setting and have successful healthcare visits. As is also the case with patients who are typically developing, high-quality outpatient medical

Y. J. Howe (✉)
Developmental-Behavioral Pediatrics, Massachusetts General Hospital, Lurie Center for Autism, Lexington, MA, USA
e-mail: yhowe@mgh.harvard.edu

P. Bartel
University of Pittsburgh School of Medicine, Pittsburgh, PA, USA
e-mail: wpb17@pitt.edu

R. E. Accordino
Child and Adolescent Psychiatry, Massachusetts General Hospital, Boston, MA, USA
e-mail: raccordino@mgh.harvard.edu

E. P. Hazen, C. J. McDougle (eds.), *The Massachusetts General Hospital Guide to Medical Care in Patients with Autism Spectrum Disorder*, Current Clinical Psychiatry,
https://doi.org/10.1007/978-3-319-94458-6_2

care is dependent upon developing relationships with patients over time in order to best understand and treat their individual healthcare needs. Making small changes to how the clinical space is arranged and the clinical visit is structured can help patients feel more comfortable in an ambulatory medical care setting.

In this chapter, we discuss the specifics of how to approach care for individuals with ASD in an outpatient medical setting. The first part of the chapter is focused on care of children and adolescents, and the second part of the chapter focuses on care of adults.

Pediatrics

Preparing the Office

Careful preparation of the clinical space ahead of time is key to helping individuals with ASD feel comfortable in an outpatient medical setting. The use of clear visuals (such as labels for each room, posting pictures and names of office staff, clearly marked bathrooms and exits, etc.) can be helpful for patients to understand the clinic flow and learn common routines. Most practices that see pediatric patients are already attuned to the needs of infants, toddlers, and young children with regard to safety concerns and the need for engaging toys and activities in the waiting room and clinical space, but with individuals who have developmental delays or intellectual disabilities, many of these considerations may still apply even as they mature. It is important to keep a range of items for those whose play interests may be more mature than their communication level would suggest. In addition, so-called "sensory" toys, such as rain sticks, soft squeezable balls, and simple cause-effect toys, are appealing to many children with ASD and are sometimes effective in relaxing distressed patients.

Although it is not possible to provide an exhaustive list, in Table 2.1, we present behavioral

Table 2.1 Office adaptations as related to specific symptoms associated with autism spectrum disorder (ASD)

Clinical symptoms frequently seen in ASD	Adaptation
Pica (repeated ingestion of nonnutritive substances)	Items in the waiting room and throughout the office should be safe for mouthing, and the waiting room should be monitored frequently for hazards
	Furniture should be hard and not excessively upholstered, as many patients may pick apart materials to mouth or swallow
	Paint should not be peeling
Swiping tabletops	Tabletops should be free of clutter, or items should be easy to pick up
Flailing or swinging arms	Pictures should be securely fastened to the wall
	Any glass (pictures, doors, windows) should be shatterproof
Bolting (leaving suddenly)	This possibility should be discussed beforehand. Door safety and parking lot safety should be considered for individuals who may lack environmental safety awareness
Ripping (usually paper)	Keep only a few magazines and handouts available at a time
Visual stimulatory behaviors (repetitive behaviors seeking visual stimuli)	Light switches ideally should be out of reach or at least safe if repetitively turned on and off
	Blinds or window coverings should be safe; hanging strings should be secured
Visual avoidant behaviors (patients may be bothered by very bright lights)	Dimmable light switches are preferred
	Providers should be adaptable to having lights off, if able
	Flickering lights should be avoided
Auditory avoidant behaviors (patients may feel overwhelmed in loud or busy settings or have discomfort in crowds)	Schedule patients at times when there are fewer patients in the waiting room
	Identify a quieter area in the office where patients can wait away from other patients
	Ideally toilet flushes in patient bathrooms should not be too loud, and paper towels should be offered as an alternative to loud hand driers
	Phones should not be excessively loud, and providers should be aware of pagers or put them on vibrate mode
	Patients should be warned in advance of sudden loud noises when possible

issues frequently encountered in patients with ASD and adaptations and modifications to an office space that could be considered. General "child-proofing" principles should be followed (i.e., covering electrical outlets, avoiding window coverings with long strings, keeping objects that are common choking hazards out of reach, and avoiding shelving that can tip over or that encourages climbing). Sensory sensitivities should be considered. It is often helpful to have dimmable lighting for those who are bothered by bright fluorescent bulbs and a quiet area for patients who are bothered by loud noises. Warnings should be given in advance if sudden noises are anticipated. Bathroom areas should also be evaluated for how accommodations might be made for those who are afraid of public restrooms, which is sometimes due to an aversion to loud automatic flushing toilets or hand dryers.

In addition, ASD-specific training of staff or physicians may be needed as familiarity with and understanding of developmental disabilities can vary a great deal among those who work in medical settings. Caregivers are often concerned about how the patient may be perceived by others, and staff should be reminded to be respectful and courteous, remain calm, and use "people-first language" (i.e., addressing an individual patient with ASD, not an "autistic patient").

Before the Visit

Making sure that the clinical staff are aware of an individual's needs ahead of the visit is helpful in order to prepare how care should be provided and what safety measures may need to be put in place. Ideally, when scheduling an appointment, a clearly outlined system should be in place so that caregivers can relay their child's specific needs. This can be done over the phone with scheduling staff or through intake paperwork. Providing a structured questionnaire can inform providers of an individual patient's needs during a visit. In addition to general birth, medical, and developmental history, this questionnaire should include information about how the individual communicates needs or wants, how he expresses pain, any specific sensory accommodations needed to ensure comfort and compliance, and any safety considerations for the healthcare visit. "Health Passports" or informational cards can help facilitate communication with healthcare providers [6, 12]. At the Massachusetts General Hospital (MGH), we encourage patients to complete the Autism Care Questionnaire [13, 14], which is discussed in more detail in Chap. 5.

Providing patients with visual instructions and materials ahead of time can be helpful in preparing them for what is to be expected at the time of the visit. Having materials online, such as pictures of the outside of the building, the waiting room, and people they will meet, is one way to do this. An online video tour of the office and a pre-appointment visit are also ways that patients can prepare for a visit. If a patient with ASD has difficulty with crowds or needs an extended amount of time to complete vital signs, staff should schedule the patient at times when the clinic is typically more quiet.

For individuals with ASD who are unable to communicate for themselves, it is imperative that a knowledgeable caregiver accompany them to the visit. For individuals living in foster care or in a group living situation, it is often important to make this clear before the visit, as many lay people may not realize the importance of collecting an accurate history in understanding medical illness. If an individual with minimal information about the patient's medical history accompanies the patient to the visit, it may not be productive for anyone.

If the patient is known to exhibit unsafe behaviors such as aggression toward others, behavioral support staff or additional family members or caregivers should be made available to accompany the individual to the clinical visit. It is rare for individuals with ASD to exhibit severe aggression, but it is useful to have an emergency plan in place for patients who become agitated or aggressive during a clinical encounter. Attunement to a patient's body language is important for caregivers in allowing them to anticipate what may be upsetting the patient and adjusting the environment to accommodate to their needs, as mentioned above. Avoid physical restraint if at all possible, as this tends to escalate rather than help a situation.

Using visuals supports and simple language while escorting patients to a pre-identified safe space can also be helpful [15].

During the Visit

Developing a predictable and consistent routine for the office visit allows individuals with ASD to become more comfortable in a clinical setting. At the start of the clinical encounter, it is helpful to tell the patient what is to be expected in clear, concrete terms appropriately adapted to the patient's developmental level (e.g., "First I am going to talk with your parents, then we will do a check up, then we will talk some more, and then we will be all done.") The use of a visual schedule can help patients with limited receptive language skills understand what they should expect during the visit (see Fig. 2.1).

Although routines are very helpful in mitigating anticipatory anxiety that the patient may experience, it is important to realize that patients with ASD may very quickly become accustomed to routines and, as a result, can have a very difficult time when routines are disrupted. Making patients aware ahead of time of any changes in clinic routines, such as the order of when vitals are collected or the length of wait times, can help prevent any undue anxiety.

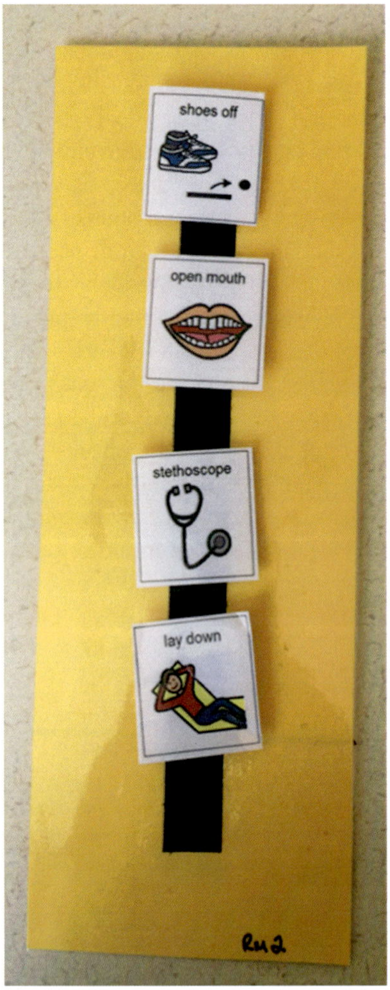

Fig. 2.1 Example of a visual schedule for physical examination

History

In this section, we will highlight key questions important to consider in taking the medical history of children and adolescents with ASD. A careful medical evaluation of patients with ASD should include taking a developmental history in addition to past medical history and social and family history.

Developmental History

Understanding baseline developmental abilities and behavioral needs can help the clinician learn of any changes in behavior, temperament, or developmental trajectory and determine whether further medical or psychiatric workup is indicated. The clinician should be aware of the typical progression of developmental skills and elicit historical information to assess the individual patient's abilities. Table 2.2 gives examples of questions that elicit information about an individual's developmental abilities as they pertain to ASD. Any loss of skill or developmental regression with illness could be a sign of a metabolic or mitochondrial disorder and may prompt further workup.

Past Medical History

As for all children, a careful birth and medical history should be obtained, as well as details of past medical or psychiatric hospitalizations and surgeries. In particular, gastrointestinal

Table 2.2 Questions pertaining to developmental abilities in patients with ASD

Developmental domain	Questions to ask
Communication	Does he/she use spoken language to communicate?
	How does he/she best communicate?
	Are any special devices (iPad apps, etc.) needed to help him/her communicate?
	Was there ever a history of language loss or other developmental regression?
	Are any repetitive speech patterns used?
Cognition	Does the patient have a developmental delay or intellectual disability?
	Has formal cognitive testing been performed?
	Can he/she read or write?
	What supports are needed for him/her in school or at work?
Play/leisure	What does he/she do for fun?
	Does the patient have any specific areas of interest or preoccupations?
	Does the patient have any friends?
	Does the patient have any repetitive forms of play?
Motor	Does he/she have fine or gross motor impairments?
	Do motor delays or hypotonia impact self-care skills?
	Does the patient have any abnormal voluntary or involuntary motor movements?
Sensory	What sensory-seeking or sensory-avoidant behaviors does the patient exhibit?
Emotional/behavioral	Does the patient have any comorbid psychiatric diagnoses?
	Does the patient have any aggressive or self-injurious behaviors?
Self-care	Is he/she toilet trained?
	Is he/she able to eat independently?
	Can he/she dress independently?
	Do difficulties with organization hamper independence?

(GI) [16, 17] and sleep complaints are common among patients with ASD [18]. Concern for possible seizure activity should also be considered. These medical comorbidities are discussed in subsequent chapters of this book, including "Neurological Disorders" (Chap. 6), "Pulmonology and Sleep" (Chap. 11), and "Gastrointestinal Disorders" (Chap. 12).

Social and Family History

A thorough social and family history should be obtained to determine what further supports are needed and to guide genetic workup. Drawing a family pedigree can be a useful way to elicit this information. Below are additional topics and questions to be considered as part of a detailed history in individuals with ASD or related conditions.

(i) Living situation: With whom and in what type of setting does the individual live?
(ii) Educational history: For children under the age of 3 years, it is important to elicit whether they are enrolled in early intervention (EI), Birth-to-Three, or other developmental support services. From age 3 until the age of 22 years, individuals may qualify for special education services under an Individualized Education Program (IEP) through their local school district (see the Center for Parent Information and resources for more information: http://www.parentcenterhub.org/repository/idea/). With EI and school services, it is important to understand what services are being provided (e.g., speech therapy, occupational therapy, behavioral therapy) and the goals of these services, the training background of service delivery providers, how many hours of services are being provided, as well as where the services are being delivered. If the individual is in a school setting, the provider may ask questions about class size, whether the child has an IEP, whether it is a private or public school, the ratio of teachers to students, and where the child receives instruction (e.g., at home, in a general education setting, in a smaller separate

special education classroom, or individually at school). Educational and behavioral treatment services provide rehabilitative and primary treatment for ASD. Regression in developmental skills or behavioral regulation abilities can be seen with changes in the quality or quantity of services provided. Changes in sleep and eating behaviors can also occur as a result of stress in the home or school environments.

(iii) Vocational history: At age 14 years, schools should start planning the transition from adolescent to adult services, as well as planning for vocational training needs. Neuropsychological, educational, and/or vocational evaluations may be needed to inform transition planning. For those who are working, what level of supervision and independence does the patient have at work, and what supports are in place to ensure success?

(iv) Additional supports and services: Individuals with ASD may receive funding or other supports through the state's Department of Developmental Services (or Department of Mental Retardation). Considering whether the individual has been able to receive health insurance through local Medicaid or supplemental insurance is also important to understand what further resources may be available. In some states, some individuals with ASD may qualify for Katie Beckett Medicaid waivers, which allow the state to ignore family income in considering whether an individual may be qualified to receive Medicaid.

(v) Legal history: Has the child or young adult ever been arrested or had interactions with the law?

(vi) Safety: Consideration of the safety of the individual's environment in all settings is important. For example, individuals who lack safety awareness may try to escape from the home or may be at higher risk for falls if they recklessly climb up on high places such as counters or windows, and additional locks or other safety measures may be needed. Special car seats or harnesses may be needed to ensure safety in vehicles. Individuals with ASD or other developmental disabilities are also particularly prone to become targets of bullying or teasing. Furthermore, as for all individuals, eliciting whether the individual may have witnessed violence or they themselves may have been victims to physical and sexual abuse is an important consideration and can lead to changes in behavior patterns [19].

(vii) Sexual history: Issues of sexuality should be addressed as for all individuals, with the knowledge that individuals with intellectual disabilities may require specific training in understanding appropriate relationships and boundaries.

Physical Examination

When conducting a general physical examination, gradual exposure to medical equipment and the routines of medical visits and examinations may be needed to help patients tolerate procedures which may be stressful. Recruiting the help of local behavioral therapists, school nurses, and other professionals for medical desensitization may be needed to train individuals in tolerating specific procedures, such as blood pressure readings, blood draws, and other dental or medical procedures. Pill swallowing may also require specific teaching. Many online resources exist for patients, including the Autism Speaks website toolkits (https://www.autismspeaks.org/family-services/tool-kits). Additional discussion of strategies to help with the physical exam and other medical procedures is included in Chap. 4.

Following a strict routine for examination, asking the patient's permission before examining, explaining to the patient as clearly as possible what is happening and why, and following the patient's lead are all helpful techniques for conducting a physical examination. The physical examination is often normal in individuals with ASD. However, the physician should be alert to any signs of a genetic or metabolic etiology for developmental delay, such as unusual facial features, enlarged liver or spleen, or neurofibromas, as well as physical conditions that can be caused by repetitive and restricted patterns of behavior (e.g., hair pulling, skin picking, callous formation from repetitive biting of hands, constipation from stool withholding or toileting avoidance, or tightened heel cords from toe walking). Seeing patients for more frequent visits when they are not acutely ill can also help them get more accustomed to medical routines and alert the clinician to any change in clinical status that would otherwise be difficult to detect without a preestablished relationship.

Clinical Vignette #1

Dr. JT is a primary care physician in a large community practice who is scheduled to see Dilan, an 8-year-old boy with ASD, for an initial appointment. Dilan moved to the area recently and is looking to establish care with a new provider. He has a seizure disorder and chronic constipation, and he sometimes exhibits aggressive and self-injurious behaviors when in pain or when anxious in a new setting. His mother calls the office expressing concern that he has previously had difficulty tolerating office visits, and she is worried about the upcoming visit.

Dr. JT recommends that the staff schedule an appointment at the beginning of the day when the clinic is calm and quiet and recommends that Dilan's parents complete the clinic's intake forms, which contain prompts for information regarding his needs. The staff also invites Dilan and his parents to visit the clinic website and mails the family a brochure containing pictures of the staff and office site. Dilan's mother completes and sends back the intake form, which indicates that Dilan is bothered by loud noises and bright lights and that he communicates using spoken language as well as using an assistive device. His mother is advised to bring in his headphones that help him in case of any loud noises in the clinic. She is also instructed to bring his communication device, and a note is placed on his chart so that staff will be aware of these needs. Dilan's mother is notified of the general office procedures so that she can prepare her son.

Dilan and his mother were met with unexpected traffic, so he appears a little tired when they arrive at the clinic. The front staff direct Dilan and his mother to be seated in a quiet spot, and he is offered a comfortable chair and a toy. Dilan appears more relaxed at the time his vital signs are checked. He tolerates weight and height measurement with some redirection and verbal prompting. He becomes more nervous about the blood pressure cuff, but the medical assistant explains what is happening, allows Dilan to examine the cuff, and demonstrates it first on his mother. He is then able to sit quietly during the examination.

At the time of the visit, Dr. JT is prepared ahead of time and uses a calm, quiet tone of voice when speaking with Dilan and his mother. Dr. JT makes sure to greet Dilan and make eye contact and asks his mother how best to use his communication device during the appointment. Using the device, Dilan is able to request water and to play with Legos, while his mother talks with the doctor. The physical examination is unremarkable, and they review the plan for monitoring and treating constipation. Dilan's seizures are stable on his current medications. The mother is directed to the Autism Speaks website for information on constipation and also referred to a local neurologist to oversee seizure management. They also develop a plan to work with the school nurse and behavioral therapists on practicing tolerating blood pressure checks. Dilan's mother expresses feeling overwhelmed with coordinating multiple medical appointments. Dr. JT suggests that she meet with the practice's nurse after the appointment to review local support groups for families of individuals with ASD and special education advocacy groups and to assist with scheduling and care coordination. They also discuss how to contact the practice when Dilan is not feeling well and outline emergency procedures.

With patients such as Dilan, the goal of routine health visits is not only to monitor medical health and oversee care, but also to establish rapport with the patient and family and for the physician to understand Dilan's needs when he is well. This approach will serve to prepare all members of his care team for times of crisis.

Healthcare Transition

Efficient healthcare transitioning (HCT) is key to coordinating the care of children with ASD as they mature into adulthood. HCT is an active process that seeks to meet the medical, psychological, social, and educational needs of adolescent patients who are bridging the gap between child-focused and adult-focused healthcare systems [20, 21]. Ongoing developmental disabilities and the high frequency of comorbid conditions seen in individuals with ASD often lead to high utilization of medical services throughout the patient's lifetime; thus it is important to ensure that the needs of adolescents with ASD are addressed during this critical period of transition [20].

For proper HCT to occur, physicians must discuss with their patients how to shift to adult care and address many of the changes that will be occurring in the coming years. Some important topics to include in this discussion are (1) identifying and transitioning to a new physician qualified to care for adults with ASD, (2) the actual healthcare needs of the adult patient, (3) health insurance and its retention, (4) possible need for guardianship for some patients and the process for pursuing this, and (5) encouraging the patient to take increased responsibility over their healthcare needs as adulthood approaches to the extent that is developmentally appropriate [20, 22]. It is suggested that physicians begin these discussions with patients and their families when they reach the age of 12 years and to revisit these topics each year thereafter in greater depth [20, 23, 24].

Unfortunately, it is reported that youth with ASD receive HCT services at a much lower rate than youth with other special healthcare needs [25]. A study found that only 14% of youth with ASD spoke with their doctor about finding an adult provider, less than 25% spoke about health insurance retention, and less than 50% spoke about adult healthcare needs or how to take on greater responsibility for their care [25]. Moreover, it was found that youth with ASD who suffer from comorbid medical conditions have a greater risk of not receiving appropriate HCT [25]. It is clear that many of the patients who most need this service are falling through cracks in our healthcare system. As such, pediatricians who treat youth with ASD should ensure that these conversations are taking place at the appropriate time, with the appropriate people (caretakers and patients), and with sufficient frequency to allow their patients to experience the smoothest possible transition to adult care.

Outpatient Care of Adults with ASD

Although much of the world's focus is on children with ASD, the prevalence rate in adults is estimated to be as high as 1% of the adult population [26]. Much like children with ASD, adults with ASD are more likely to have unmet medical needs, difficulties accessing care, lower utilization of preventative care, and an increased risk of emergency department visits when compared to unaffected adults [27]. As adults with ASD have an increased risk for numerous medical conditions, including epilepsy, GI disorders, nutritional deficits, metabolic disorders, sleep disturbances, and mental health issues, it is critical to improve the quality and accessibility of healthcare for this population [27]. Many of the hallmark traits of ASD, including communication deficits, hyper-/hyposensitivity to sensory stimuli, and impaired executive function, complicate effective healthcare delivery and pose a significant challenge for physicians to overcome.

Unfortunately, many physicians who treat adults are underprepared to serve the ASD population, making an already challenging problem even more difficult. A study in Germany found that general practitioners did not have a significantly greater understanding of ASD than the general population [26, 28]. Another survey of adult healthcare providers at Kaiser Permanente Northern California showed that not only did providers lack the skills, training, and tools to effectively treat adults with ASD, but also many providers were not even aware that their patients had ASD [29]. This study reported that all physicians included had received little or no training during medical school or residency on how to care for patients with ASD, with the exception of one physician who had trained in both pediatrics and internal medicine. This lack of training and exposure explains why this study found that these physicians were often frustrated, and sometimes uncomfortable, during their work with adults with ASD [29]. It is thus unsurprising that a survey of adult patients with and without ASD revealed that adults with ASD were significantly less satisfied with the medical care they received [30]. Another survey found that many patients with ASD reported the impression that their physicians were unaware of what ASD entailed and were unfamiliar with how to treat individuals with ASD [31].

ASD does not represent an insurmountable obstacle to care. Although there are numerous challenges to treating adults with ASD, significant strides can be made in healthcare efficacy simply by providing physicians with the knowledge and tools to better help their patients with ASD. This section of the chapter will focus on specific strategies and approaches pertaining to outpatient medical care of adults with ASD.

Preparing the Office

As in pediatrics, proper consideration to creating a comfortable and safe environment for the patient goes a long way. Unfortunately, while the "child proofing" of pediatric practices creates an environment that is suited to the care of individuals with intellectual disability and developmental delays, such office alterations are impractical for most internal medicine practices. Since many adults with ASD and their caretakers prefer to wait in examination rooms instead of the waiting room to reduce social and sensory stressors, ensuring that at least one examination room meets the standards offered in Table 2.1 will adequately prepare most practices. Alternatively, scheduling patients with ASD at the beginning of the clinic day preferentially can avoid longer wait times.

While many adults with ASD or their caretakers will bring along items or toys suitable for their entertainment if necessary, it is still a good idea to keep a few of the previously mentioned "sensory" toys on hand, especially stress balls. Heavy work, defined as any activity that provides resistance to the muscles and joints of the body, is a popular method used by occupational therapists to alleviate sensory defensiveness [32]. As such, having a stress ball on hand for the patient to use during the examination can ameliorate stressful situations.

It is also important for the clinical staff to be properly trained to communicate with individuals with ASD and to address any stereotypes they may have. Staff should recognize that adults with ASD are often capable of independence, even if a caretaker or supporter is present. Many adults with ASD express frustration when healthcare professionals address their supporter before them and dislike the immediate assumption that they are incapable of understanding or making decisions about their body [31]. Only when it is clear that a patient is not able to answer a question should physicians or staff turn to the caretaker for answers.

Before the Visit

Many people conceive of ASD as a spectrum disorder, but it is in reality much more complicated than a line with "high functioning" on one end and "low" on the other [30]. A more useful conceptualization of ASD is as spectra on multiple axes, including communicative abilities, cognitive capabilities, need for consistency, sensory responsiveness, and many others. Communication is key, as only through effective discourse with patients or their caretakers will physicians be able to elicit the individual needs of their patient and develop a plan of effective healthcare before the visit takes place.

For example, a patient may communicate that issues with auditory stimulation are more of a problem than olfactory or physical stimulation. This information allows the physician to prepare a hospitable environment for their examination. Similarly, if a patient is prone to challenging behavior such as aggression or self-injury, communicating with his caretaker beforehand may help to develop a plan to calm him. This is much easier than attempting to create a response spontaneously during the visit when a problem arises. A willingness to accept that each patient is an individual with unique needs and the flexibility of physicians to change their examination styles to accommodate these needs after they have been communicated are the first steps to overcoming the challenges in treating an adult with ASD.

Offices should have a system in place that allows patients or their caretakers to outline their specific needs and unique considerations. As many adults with ASD have specific preferences as to how they wish to communicate, a flexible system that allows patients to submit this information online or via phone, fax, or email ensures that patients or their caretakers will be able to find a way to convey their needs with the office. In the same vein, allowing patients to schedule appointments through multiple channels and mediums will help patients to feel more at ease with managing their visits and reduce barriers to care [31].

Many patients express discomfort related to unfamiliarity with the staff and the office space. As such, being willing to send pictures of the staff, pictures of individual rooms, and a layout of the building, or having all of these present on the office website, can help patients to feel more comfortable before their first visit [26].

During the Visit

The quality of physician-patient communication positively correlates with health outcomes even in the general population and is just as important when dealing with adults with ASD [27, 31]. Healthcare professionals should respect requests for alternate forms of communication (e.g., written notes, use of communication devices) even when adults with ASD are capable of fluent verbal communication. Some patients, though capable of articulate speech, may find this method of communication stressful to the point that it hampers their ability to convey their healthcare needs effectively or understand the options of treatment presented to them [31]. As such, the clinical staff should be receptive to using whatever form of communication makes the patient most comfortable.

Physical Examination

Adults with ASD can benefit from many of the same strategies discussed in the pediatric portion of this chapter. Providing a clear description of what will happen during the visit and developing a routine over time are both ways to help adults with ASD feel more comfortable in the clinical environment. Before the examination, the physician should figure out the most effective form of communication for the patient so that he is comfortable giving and receiving information [27, 31].

Use literal and direct language where possible, as adults with ASD often have difficulties interpreting figures of speech or answering broad, open-ended questions [31]. An inability to answer certain questions with complete accuracy can be a source of stress for patients. Offering multiple choice answers or reassuring them that 100% accuracy is not necessary can facilitate communication [27]. It is important not to force eye contact on a patient who seems unwilling, as this may cause stress and an inability to communicate comfortably.

In a survey conducted to better understand the experiences of adults with ASD in the healthcare setting, one patient stated, "I am not able to bring up my concerns because it is all I can manage to figure out what the doctor is saying so I can respond to his questions [31]. Another study noted that many adults with ASD "report[ed] insufficient time to indicate that an area [was] tender before the provider began palpitating a different area [27]. These experiences highlight that many individuals with ASD need more time to process information than physicians are used to giving. Slowing down examinations allows sufficient time for patients to work through stimuli and questions and accurately voice their concerns and answers. It is also helpful to have patients repeat important information back to the physician as a way to confirm comprehension, as well as to write it down for their later review.

Table 2.3 contains a few suggestions on how to facilitate the physical examination and procedures for adults with ASD.

Table 2.3 (Adapted from *Primary Care for Adults on the Autism Spectrum*, 2014 [30]) – Strategies for successful physical examination, tests, procedures, and phlebotomy

Physical examinations, tests, and procedures
Explain procedures before beginning
Show and demonstrate equipment to patient before procedure where possible
If possible, walk the patient through a mock procedure for especially difficult examinations
Always announce the intention to touch patients before doing so, and give them time to process this information
Minimize how long patients must be undressed or in a gown
Allow extra time for patients to process information, and allow ample time for a response so they do not feel rushed
Use literal language when asking questions, and be aware that relevant information might not be provided unless specifically elicited
Prepare a signal beforehand to show that patients need a break
Offer patients a stress ball to distract their attention, and decrease sensory overstimulation through heavy work
Phlebotomy
Do the minimum amount of required blood work, and group tests together to minimize number of blood draws
Permit the patient to lie down during blood drawing
If the patient can tolerate the sensation, use a numbing spray or cream for blood work
Give a precise indication of how long it will take, i.e., how many tubes of blood you need
Consider anti-anxiety medication on a case-by-case basis
Allow patients to prepare themselves by giving sufficient warning before beginning

Clinical Vignette #2

Dr. WB is a primary care physician scheduled to see Michael, a 25-year-old man with ASD who lives independently, for his first appointment. Michael has recently changed insurance and is looking to build a relationship with a new, in-network healthcare provider. Although Michael contacted the office over the phone, he expressed a preference for communication via email, and all subsequent communication has been electronic. Michael has hypertension and gastrointestinal (GI) issues (both gastroesophageal reflux and an intolerance to certain textures of foods). The distress from his GI problems has prompted this visit. Before scheduling his appointment, Michael submits an online survey in which he reports intense auditory and temperature sensitivities, his preference to communicate through written notes, and severe anxiety caused by needles. He also mentions that being in unfamiliar places with people he does not know is difficult for him.

Dr. WB decides to schedule Michael's appointment for the beginning of the day, when the office is quieter, and to minimize wait times. Prior to the appointment, Dr. WB sends Michael photos of the office and the examination room they will be in, along with pictures of the staff who will be working the day of his appointment, and he makes a note in Michael's chart that the patient prefers to communicate through writing.

When Michael arrives on the day of his appointment, the front staff who have been previously notified of his preferences show him to the examination room, and they lower the air conditioner, so it is not too cold for Michael in the room. Michael seems calm in this environment. The nurse in the office patiently waits and reads Michael's written note and is able to complete height, weight, heart rate, and blood pressure measurements. She tells Michael that Dr. WB will be in to see him in 10 min.

Dr. WB makes sure to not keep Michael waiting longer than 10 min, aware that indefinite waiting times and uncertainty are sources of stress for many patients with ASD. When Dr. WB enters the room, Michael seems apprehensive of the coming tests. Michael does not seem to want to make eye contact, and Dr. WB respects his wishes. Dr. WB engages Michael, asking him about his interests to create familiarity and help him to feel comfortable. After a brief exchange about the Pittsburgh Steelers (Michael is a huge fan), Dr. WB clearly outlines the procedures and the structure of the examination, making sure to give Michael time to ask any questions he might have. He also asks Michael to write down a note that says "Stop!" which he tells Michael to hold up anytime he feels he needs a break from the exam.

When Michael indicates that he is ready to proceed, Dr. WB begins the examination. He is careful to announce his intent to touch Michael whenever he does and to leave sufficient time for him to understand such a request. He shows every instrument used in the exam to Michael and demonstrates how it is used before employing it. Michael holds up the "Stop!" card when Dr. WB begins to check his heart. Dr. WB stops his examination and gives Michael time to compose himself. Michael writes a note that the stethoscope is too cold for him to tolerate. Dr. WB takes a moment to warm the stethoscope in his hand and apologizes to Michael for causing him discomfort. Dr. WB offers the warmed stethoscope to Michael, who indicates that it is an acceptable temperature, and the exam proceeds.

When it is time to draw blood, Dr. WB asks Michael if he has had an experience with EMLA cream as a means of dealing with his phobia of needles. Michael writes that the cooling sensation of EMLA cream is difficult for him and that he prefers to proceed without it. Dr. WB offers him a stress ball, suggesting that it might help to distract him from the procedure. Michael accepts it. Dr. WB tells Michael exactly how many vials of blood they have to fill and runs through the procedure. He lets Michael lie down and gives him time to prepare himself before starting.

After the exam is over, they develop a plan of care to begin monitoring Michael's GI problems. Before ending the examination, Dr. WB asks Michael to repeat the plan to him to make sure Michael has fully understood it and then asks Michael if he has any further questions or concerns. Michael writes that he is worried about navigating his new insurance. Dr. WB offers to introduce Michael to the social worker in the office, who can assist him with his difficulties understanding his insurance.

Clinical Pearls

- ASD is a lifelong neurodevelopmental condition that affects an individual's ability to communicate and interact with others and can affect the quality of care they receive. It is therefore necessary for all pediatric, adolescent, and adult providers to be aware of the needs of individuals with ASD.
- Asking for specific information before the clinical encounter about the individual patient's specific needs, including preferred communication methods, can help prepare staff to care for individuals with ASD.
- Preparation of the clinical space with regard to safety and sensory stimuli can help patients with ASD feel more comfortable in an outpatient medical setting.
- Providing patients with visual information about routine clinic procedures ahead of time can help patients with ASD learn what to expect and alleviate any anxiety they may have about what will happen during their appointment.
- Following a clear, consistent, and predictable routine can also help patients with ASD feel more comfortable during an outpatient encounter.
- Seeing patients with ASD more frequently for shorter encounters and asking questions about developmental skills can alert clinicians to worsening or regression at times of stress in addition to nurturing the patient-provider relationship.
- In adolescence, it is critical that physicians address healthcare transition needs in order to prepare patients for the shift from pediatric to adult medical care.
- For adolescents and adults, it is important to address the individual with ASD first and then turn to the caregiver (if applicable) only if the individual is not able to answer a specific question.
- With individuals with ASD who have difficulty with abstract or nuanced language, use literal and direct language, avoid figures of speech wherever possible, and be aware of

when closed-ended questions may be needed for those who feel the need to answer questions accurately.

- Speak slowly with patients who have trouble processing language, give plenty of time for a response, and confirm comprehension.

Conclusion

ASD is a lifelong condition that affects the way an individual interacts with people in all settings and, in particular, can lead to difficulty with completing a medical encounter, affecting the quality of care individuals with ASD receive. In this chapter we have presented specific suggestions for accommodating the clinical environment and structuring the medical encounter that healthcare providers can use in the outpatient medical setting when caring for individuals with ASD. Though presented in the context of care for patients with ASD, many of these accommodations are relevant to the general population and could improve the healthcare experience for all patients.

References

1. American Psychiatric Association. Diagnostic and statistical manual of mental disorders: DSM-5. 5th ed. Washington, D.C: American Psychiatric Association; 2013.
2. Baio J, Wiggins L, Christensen DL, Maenner MJ, Daniels J, Warren Z, et al. Prevalence of autism spectrum disorder among children aged 8 years –autism and developmental disabilities monitoring network, 11 sites, United States, 2014. MMWR Surveill Summ. 2018;67:1–23.
3. Howlin P, Moss P, Savage S, Rutter M. Social outcomes in mid- to later adulthood among individuals diagnosed with autism and average nonverbal IQ as children. J Am Acad Child Adolesc Psychiatry. 2013;52(6):572–81. e1.
4. McDougle CJ. Sounding a wake-up call: improving the lives of adults with autism. J Am Acad Child Adolesc Psychiatry. 2013;52(6):566–8.
5. Allely CS. Pain sensitivity and observer perception of pain in individuals with autistic spectrum disorder. Sci World J. 2013;2013:916178.
6. Bultas MW, McMillin SE, Zand DH. Reducing barriers to care in the office-based health care setting for children with autism. J Pediatr Health Care. 2016;30(1):5–14.
7. Raymaker DM, McDonald KE, Ashkenazy E, Gerrity M, Baggs AM, Kripke C, et al. Barriers to healthcare: instrument development and comparison between autistic adults and adults with and without other disabilities. Autism. 2016;21:972–84.
8. Zuckerman KE, Lindly OJ, Bethell CD, Kuhlthau K. Family impacts among children with autism spectrum disorder: the role of health care quality. Acad Pediatr. 2014;14(4):398–407.
9. Kogan MD, Strickland BB, Blumberg SJ, Singh GK, Perrin JM, van Dyck PC. A national profile of the health care experiences and family impact of autism spectrum disorder among children in the United States, 2005–2006. Pediatrics. 2008;122(6):e1149–58.
10. Golnik A, Ireland M, Borowsky IW. Medical homes for children with autism: a physician survey. Pediatrics. 2009;123(3):966–71.
11. Davignon MN, Friedlaender E, Cronholm PF, Paciotti B, Levy SE. Parent and provider perspectives on procedural care for children with autism spectrum disorders. J Dev Behav Pediatr. 2014;35(3):207–15.
12. Browning A. My hospital passport: the National Autistic Society; 2016. Available from: http://www.autism.org.uk/about/health/hospital-passport.aspx.
13. Massachusetts General Hospital Lurie Center Autism Care Questionnaire. Available from: http://www.massgeneral.org/children/services/luriecenter/Autism-Care-Questionnaire.aspx.
14. Broder-Fingert S, Shui A, Ferrone C, Iannuzzi D, Cheng ER, Giauque A, et al. A pilot study of autism-specific care plans during hospital admission. Pediatrics. 2016;137(Supplement 2):S196–204.
15. McGuire K, Fung LK, Hagopian L, Vasa RA, Mahajan R, Bernal P, et al. Irritability and problem behavior in autism spectrum disorder: a practice pathway for pediatric primary care. Pediatrics. 2016;137(Suppl 2):S136–48.
16. Coury DL, Ashwood P, Fasano A, Fuchs G, Geraghty M, Kaul A, et al. Gastrointestinal conditions in children with autism spectrum disorder: developing a research agenda. Pediatrics. 2012;130(Suppl 2. United States):S160–8.
17. Buie T, Fuchs GJ 3rd, Furuta GT, Kooros K, Levy J, Lewis JD, et al. Recommendations for evaluation and treatment of common gastrointestinal problems in children with ASDs. Pediatrics. 2010;125(Suppl 1):S19–29.
18. Elrod MG, Hood BS. Sleep differences among children with autism spectrum disorders and typically developing peers: a meta-analysis. J Dev Behav Pediatr. 2015;36(3):166–77.
19. Mandell DS, Walrath CM, Manteuffel B, Sgro G, Pinto-Martin JA. The prevalence and correlates of abuse among children with autism served in comprehensive community-based mental health settings. Child Abuse Negl. 2005;29(12):1359–72.
20. Cheak-Zamora NC, Farmer JE, Mayfield WA, Clark MJ, Marvin AR, Kiely Law J, Law PA. Health care transition services for youth with autism spectrum disorders. Rehabil Psychol. 2014;59(3):340–8.

21. Billstedt E, Gillberg C, Gillberg C. Autism after adolescence: population-based 13- to 22-year follow-up study of 120 individuals with autism diagnosed in childhood. J Autism Dev Disord. 2005;35:351–60.
22. Child and Adolescent Health Measurement Initiative. National profile of children with special health care needs and autism spectrum disorder: Key findings from the 2009/10 NS-CSHCN & 2007 NSCH. 2012. Retrieved from http://www.childhealthdata.org/docs/drc/asd-databrief_4.2.12.pdf
23. Holtz K, Owings N, Ziegert A. Life journey through autism: a guide for transition to adulthood. 2006. Retrieved from: http://www.researchautism.org/resources/reading/documents.
24. Lotstein DS, Ghandour R, Cash A, McGuire E, Strickland B, Newacheck P. Planning for health care transitions: results from the 2005–2006 national survey of children with special health care needs. Pediatrics. 2009;123:e145–52.
25. Raymaker DM, McDonald KE, Ashkenazy E, Gerrity M, Baggs AM, Kripke C, et al. Barriers to healthcare: instrument development and comparison between autistic adults and adults with and without other disabilities. Autism. 2017;21:972–84.
26. Dern S, Sappok T. Barriers to healthcare for people on the autism spectrum. Adv Autism. 2016;2:2–11.
27. Nicolaidis C, Kripke CC, Raymaker D. Primary care for adults on the autism spectrum. Med Clin N Am. 2014;98:1169–91.
28. Kirchner J, Appelmann S, Chiewkowsky C, Dern S, Dohle R, Elias R, Gotz E, Gottschlich R, Grambert CN, Kliemann D, Melzow F, Speer O, Purwins S, Dziobek I. Wissen und Unwissen uber Autismus. Poster presented at the 3rd Scientific Meeting for Autism Spectrum Conditions (WTAS) February 18–19th 2010, Frankfurt am Main.
29. Zerbo O, Massolo ML, Qian Y, Croen LA. A study of physician knowledge and experience with autism in adults in a large integrated healthcare system. J Autism Dev Disord. 2015;45:4002–14.
30. Nicolaidis C, Raymaker D, McDonald K, Dern S, Boisclair WC, Ashkenazy E, et al. Comparison of healthcare experiences in autistic and non-autistic adults: a cross-sectional online survey facilitated by an academic-community partnership. J Gen Intern Med. 2013;28:761–9.
31. Nicolaidis C, Raymaker DM, Ashkenazy E, McDonald KE, Dern S, Baggs AE, et al. "Respect the way I need to communicate with you": healthcare experiences of adults on the autism spectrum. Autism. 2015;19:824–31.
32. Kuhaneck HM, Chisholm EC. Improving dental visits for individuals with autism spectrum disorders through an understanding of sensory processing. Spec Care Dentist. 2012;32:229–33.

3 Inpatient Medical Care

Ann Kao and Jocelyn Carter

Pediatric Inpatient Care

Clinical Vignette # 1

TJ is a nonverbal 5-year-old male with a diagnosis of ASD who is admitted to the inpatient unit of a pediatric hospital for food refusal and increased intermittent bouts of agitation, which consist of head banging and grunting.

He was initially seen in the emergency department (ED), where he had an expedited workup and admission after his gastrointestinal (GI) specialist phoned the ED doctor and explained that he would need an inpatient workup. He did not allow the nurses to take vital signs or anyone to examine him despite coaxing and coaching from his parents.

On the floor, TJ continued to cry and was resistant to examinations. An X-ray showed significant stool burden, but he refused all oral intake and gagged and vomited when passage of a nasogastric tube (NGT) was attempted. Given his refusal of oral intake and the inability to administer medications, the decision was made to take him to the operating room under general anesthesia for a cleanout and NGT placement.

The day prior to the intervention, several consults were placed including a consult to occupational therapy (OT) to help with coping. The OT was able to discuss preferred calming mechanisms, what types of enhanced communication the child used at home (picture cards), as well as preferred foods and methods of eating and drinking.

The OT crafted a care plan in coordination with child psychiatry, child life, and speech and language pathology that included enhanced communication, tablet computers with music and pictures for distractions, pureed foods with a special cut nipple bottle, and limiting care providers to one at a time with TJ's mother facilitating exams. He was also given a veil-enclosed bed and a weighted blanket.

TJ was able to take a few doses of MiraLAX and liquid stool softeners that night and tolerated a Fleets enema administered by his mother while playing an interactive game on the tablet.

The GI team was able to defer the general anesthesia evaluation. TJ progressively improved after a large stool output and was able to be discharged home on hospital day 5.

A. Kao
Department of Pediatrics and Internal Medicine, Massachusetts General Hospital, Boston, MA, USA
e-mail: akao@mgh.harvard.edu

J. Carter (✉)
Department of Medicine, Massachusetts General Hospital, Boston, MA, USA
e-mail: jcarter0@mgh.harvard.edu

E. P. Hazen, C. J. McDougle (eds.), *The Massachusetts General Hospital Guide to Medical Care in Patients with Autism Spectrum Disorder*, Current Clinical Psychiatry,
https://doi.org/10.1007/978-3-319-94458-6_3

Background

Challenges for Pediatric Patients with ASD in the Inpatient Setting

Caring for children with ASD in the hospital raises unique challenges for care providers. There have been very few studies of in-hospital care of children with ASD. Several surveys of caregivers, including physicians, nurses, and parents, have documented the increased stress of parents and lack of comfort of providers in caring for patients with ASD [8].

Inpatient care can be particularly challenging for children with ASD. Children with ASD are disproportionately affected by the disruption of routines, including sleep, and the absence of a familiar environment associated with hospitalization. Difficulties with communication and sensory integration issues can also make the hospital setting quite traumatic for children with ASD [16]. At the same time, patients with ASD have a higher rate of overnight hospitalizations. On average, children with ASD had 4 times as many inpatient hospital days and 12 times as many psychiatric inpatient hospital days as children without ASD in one large Kaiser Permanente study [4]. In another large study of all patients with ASD (both children and adults), length of stay was also increased: 1.5 times higher for individuals with ASD compared to a control group [10].

Lack of ability to effectively communicate with children with ASD can lead to missed or delayed diagnosis as well as the use of potentially avoidable procedures and tests [16]. In a survey of parents of 80 patients with ASD affiliated with Massachusetts General Hospital, 63% under the age of 5 years communicated using only sign language or gestures, and patients of all ages were likely to use communication devices [8].

Strategies for Improving Care of Pediatric Patients in the Inpatient Setting

There is a lack of literature on effective interventions in the inpatient setting to improve quality and perception of care for pediatric inpatients with ASD. Checklists and audits have been proposed as quality improvement processes for care of patients in the hospital with ASD [14]. One pilot study done at Massachusetts General Hospital for Children (MGHfC) by Broder-Fingert et al. showed a better general hospital experience and improved perception of staff attention to their children's ASD-specific needs with the use of an autism-specific care plan [1].

The MGHfC Experience

In our experience a multidisciplinary framework is the key to care of children with ASD. Buy-in from leadership of different departments including emergency, inpatient, subspecialties, nursing, child life, dietary, OT, physical therapy (PT), psychiatry, and radiology areas is crucial. Providing physicians and nurses with a foundation of knowledge in care of patients with ASD is also essential.

Our institution has advanced efforts to minimize ED time and to arrange for direct admission to the inpatient units whenever possible for children with ASD. Patients in the emergency room are identified based on a diagnosis of ASD listed in the problem list of their Electronic Health Record (EHR). The institution is in the process of developing an icon to appear in the header of the EHR in order to notify providers more quickly so that appropriate accommodations can be initiated early in the hospital stay. When a patient in the emergency room is determined to be in need of medical admission, all efforts are made to expedite bed placement through direct communication with the resource nurse on the inpatient unit as well as the admitting team as early as possible. Our units do not solely contain private rooms, and placement with a roommate can be challenging. There is a process of individual evaluation in conjunction with parents, nursing, and clinicians to optimally place a patient either in a private room or with a compatible roommate. When there are needs for specialized equipment such as veil beds and weighted blankets, these are made available as early as possible in the hospitalization. Child life and OT work together to create an individualized toolkit for each patient including sensory and communication equipment.

If a patient's admission is scheduled, an attending nurse (a nurse who is specialized in coordination of care for the unit) is notified, and she ensures that there is an Autism Care Questionnaire completed in the chart. If one has not been done, the attending nurse will contact the parents to have one filled out to facilitate staffing and planning.

We have created a specialized order set in the EHR to facilitate admission of patients with ASD. This prompts the clinician to remember to order an OT consult, look for the Autism Care Questionnaire, and to consider other multidisciplinary team care members such as nutrition, child life, psychiatry, and social work. Using input from the multidisciplinary care team, our Autism Care Questionnaire is then crafted into an Autism Care Plan, which is posted in the chart as well as on the wall above the patient's bed so that all care providers can refer to it when interacting with the patient.

In order to reduce the stress on patients with ASD, physician teams modify the structure of rounds including minimizing the number of care providers entering the patient's room and avoiding unnecessary repetition of physical examinations. Nursing also considers modification of the schedule for recording vital signs when appropriate. Close and frequent communication with the parents and outpatient providers is crucial in aiding the transition both into and out of the hospital, and hospital care plans are modified in order to allow the patient to return home to their familiar environment as expediently as possible. The dosing schedule of medications and the mechanism of administration of medications are agreed upon in advance with partnership with the families and help from child life and OT. Home communication devices and familiar toys, clothing, and music can all aid in a successful transition to the hospital. Our medical team aims to limit the introduction of any new medications, as unanticipated medication effects can be problematic in the ASD population given the likelihood of medical comorbidities and polypharmacy.

Further study on the Autism Care Plan and other inpatient interventions such as checklists and audits is sorely needed in order to guide care of this patient population.

Adult Inpatient Care

Clinical Vignette #2

AB was a 21-year-old nonverbal woman with ASD who presented to an ED with abdominal pain with decreased appetite. Due to high patient volumes in the ED, the patient was placed in the hallway until a private bed may become available. Intravenous (IV) antibiotics were started for a presumed urinary tract infection. Multiple nursing and physician evaluations occurred in the course of her ED stay. Over time, the patient became increasingly agitated and uncooperative, and she was given IV haloperidol to manage her agitation. After an additional 4 h, a bed on an inpatient floor became available, and the patient was transported with her mother to the inpatient medicine unit for admission. Because a private bed was not available, the patient was placed in a double room with a patient suffering from delirium due to alcohol withdrawal. A nursing intake was completed with the patient's mother present, and her mother answered all of the questions regarding the patient's social habits and family history. Following admission, repeat blood work with additional nursing and physician evaluations was performed, and the patient exhibited worsening agitation with self-removal of multiple IV lines throughout the day. Per nursing request, a soft restraint was placed to preserve the IV access for fluids and antibiotic therapy.

The patient's mother became upset that the patient was being restrained and requested a different nurse. Multiple subsequent nursing reassignments had to be made to accommodate this request, resulting in disruption and delayed care throughout the floor. After a meeting with the patient's mother, attending physician, and the nursing unit director, an agreement was reached on ways of improving communication with the patient and her mother. On the day of discharge, the group home director arrived and completed an individual assessment of the patient and reviewed the hospitalization events. The group home director asked the physician and case manager to document all new medications, follow-up appointments, and discharge instructions on the group home forms prior to accepting the patient back to the group home as a resident. Due to these unanticipated documentation requests, the patient was discharged after a 5-h delay.

This vignette illustrates how even a relatively simple clinical diagnosis can turn into a complex hospitalization for some patients with ASD. Minimizing environmental auditory and visual stimuli, reducing nonessential testing or diagnostics, understanding the patient and guardian's expectations for care, and better preparation for discharge could have improved the patient care experience. This case underlines key phases of care for patients with ASD and demonstrates how routine inpatient practices can have a negative outcome for patients with ASD.

Caring for Those with ASD in the Hospital: What Is Known

While there is a clear dearth of evidence-based literature on adults with ASD, the majority of best practices in inpatient care delivery for adults with ASD have been adapted from the pediatric literature. Venkat and associates [17] provide key recommendations for providers in acute care settings that may encounter adult patients with ASD. These include patient-centered preparation of the care environment, engaging caregivers and patients, and the use of patient-centered communication to assist in care delivery at outpatient clinics, emergency departments, and inpatient settings.

Despite the focus on developing practices in pediatric settings for ASD patients, planning for the transition to adult health services occurs only about 20% of the time [9]. Cheak-Zamora and associates [2] surveyed a cohort of 101 parents of young adults with ASD transitioning to adult ASD health care and found that fewer than 15% had received health-care transition services. This was in stark contrast to approximately 50% of youth with other special health-care needs that receive health-care transition services based upon the data collected in the 2005–2006 National Survey of Children with Special Health Care Needs [3]. A lack of focus on the careful transition of those with ASD from pediatric to adult health-care services can only expose patients to additional risk of being lost to follow-up, generating ever-widening gaps in care. There are no systematic reviews of medical home use in transitioning adolescents with ASD to adult care, as underscored by Rogers and colleagues [15]. This drives home the lack of research done in this area and the growing need for studies focused on services for adolescents as they mature into adults.

Innovation in Care Delivery for Inpatients with ASD

In terms of intervention and strategies to address the lack of transition programming in place for adolescents with ASD as they transition to adulthood, a number of tactics were proposed by an expert panel of pediatric providers surveyed on their perspectives on key practices in transitioning youth to adult ASD care [9]. Recommendations included providing written medical summaries to adult providers detailing past pediatric medical profiles, compiling lists of available adult providers or community resources for patients and parents of patients with ASD to consider as adult providers, coordinating care and communication between individual pediatric and adult providers, making or assisting patients in making transition-specific appointments, and using checklists to track transition progress. Informational workshops were also suggested to help families and youth prepare for this transition. Additional education for adult providers and medical students was another recommendation that providers offered. Some respondents also identified the need for a transition center where all services could be coordinated in one place.

As the number of primary care providers and generalists taking care of adult patients with ASD increases, growing attention has been placed on the ability of providers to care for adults with ASD. Warfield and colleagues took a close look at primary care physician perspectives on providing care to adults with ASD [18]. Health-care providers indicated that there are a number of challenges in care delivery to adults with ASD in terms of gaps in provider training and a lack of resources for adults with ASD. A survey of adult health-care providers in the Kaiser Permanente Northern California system demonstrated that most providers lacked clinical skills, knowledge, educational training, and resources needed to care for adults with ASD optimally [19].

The perspectives of adult patients with ASD are increasingly providing evidence of need for improvement in inpatient medical care delivery for adults with ASD. Online surveys of adults with ASD and their guardians demonstrated unmet needs in health-care access as well as a multitude of domains related to social determinants of health [7]. A survey of adults with and without an ASD diagnosis demonstrated that patients with ASD had lower rates of satisfaction with patient-provider communication and higher rates of unmet health-care needs related to physical health and mental health. Not surprisingly, adults with ASD report higher rates of ED use.

In addition, studies focused on adults with ASD show increased predominance of coexisting conditions as compared to those without ASD. According to Fortuna and colleagues, adults with ASD have higher rates of seizure disorder and depression (in adults 18–29 years and adults over 40 years old, respectively). In those over 40 years of age, only 43–54% could independently perform their activities of daily living, and 91% of those with IQ scores available had intellectual disability (IQ<70) [5]. Significantly increased rates of psychiatric disorders, as well as diabetes, hypertension, GI disorders and stroke, have been found in a population of adults with ASD as compared to a cohort of adults without ASD. Ironically, members of the adult ASD population who clearly have an increased risk for comorbid conditions may be less likely to have these needs met due to a lack of transition care planning as described above.

Few studies describing implementation of best practices in caring for adults in inpatient settings exist. Some examples include those characterized by McGonigle and colleagues in the development and evaluation of educational materials for ED staff and providers [11, 12]. McGonigle and associates also made similar recommendations for optimal management of inpatient pediatric, adolescent, and adult patients based on expert experiences in this area [11, 12]. The lack of patient-centered hospital care in adults with ASD is mirrored to some extent in the pediatric literature focused on unmet needs for inpatients with ASD. Pediatric qualitative survey studies demonstrate an ongoing need for inclusion for youth and parent preferences in the construction of inpatient care plans [13].

Case Study at the Massachusetts General Hospital: Improving Medical Care for Adults with ASD

In an effort to rise to this developing imperative, the Massachusetts General Hospital sought to improve the delivery of high-quality care to adult inpatients with ASDs in 2015. As emphasized in Clinical Vignette #2 presented above, most of the standard practice for inpatient adult care falls woefully short when caring for patients with ASD. To better address the needs of adults with ASD and redefine the evolving standard of care for inpatient adults with ASD, a group of providers and caregivers came together with the global aim of improving care delivery for adult inpatients with ASD as well as their families from admission to discharge. This group included experts in ASD, pediatricians, case managers, nurses, internal medicine hospitalists, social workers, occupational therapists, physical therapists, speech therapists, and parents of patients with ASD. Specific aims included the following:

1. Educating inpatient clinical providers as well as nonclinical staff about ASD and the individual communication and sensory needs of patients while hospitalized
2. Creating a battery of tools that could be used in real time to assist providers both in basic clinical care and challenging clinical scenarios
3. Developing informational and educational resources for patients and families to optimize the inpatient care experience as well as the transition out of the acute care setting

Deliverables to aid the effort became defined as a toolkit which was comprised of the following: educational videos for clinical and nonclinical providers unfamiliar with ASD, an Autism Admission Basics Checklist (Fig. 3.1), an Autism Clinical Care Algorithm (Fig. 3.2), an Autism Care Questionnaire (Fig. 3.3), an Autism "What to expect as an inpatient" Informational Guide (Fig. 3.4), an Autism Case Management Resource (Fig. 3.5), an online Inpatient ASD Image Gallery to help prepare patients for admission, and an Autism Order Set.

MGH Autism Toolkit Components

The admission basics checklist for unplanned admissions (Fig. 3.1) was designed to aid providers as they prepare for a patient with ASD in the ED or on the inpatient medical unit. Avoiding sensory overload by reducing bright light and loud noises can help create a less stressful environment for inpatients with ASD [6]. Alternatively, eliminating what may be unnecessary vital sign checks, diagnostics, monitoring, and lab draws can help reduce the flurry of activity that can contribute to stress. This type of admission tool is particularly valuable in that it may serve as a checklist of sorts for providers who may have limited bandwidth as they juggle their many clinical duties. This tool also can serve as a helpful foundation for a standardized approach to care in a number of different settings that welcome patients with individualized communication preferences and sensory sensitivities.

The clinical care algorithm (Fig. 3.2) is another helpful piece of the autism toolkit. This algorithm gives providers stepwise guidance to help provide the best care possible to adult

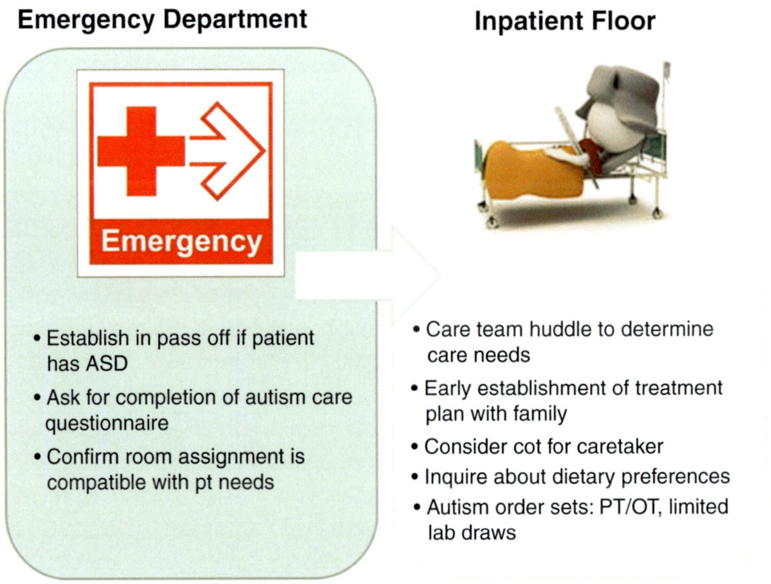

Fig. 3.1 The admission basics checklist

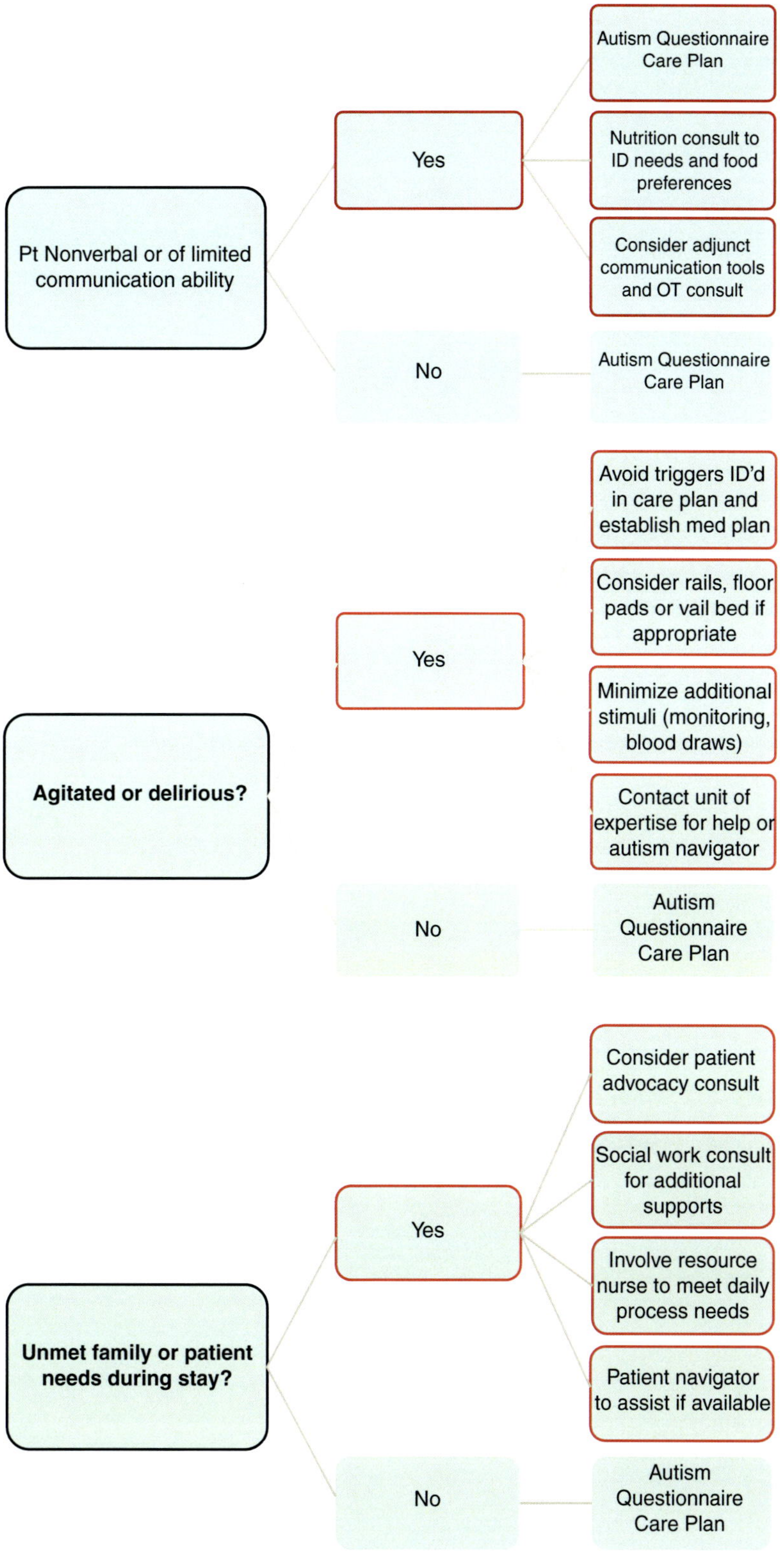

Fig. 3.2 The clinical care algorithm

Autism Care Questionnaire (ACQ)

We want to make sure this hospital visit is a positive experience. Please fill out this form to help us learn about you/the patient so we can better meet your/the patient's needs.

Patient Information

Date: ______________________________
Patient's name: ______________________________
Patient's date of birth: ______________________
Patient's age: ______________________________

Name of person completing this form:
What is your relationship to the patient? ______________________________

Does the patient have a guardian (circle one)? Yes No
Guardian's name:
Guardian's contact information:
If the guardian is appointed by the court, a copy of the guardianship should be submitted to the hospital.

Does the patient have a health care proxy (circle one)? Yes No
Health Care Proxy's Name: ______________________________
Health Care Proxy's contact information: ______________________________

Communication:

1) How does the patient prefer to communicate needs/wants? (check one)

☐ Talking
☐ Making sounds, grunting, yelling
☐ Sign language
☐ Pointing/gesturing
☐ Pictures or symbols
☐ Pictures with words
☐ Typed words
☐ Handwritten words
☐ Using tablet or communication device
☐ Facial expressions (smiling, frowning, etc.)
Other: ______________________

2) What other ways will the patient tell us what he/she needs/wants? (check all that apply)

☐ Talking
☐ Making sounds, grunting, yelling
☐ Sign language
☐ Pointing/gesturing
☐ Pictures or symbols

Fig. 3.3 The Autism Care Questionnaire for patients and families

- ☐ Pictures with words
- ☐ Typed words
- ☐ Handwritten words
- ☐ Using tablet or communication device
- ☐ Facial expressions (smiling, frowning, etc.)

Other: ______________________________

3) How does the patient communicate "yes" or "no" when asked a question?______________________________

____

4) How does the patient learn new information or instructions (Check all that apply)?

- ☐ Talking
- ☐ Sign language
- ☐ Pictures or symbols
- ☐ Pictures with words
- ☐ Typed words
- ☐ Handwritten words
- ☐ Stories
- ☐ Using tablet or communication device
- ☐ To Do/finished boards
- ☐ First/then boards
- ☐ Other: ________________________

5) How does the patient know that time is passing?

- ☐ Using a clock or watch
- ☐ Using a timer
- ☐ Using schedule boards
- ☐ Counting aloud
- ☐ Other:_____________________

6) What is the best way for us to tell the patient how long he/she will be sitting in the waiting room, waiting for a test, or how long the test will take?

____

____

7) How will the patient tell us that he/she has to go to the bathroom?

____

____

8) How will the patient tell us if he/she is hungry or thirsty?

____

____

9) How will the patient let us know if he/she is in pain (Check all that apply)?

- ☐ Talking
- ☐ Making sounds, grunting, yelling
- ☐ Crying
- ☐ Sign language
- ☐ Pointing/gesturing
- ☐ Pictures or symbols

Fig. 3.3 (continued)

- ☐ Pictures with words
- ☐ Typed words
- ☐ Handwritten words
- ☐ Using tablet or communication device
- ☐ Facial expressions (frowning, etc.)
- ☐ Hitting or hurting self
- ☐ Hitting or hurting others

10) Are there other clues that will let us know if the patient is in pain?

____

The Hospital Visit and Examination

1) How should we greet the patient?______________________________________

2) What is the best way for us to examine the patient (Check all that apply)?

- ☐ Communicate with the patient (using the favored communication method) before each step of the exam
- ☐ List or count things that the doctor needs to do (i.e. 1-look at eyes, 2-look in ears, 3-listen to heart, etc.)
- ☐ Allow the patient to touch any instruments (i.e. stethoscope, blood pressure cuff) him or herself
- ☐ Hide instruments until their use becomes necessary
- ☐ Do parts of the exam on someone else first
- ☐ Distraction
- ☐ Other:

3) Is there a part of the exam that the patient will not like (Check all that apply)?

- ☐ Using a stethoscope to listen to lungs
- ☐ Checking blood pressure with the cuff
- ☐ Eye test
- ☐ Ear test
- ☐ Looking in mouth/throat
- ☐ Belly exam
- ☐ Testing reflexes
- ☐ Other:

4) Will the patient wear a hospital gown (circle one)? Yes No
If no, what would the patient want to wear?___________________________

5) Will the patient wear a hospital ID band on their wrist (circle one)? Yes No
If no, please let us know before the patient comes to the hospital if possible.

Comfort and Safety

1) Is the patient sensitive to (Check all that apply):

- ☐ Loud noises
- ☐ Unexpected noises
- ☐ Bright lights

Fig. 3.3 (continued)

- ☐ Specific colors
- ☐ Fragrances/smells
- ☐ Textures
- ☐ Touch
- ☐ Specific types of touch

2) How long does the patient usually sleep at night?____

3) Will a sitter be used to help ensure that the patient is safe (circle one)? Yes No
If yes, what hours will the sitter be at the hospital?_________________________________

4) Does the patient have any food allergies (circle one)? Yes No

If yes, what are the allergies?____

5) Is the patient on a special diet (circle one)? Yes No

If yes, what type?____

6) Are there special times of the day that the patient eats snacks or meals (circle one)? Yes No

If yes, what times?____

7) Does the patient like to separate food on a plate or use different plates for different foods (circle one)? Yes No

If yes, what does the patient like?____

8) Are there any words, phrases or actions that will upset the patient (circle one)? Yes No
If yes, what are they?

____

____

9) How will the patient let us know if he/she is upset/anxious (check all that apply)?

- ☐ Talking
- ☐ Making sounds, grunting, yelling
- ☐ Sign language
- ☐ Pointing/gesturing
- ☐ Pictures or symbols
- ☐ Pictures with words
- ☐ Typed words
- ☐ Handwritten words
- ☐ Using tablet or communication device
- ☐ Facial expressions (smiling, frowning, etc.)
- ☐ Physical motions (rocking, flapping, squeezing hands)
- ☐ Hitting or hurting self
- ☐ Hitting or hurting others

Fig. 3.3 (continued)

10) What are the first things we should do if the patient is upset/anxious (check all that apply)?

- ☐ Leave him/her alone
- ☐ Give him/her some space
- ☐ Talk to him/her
- ☐ Other

11) Would any of these help us decrease the patient's anxiety (check all that apply)?

- ☐ A map of the hospital
- ☐ An escort that will help the patient around the hospital
- ☐ Low lighting
- ☐ Sunglasses
- ☐ Headphones to decrease noise
- ☐ A heavy blanket
- ☐ Music
- ☐ Videos
- ☐ Puzzles/games
- ☐ Other

12) Are there any other safety concerns we should know about (circle one)? Yes No
If Yes, what are the concerns?

____

____

13) Is there anything else we should know about so we can make the patient's hospital visit as positive as possible?

____

____

Fig. 3.3 (continued)

patients with ASD. It includes recommendations about approaches to the management of agitated patients, distressed patients and families, and patients with significant communication impairments. While this algorithm is only focused on a few core domains, having access to a guide to approaching more commonly occurring challenges may serve as an impetus to expand this approach as needed in individual institutions.

The Autism Care Questionnaire (ACQ; Fig. 3.3) is another valuable component of the toolkit. Based on a pediatric care plan [1], the ACQ creates a platform for clinical encounters with ASD patients and their families. The ACQ helps providers in clinical settings attain important information about the patient's ideal means of communication, sensory and behavioral needs, potential triggers for anxiety or agitation, effective soothing strategies, and other individual care preferences. Given the uniqueness and variability of patients with ASD, having a road map of pre-existing needs and capabilities as well as potential situations that trigger agitation or cause stress is invaluable.

As presented in the Clinical Vignette #2 above, effective adult inpatient care for ASD patients can be thwarted by failing to partner with ASD patients and families early on, resulting in communication breakdown that can ultimately impede clinical care. In order to avoid putting patients at risk, a care plan such as this one can give patients and families a clear and proactive voice upon which a patient-centered care plan can be built. While preferably this tool would be completed in the outpatient setting and could already be a part of the patient profile at the time of an ED visit or inpatient admission, this tool can be completed in the

ED or on the inpatient unit floor as well. The earlier that the care plan is completed, the sooner the care team providers can review the domains describing typical patient behaviors, communication practices, social cues, sensory tolerances, safety protocols, and individual triggers and incorporate them into the care plan moving forward.

In contrast to the heavy reliance of inpatient clinical providers on patient feedback for clinical symptoms, inpatient encounters with patients with ASD who may have limited verbal language-based communication require a care plan up-front that is inclusive and respectful of pre-existing patient-specific norms. While there can be no substitute for bedside exam and patient interaction, a care plan such as this one can be critical to avoiding individual patient triggers that can easily derail the clinical encounter. At the same time, a pre-existing care plan may not

What to Expect When An Adult with Autism Is Admitted to MGH

We understand that being admitted to the hospital may be a new experience and this informational has been developed to help patients and families understand what types of activities and interactions to expect. If family/caregivers would like to be present for any part of the care delivery (including daily rounds or testing), please notify the doctors and nurses in the care team. Also, if any questions arise, please do ask the nurses and doctors involved at your earliest convenience.

Patient-Centered Daily Rounds

Each morning the care team of doctors, nurses and any involved care providers will come to the patient's room to speak with the patient/family and examine the patient, discuss any updates in laboratories, imaging tests or other results, review vital signs/ medications, and establish the plan for the day (including additional testing, radiology, or procedures).

While rounds may occur at different times in the morning depending on which floor the patient is assigned to (between 8 am-12 pm), you may always ask your nurse or doctors to arrange a time to speak with you about any questions or concerns that you have at any point in the hospital stay. Also, rounds may be modified in order to meet the needs of the patient/family. Please discuss this with the assigned nurse/doctors if this is desired.

Your Role as a Team Member

Since both patients and patient family members may be very well acquainted with the patient's needs and behaviors, **please be sure to share your knowledge with the nurse and doctors** taking care of the patient. Adjustments may always be made to best serve the patient. Also, please consider the following:

-Be sure to fill out an **Autism Care Questionnaire (ACQ; previously the Acute Care Plan)** and bring this with you to the hospital

Fig. 3.4 What to expect when an adult with autism is admitted

-If you are unable to bring a copy of the ACQ, please ask your nurse or doctors in the Emergency Department or on the medical floor for a copy of the ACQ so that you can complete this to help guide the hospitalization.

-If there are **specific behaviors or activities that make the patient uncomfortable** (like having blood drawn or having a group of people like the rounding care team come to their room), please be sure to express this to your nurse and care team early on.

- **If comforting to the patient, we encourage a patient family member or guardian to stay overnight with the patient during hospitalization**. If you are able to stay, please notify your nurse or care team so that a bed may be ordered for you to stay in the room with the patient.

-**If there are specific foods or nutrition that the patient prefers, please notify the nurse and care team early on.** Also, if you have brought specific foods with you to the hospital that the patient favors, please discuss this with the nurse and care team prior to giving the patient any food from home.

Additional Resources

We understand that it can often be challenging to know what resources are available in the hospital. Please consider the following as additional resources during the hospitalization and feel free to let your nurse and care team know if you'd like to connect with one of the individuals listed below.

- **Physical Therapy**- this is a resource for assistance with walking, balance and movement
- **Occupational Therapy**- this is a resource for assistance with daily routine and managing hospital surroundings (call buttons, lighting, auditory/ tactile sensitivity)
- **Speech Therapy**- this is a resource for assistance with communication
- **Case Management**- this is a resource to clarify insurance coverage questions, needs for rehabilitation, barriers to discharge or additional support needed at home for the patient. Case management may also assist with transportation home at the end of the inpatient stay
- **Social Work**- this resource helps connect to additional disability services or community services for support within the patient's community. They may also assist with parking costs for a caregiver or guardian staying with the patient during hospitalization.
- **Patient Advocacy**-this is a resource for assistance in communicating important needs to the care team and resolving any miscommunication. Patient advocates can also act as a liaison to ensure that the diagnosis and care plan are clearly stated.

Fig. 3.4 (continued)

always guarantee rote adherence for providers that may have to utilize their best clinical judgment for acute treatment but functions more as a window to awareness and discussion for patients, families, and providers. The care plan can also help to set expectations for patients, families, and providers so that all parties are on the same page.

The patient and family informational guide "What to expect when a patient with ASD is admitted" (Fig. 3.4) is a helpful way to introduce patients with ASD and their families to the inpatient realm. By describing the routine of the day and addressing common questions and concerns, this information can be an important part of learning about how the inpatient care delivery experience will unfold. The guide also invites patients and families to ask questions and seeks to create a culture of inclusion for patients and families while hospitalized.

The Autism Case Management Tool (Fig. 3.5) is a helpful resource for case managers taking care of adult patients with ASD. There is strong evidence that additional support for patients and families at the time of discharge is one of the most impactful interventions in existence for adult patients with ASD. Although many case managers are familiar with local post-acute facilities that may provide additional care to adult patients being discharged with rehabilitation needs due to acute injury or needs for long-term placement due to conditions associated with advanced aging or dementia,

Autism Resource Guide for Case Management

I: Services

The
Bridgewell
Contact Grace Martin, RN at (781) 593-1088

Provides comprehensive services for individuals with disabilities and other life challenges. Services include day care, residential and recreational programming.

May Institute of Boston
Contact Donna Chiacha, RN at (617) 325-6700

Provides educational and physical/behavioral therapy programming services for adults with autism.

II: Education/Support

MGH Resources

The Blum Center
Contact Brian French at (617) 724-7352

Resource center for patient and family learning.

The Lurie Center
(781) 860-1700

The Lurie Center is a multidisciplinary program designed to evaluate and treat children, adolescents and adults with a wide variety of conditions including autism and autism spectrum disorder, Asperger's disorder and developmental delays.

The Bressler Foundation
Contact Alyssa Bertolon at (617) 726-7899

The Alan and Lorraine Bressler Clinical and Research Program for Autism Spectrum Disorders is dedicated to the evaluation and care of children, adolescents, and young adults with ASD.

Fig. 3.5 Case management resource guide

State/City Resources

Massachusetts Department of Developmental Service (www.mass.gov/eohhs/gov/**departments**/dds/)

Agency dedicated to supporting individuals with intellectual disabilities. Online resources include a list of Massachusetts autism support centers, services available when individuals with disabilities turn age 22 years and family support resources

Autism Support Center Boston (www.tillinc.org/**autism_support**.html**)**
Contact Josh Lyons at (781) 302-6000

TILL has been chosen by the Department of Developmental Services as the Autism Support Center for the Boston Metro Region and offers activities and resources that provide information and empowerment to families caring for individuals with autism.

National Rehabilitation Information Center (www.naric.com/)
(800) 346-2742

Online resource for disability, rehabilitation, advocacy, education, benefits and financial assistance information.

Advocates for Autism in Massachusetts
Contact Judy Zacek at (781) 891-6270

Agency devoted to support, inclusion and engagement of individuals with autism through policy and advocacy for human and civil rights.

Massachusetts Guardianship Association (www.massguardianshipassociation.org)

A non-profit organization offering information and resources on guardianship in Massachusetts.

III. Financial Resources

Social Security Administration (www.socialsecurity.gov/disability/)
(800) 722-1213

Provides cash benefits to people with physical or mental disability that prevents them from working and is expected to last at least one year. Additional benefits may include Medicaid insurance support or food vouchers.

Fig. 3.5 (continued)

few are aware of post-acute care facilities that include the ability to support the care of patients with ASD. Tragically, this can be compounded by the dearth of post-acute facilities capable of meeting the needs of patients with ASD. Identifying current resources or potential post-acute care facilities that provide appropriate levels of care for adult ASD patients being discharged from the hospital can have great value in terms of underlining potential gaps in community needs in this area. Furthermore, case managers can also serve as a resource to families that are in need of additional social, emotional, or financial support. While some may assume that adults with ASD already have appropriate support and program partnering at the community level by the time that they are seen in the hospital, studies suggest that this is not the case and that there are many patients and families that have little knowledge of the resources that may be available to them. While many of the resources that we present here are specific support systems in the area of our institution, it is provided as a model for individual institutions to create similar lists of resources tailored to meet the needs of adult patients with ASD in the communities they serve.

The Inpatient Image Gallery for Patients with ASD is an online series of images taken in areas that are commonly visited during hospitalization. This resource allows individuals with ASD who are uncomfortable in unfamiliar environments to familiarize themselves with areas that they may visit during an admission. Some patients may feel less anxious by having access to such an image gallery before and even during hospitalization. This resource is particularly useful for planned admissions, but even patients with chronic medical issues may view these images proactively in anticipation of a possible unexpected admission and then review them again at the time of admission. Key areas that are highlighted include the entrance leading to the hospital, the ED, the major hallways leading to typical unit floors where patients are admitted, and the X-ray, CT scan, interventional radiology, and MRI areas. Individual institutions may identify a number of additional areas that would be beneficial for patients to visualize and include them in a similar tool.

We also developed a series of educational videos about ASD designed for both clinical providers and nonclinical hospital employees such as hospital maintenance, food service, and transportation staff. This series of videos was developed to provide an overview of ASD as a condition, educate staff about the best practices in engaging with individuals with ASD, and provide information to clinicians about the best practices for caring for patients with ASD. Individual institutions may consider similar tools as an in-service or learning competency requirement for employees, both clinical and nonclinical, which may come into contact with individuals with ASD.

Through these resources, the Autism Care Committee at MGH is taking strides to create solutions and bridge the gaps identified in the literature regarding inpatient care of both children and adults with ASD. While these toolkit resources are not a panacea for solving all of the challenges in ASD inpatient care delivery, they recognize the historical lack of ASD patient-friendly care environments and specifically seek to address:

- The general paucity of educational and training materials introducing the basics of ASD to clinical and nonclinical providers
- The need for a partnership between patients/families and providers in creating care plans that reflect patient needs and preferences
- The need for better messaging on the provider-patient/family interface that prepares patients and families for the inpatient setting by establishing general expectations and encouraging iterative communication to optimize care
- The lack of available clinical care guidelines to aid smooth transitions to the inpatient setting and prompt providers to design optimal care in busy inpatient settings
- The need for clinical care algorithms to help providers partner with patients/families to create timely solutions to challenges impeding clinical care in real time
- The need for additional case management resources for post-acute care as well as social

and financial support for families of patients with ASD
- The lack of visual aids to assist patients with ASD to begin to familiarize themselves with common inpatient settings prior to admission

Clinical Pearls and Future Directions

- Using direct admission to the hospital is preferred when possible.
- Using a care questionnaire and/or hospital care plan can improve communication, care quality, and patient satisfaction with care.
- A multidisciplinary approach that includes occupational therapy and child life specialist staff is essential to ensuring that needs of hospitalized patients with ASD are met.
- Using cross specialty care (e.g., sending a pediatric nurse or child life specialist to adult units when needed).
- Limiting vital signs and unnecessary medical interventions can improve outcomes.
- Allowing the patient's caregiver to stay overnight in the room with the patient when appropriate can help to normalize the hospital environment.
- Creating a Family Advisory Council and using the input of family members of those with ASD can help guide care improvement.
- Creating an Electronic Health Record Icon to "flag" patients so care providers can be immediately aware of the ASD diagnosis can help improve team awareness and communication when ASD patients are admitted.
- Utilizing the Electronic Health Record to create specialized order sets for patients with ASD can create a systematic approach to caring for patients with ASD in hospitalized settings.

References

1. Broder-Fingert S, Shui A, Ferrone C, Iannuzzi D, Cheng ER, Giauque A, Connors S, McDougle CJ, Donelan K, Neumeyer A, Kuhlthau KA. Pilot study of autism-specific care plans during hospital admission. Pediatrics. 2016;137(Suppl 2):S196–204.
2. Cheak-Zamora NC, Farmer JE, Mayfield WA, Clark MJ, Marvin AR, Law JK, Law PA. Health care transition services for youth with autism spectrum disorders. Rehabil Psychol. 2014;59(3):340–8.
3. Cheak-Zamora NC, Yang X, Farmer JE, Clark M. Disparities in transition planning for youth with autism spectrum disorder. Pediatrics. 2013;131(3):447–54.
4. Croen LA, Najjar D, Ray T, Lotspeich L, Bernal P. A comparison of health care utilization and costs of children with and without autism spectrum disorders in a large group model health plan. Pediatrics. 2006;118(4):e1203–11.
5. Fortuna RJ, Robinson L, Smith TH, Meccarello J, Bullen B, Nobis K, Davidson PW. Health conditions and functional status in adults with autism: a cross-sectional evaluation. J Gen Intern Med. 2016;31(1):77–84.
6. Giarelli E, Nocera R, Turchi R, Hardie TL, Pagano R, Yuan C. Sensory stimuli as obstacles to emergency care for children with autism spectrum disorder. Adv Emerg Nurs J. 2014 36(2), 145-163.
7. Gotham K, Marvin AR, Taylor JL, Warren Z, Anderson CM, Law PA, Law JK, Lipkin PH. Characterizing the daily life, needs, and priorities of adults with autism spectrum disorder from interactive autism network data. Autism. 2015;19(7):794–804.
8. Kopecky K, Broder-Fingert S, Iannuzzi D, Connors S. The needs of hospitalized patients with autism spectrum disorders: a parent survey. Clin Pediatr (Phila). 2013;52(7):652–60.
9. Kuhlthau KA, Warfield ME, Hurson J, Delahaye J, Crossman MK. Pediatric provider's perspectives on the transition to adult health care for youth with autism spectrum disorder: current strategies and promising new directions. Autism. 2015;19(3):262–71.
10. Lokhandwala T, Khanna R, West-Strum D. Hospitalization burden among individuals with autism. J Autism Dev Disord. 2012;42:95–104.
11. McGonigle JJ, Migyanka JM, Glor-Scheib SJ, Cramer R, Fratangeli JJ, Hegde GG, Shang J, Venkat A. Development and evaluation of educational materials for pre-hospital and emergency department personnel on the care of patients with autism spectrum disorder. J Autism Dev Disord. 2014a;44(5):1252–9.
12. McGonigle JJ, Venkat A, Beresford C, Campbell TP, Gabriels RL. Management of agitation in individuals with autism spectrum disorders in the emergency department. Child Adolesc Psychiatr Clin N Am. 2014b;23(1):83–95.
13. Muskat B, Burnham Riosa P, Nicholas DB, Roberts W, Stoddart KP, Zwaigenbaum L. Autism comes to the hospital: the experiences of patients with autism spectrum disorder, their parents and health-care providers at two Canadian paediatric hospitals. Autism. 2015;19(4):482–90.

14. Pratt K, Baird G, Gringras P. Ensuring successful admission to hospital for young people with learning difficulties, autism and challenging behavior: a continuous quality improvement and change management programme. Child Care Health Dev. 2011;38(96):789–97.
15. Rogers K, Zeni MB. Systematic review of medical home models to promote transitions to primary adult health care for adolescents living with autism spectrum disorder. Worldviews Evid-Based Nurs. 2015;12(2):98–107.
16. Sakai C, Miller K, Brussa A, MacPherson C, Augustyn M. Challenges of autism in the inpatient setting. J Dev Behav Pediatr. 2014;35(1):82–4.
17. Venkat A, Jauch E, Russell WS, Crist CR, Farrell R. Care of the patient with an autism spectrum disorder by the general physician. Postgrad Med J. 2012;88(1042):472–81.
18. Warfield ME, Crossman MK, Delahaye J, Der Weerd E, Kuhlthau KA. Physician perspectives on providing primary medical care to adults with autism Spectrum disorders (ASD). J Autism Dev Disord. 2015;45(7):2209–17.
19. Zerbo O, Massolo ML, Qian Y, Croen LA. A study of physician knowledge and experience with autism in adults in a large integrated healthcare system. J Autism Dev Disord. 2015;45(12):4002–14.

4 Medical Procedures: Challenges and Strategies

Jill Pineda and Jennifer Mullett

Introduction

Individuals with autism spectrum disorder (ASD) exhibit difficulties with social communication and may process language differently than typically developing patients seen in a medical setting. They may also exhibit highly restricted interests, difficulties with change or unfamiliar environments, and sensory sensitivities, such as under- or over-reactivity to various stimuli (e.g., loud noises, lights). Difficulties with language and social communication may directly impact their ability to understand what may be expected during medical procedures and limit their ability to advocate for themselves, making even the most routine medical procedures anxiety-provoking and challenging for both the patient and the parent or caregiver.

Furthermore, patients with ASD can have significant difficulty with flexibility and changes in routine, making it essential to plan ahead and prepare the patient for what to expect during a procedure in order to minimize anxiety and gain the patient's cooperation. This chapter provides an overview of existing literature in the approach to treatment of individuals with ASD across the lifespan and the most effective tools and strategies that can be used in a variety of clinical settings for this population of patients. Clinical vignettes are presented, and clinical pearls with suggested approaches are provided. The vast majority of available literature focuses on the care of pediatric patients with ASD. In many circumstances, similar approaches can be applied to adults or elderly patients. For this reason, general approaches for pediatric patients are addressed first, with additional information provided about considerations to make when working with adults or elderly patients.

General Principles and Approaches

Communication

Communication is one of the most important factors when providing health care to any population, but is especially critical to consider when working with individuals with ASD. Communication involves the ability to exchange information with others and may occur through a variety of modalities (e.g., verbal and gestural), or through the use of visual symbols and pictures [1]. Individuals with ASD can vary greatly in their ability to use language to communicate, which may relate to his or her intellectual and social development [15]. Some

J. Pineda
Neuropsychology Department, Kennedy Krieger Institute, Baltimore, MD, USA
e-mail: pineda@kennedykrieger.org

J. Mullett (✉)
Lurie Center for Autism, Lexington, MA, USA
e-mail: jmullett@mgh.harvard.edu

E. P. Hazen, C. J. McDougle (eds.), *The Massachusetts General Hospital Guide to Medical Care in Patients with Autism Spectrum Disorder*, Current Clinical Psychiatry,
https://doi.org/10.1007/978-3-319-94458-6_4

individuals may exhibit superior verbal skills, while others may present with few or no spoken words.

With advancements in treatment and education, there are now countless modalities through which an individual may communicate, from spoken language to alternative and augmentative communication (AAC). The latter may include using facial expressions, gestures, symbols, pictures, or technology to communicate (e.g., by typing or using a tablet computer). As medical providers, it is essential that we continue to prioritize communication with the patient, even if the modality takes a form other than spoken language. When preparing to see a patient with ASD, it is critical to assess the patient's preferred communication modality and be prepared to direct information in a way that the patient can understand. It can be helpful to collect information from a caregiver or family member to determine how the patient communicates best and to ask the patient or family to bring in any assistive devices or materials that might facilitate communication. Additionally, it can be helpful to ask caregivers or family members how much information should be shared with the patient. Some patients may benefit from more elaborate and detailed descriptions of upcoming procedures, while others may respond better to very brief or general descriptions of what to expect. For patients who have difficulty with unexpected change and unfamiliar environments, it is even more critical to communicate expectations ahead of time to minimize anxiety and unfamiliarity when possible.

Visual Supports

Many individuals with ASD are better able to process information presented visually compared to information presented in written or spoken language. Visual supports can be used not only to familiarize the patient with what to expect but to further assess which steps of a medical procedure may be more challenging for a particular person [4]. Visual supports can be a valuable tool and may include resources such as social stories containing a script of what to expect with corresponding pictures, a visual schedule of a routine (see Fig. 4.1), or a visual task analysis with pictured steps of a procedure.

A visual task analysis is created by breaking down complex medical procedures or tasks into a sequence of smaller steps or actions and incorporates pictures to help patients with ASD understand. By using a visual task analysis, providers can preview various steps of the process and evaluate how the patient may respond. For example, this may include breaking down the sequence required in a blood draw and taking a picture of each step (e.g., sit in the chair, hold out your arm, apply tourniquet, nurse cleans arm, feel a pinch when the needle goes in, etc.). This may take some prior planning to create within a clinic but can be a useful tool that can be available for patients in the future. If the patient uses spoken or signed languages or AAC devices, a provider may ask them to express how "comfortable" or "nervous" they may feel about each step by using a rating scale from one to five; for individuals who may be nonverbal or lack a primary mode of communication, providers may consider utilizing

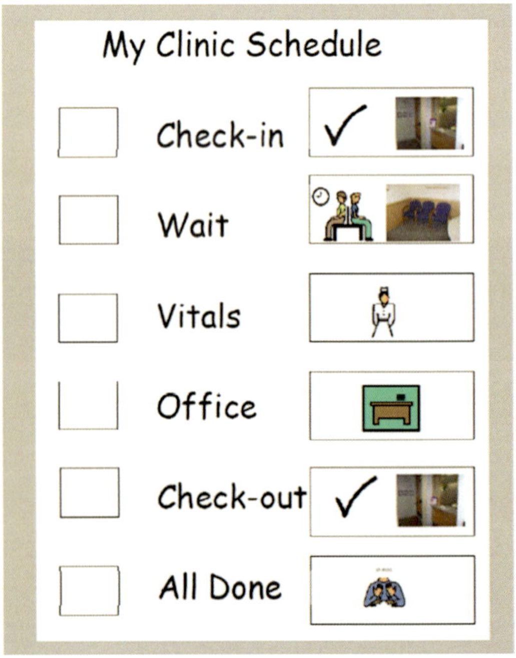

Fig. 4.1 Check-off schedule to provide visual schedule of events at an office visit [6]

visual pain scales to closely observe a patient's facial expressions or grimaces when they are shown each step of the process (e.g., Faces Pain Scale – Revised, Keck et al. [9]; FLACC Pain Assessment Scale, [14]; Individualized Numeric Rating Scale, [22]).

By gaining knowledge of steps of a procedure or exam that may be more difficult for a particular individual, medical providers can plan ahead, collaborate with family members, and determine whether other techniques will be safer and more effective in treating the patient with ASD. Finally, the use of a visual timer may be useful in helping a patient be able to monitor the time remaining in the medical procedure. Visual supports can help mitigate some of the primary difficulties in working with individuals with ASD by making information accessible despite impairments in social communication and language and familiarizing the patients with what to expect given associated difficulty with flexibility or changes in routine or unfamiliar settings or providers.

Behavioral Contingencies and Positive Reinforcement

Consistent with decades of research conducted in the field of Applied Behavior Analysis (ABA) and the establishment of ABA as an evidence-based approach in working with individuals with neurodevelopmental disorders, it is often very useful to employ behavioral contingencies and positive reinforcement when working with individuals with ASD. Behavioral contingencies include establishing "if-then" or "first-then" conditions in which the patient is expected to complete a certain action, in this case part or all of the medical procedure, and is then rewarded with a more preferred activity, such as a break, game, or snack (see Fig. 4.2).

It is important to explicitly assess preferred activities by asking the patient or caregivers what items, activities, or tangible reinforcers (e.g., foods) are most favored; it is especially important to consider introducing items that the patient

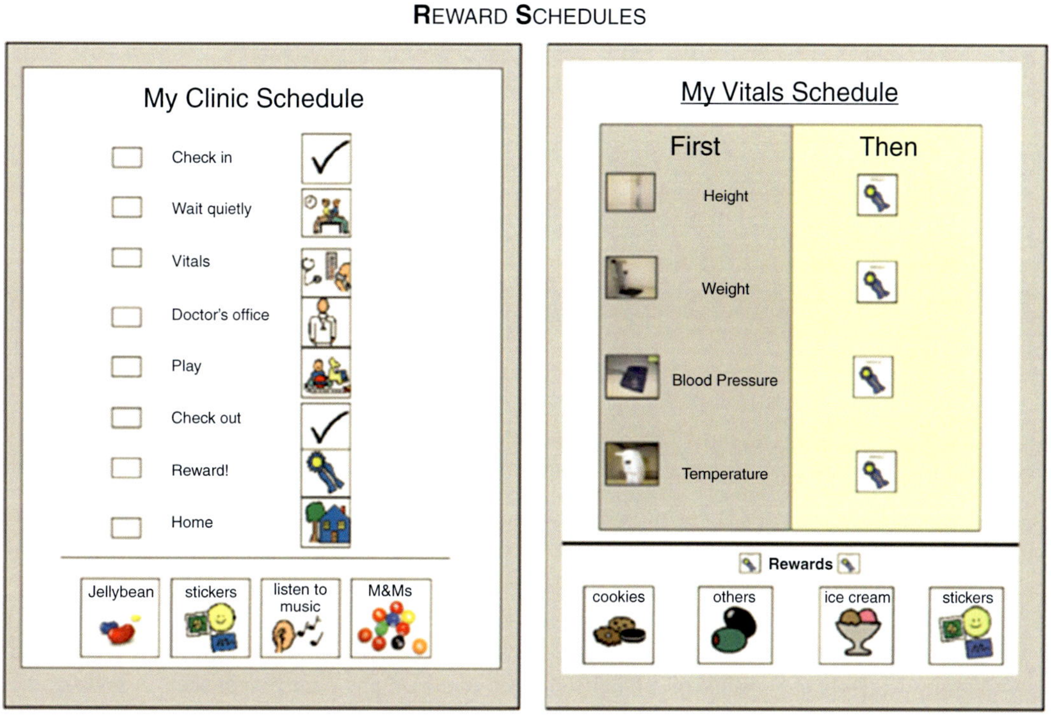

Fig. 4.2 Reward schedule for completion of pre-identified tasks [6]

does not commonly have access to in order for the motivation to obtain the reinforcer to be strong. Providing a patient with one of these preferred activities or requests following the completion of a task is considered to be one example of implementation of positive reinforcement, in which a behavior is reinforced and, as a result, is much more likely to occur again. If this contingency is set forth at the outset of the medical procedure, it is important to be consistent and follow through with the agreed-upon plan, both upholding expectations and following through with the patient's preferred activity. Doing so may increase the trust of the patient, establish a routine of expectations and reward, and improve overall compliance with the procedure in the future.

In addition, it is important for caregivers and providers to limit the attention they give to behavioral distress, noncompliance, or undesirable behaviors in order to minimize these behaviors throughout the medical procedure. While ignoring completely may be beneficial for some children, others may benefit from neutral acknowledgment or directives such as "You can do it," or "Hold out your arm," while also upholding the expectation that the individual will follow through with the expectations. While it is important to consider discontinuing a procedure when it is unsafe for the patient, caregivers, or staff, it is important to note that when providers or caregivers discontinue a procedure following refusal or behavioral distress, it is more likely that the patient will exhibit higher levels of behavioral distress when the procedure is implemented in the future.

Systematic Desensitization

Another behavioral approach that can be effective when implementing medical procedures in individuals with ASD is the use of systematic desensitization. Systematic desensitization involves stimulus fading by gradually increasing exposure to the feared stimulus and is often combined with differential reinforcement, meaning that distress is ignored and compliance is praised and reinforced [17]. Stimulus fading is especially useful in the treatment of phobias and tends to be an effective approach with individuals with ASD given inherent difficulties with tolerating unfamiliar situations, co-occurring anxiety, and, in some cases, a high level of sensory sensitivities.

An example of systematic desensitization in implementing a dental cleaning may include having the patient enter the office, showing him pictures of what is going to happen, and then asking him to open his mouth. A provider may then begin touching the patient's front teeth with a toothbrush, touching the molars with a toothbrush, and continuing to gradually introduce more invasive tools (e.g., scaler) in this manner and at a comfortable pace. While this may initially require more time, it is more likely to elicit compliance in the long term.

Individuals with ASD and other developmental disorders can show fear or avoidance reactions to medical procedures [10]. By using systematic desensitization in combination with other approaches, research suggests that medical professionals are often able to avoid more restrictive or invasive approaches such as general anesthesia, restraints, or sedation [3], which pose additional risks to the patient [12]. It can also be very helpful to implement mock trials of the procedure in order to review the steps that the patient is expected to follow and assess how approaches may need to be adjusted for the patient's individual needs. For example, a patient who requires an imaging study in a scanner could visit a mock scanner prior to the actual scan session. Similarly, a patient who requires a blood draw could be allowed to see and touch equipment that is used for blood collection including the tourniquet, gauze, Band-Aid, and a needleless butterfly needle. Mock trials can naturally decrease a patient's anxiety by introducing less invasive stimuli before carrying out the entire procedure. This may be particularly helpful when preparing for blood draws or needle sticks so that a patient's response to different aspects of the procedure can be assessed in a safe environment without the potential for mistakes when working with a real needle.

Relaxation Strategies

A number of relaxation strategies can be used to help individuals with ASD and other developmental disorders tolerate medical procedures. Effective strategies may include deep breathing, progressive muscle relaxation, visual imagery, and distraction. These relaxation techniques may need to be taught and rehearsed with caregivers ahead of time when preparing for the appointment. Distraction techniques can be useful in minimizing a patient's procedure-related distress and have been found to increase relaxation, especially when watching the procedure may contribute to higher levels of distress or anxiety (e.g., blood draws) [21, 23]. Distraction can be implemented by having a caregiver redirect the patient's attention to a preferred activity, story, or book or by playing preferred music that will help the patient minimize negative thoughts about the procedure.

Distraction can be especially useful for individuals with sensory sensitivities to certain aspects of a procedure, such as sounds that occur during magnetic resonance imaging (MRI). Distraction is also beneficial for those with chronic medical conditions and has been found to reduce self-reported pain, improve cooperation, and increase success with procedures such as needle sticks [21]. It can serve the purpose of counterconditioning by replacing a patient's fear, avoidance, or escape with a relaxation response [19, 20]. Clinics implementing medical procedures should consider creating a toolbox of various activities: sensory toys, such as ooze tubes, liquid motion timers, glitter or spinner wands, squishy or puffer balls, hand massagers, or fidget toys, or books that can be introduced to the patient to distract him from the procedure. For example, a patient who needs to have her blood drawn can be offered a choice of activities or stimuli that she would like to hold in her free hand or look at in order to minimize her attention to the needle or steps of the procedure. It is important to assess if distraction may be a helpful tool by consulting with the patient or caregivers. Some individuals may benefit from distraction techniques, while others prefer to watch the steps of the procedure to minimize their anxiety.

Collaboration with Providers and Individuals Familiar with the Patient

Despite a vast array of tools and approaches available within the medical field, one of the best resources for successful treatment includes collaboration with other providers and family members who know the patient well. Many individuals with ASD may have a history of involvement in therapeutic services with a speech-language pathologist, occupational therapist, physical therapist, psychologist, or behavioral therapist. These individuals can be helpful contacts and resources to gain more information about a patient's history of symptoms, treatment, or effective strategies for working with the patient. Many individuals with ASD may have a behavioral therapist that may be available to accompany the patient to the appointment to help coordinate and implement behavioral contingencies and provide positive reinforcement to ensure a successful procedure. A behavioral therapist may be particularly adept at handling challenging behaviors, including bolting, aggression, and self-injurious behaviors that may interfere with medical procedures.

Having parents or caregivers present during the procedure may be ideal given their knowledge of their child's individual needs or sensitivities; however, it is critical that parents are able to remain calm and encouraging, while also minimizing attention or reactions when a patient becomes distressed in order to avoid reinforcing these behaviors. If this is difficult for some caregivers, some coaching of parents can be useful or they may be asked to excuse themselves for parts of the procedures in order to maintain the patient's cooperation and relaxation. By working collaboratively as a team, providers can better individualize approaches and strategies when planning for outpatient or emergency medical procedures.

Approaches to Specific Procedures in the Outpatient Setting

The following information pertains to preparing for procedures that may be commonly addressed in outpatient settings, such as obtaining vital signs, conducting blood draws, collecting urine, administering shots or vaccines, increasing compliance with pill swallowing, and providing outpatient audiology or dental services. While the examples provided are not exhaustive, they offer strategies and approaches that can be applied to almost any medical procedure. Given the breadth of literature on pediatric approaches, these examples focus on use with children, but most can also be used with adults. Some additional suggestions on modifications for adults are offered later.

Vital Signs

Collecting vital signs is an essential part of a thorough physical assessment in any medical setting. Encouraging a patient to participate in the process at each visit will gradually desensitize him to the request. Strategies to lessen anxiety could include making the experience a game with step-by-step goals to be achieved (e.g., with stickers after each completed task and the use of visual schedules) and allowing the patient to touch and explore the equipment before it is used on him. Incorporating the measurement of a caregiver, sibling, or a favorite toy can also be effective modeling techniques to gain cooperation.

It is helpful to use child-friendly language when describing what to expect. Describing a blood pressure cuff as "a big hug on your arm" allows the patient to imagine what the sensation may feel like. Encouraging the patient to count or sing his favorite song for the duration serves as an effective distraction technique. If a patient has difficulty independently standing on a scale to measure his weight, it can be helpful for a parent or caregiver to hold him, and then the parent's weight can be subtracted; this may be especially important if you need to obtain a weight estimate for determining doses of medications. Like with many other procedures, it is important to first introduce the least invasive measure and gradually introduce other steps that may be more difficult. Learning to tolerate such measures will benefit the patient throughout the life span. It is important to consider that at times it may be necessary to bypass certain assessments due to a patient's inability to tolerate them; however, clinicians should not shy away from trying again at subsequent visits.

Blood Draws, Needle Sticks, and Shots

Hesitation and noncompliance with needle procedures are not uncommon in children with developmental disabilities, and these procedures often result in severe stress, in part due to anticipated pain, unfamiliar equipment, and difficulty inhibiting movement or tactile defensiveness [21]. Individuals with ASD are likely to require needle procedures due to associated medical conditions but may have more difficulty engaging in the procedures as a result of aspects of their disabilities, such as sensory sensitivity or impaired communication.

In order to prepare a patient for a blood draw, needle stick, or shot, it can be helpful to create an individualized visual task analysis, as previously described. Table 4.1 shows an example of a written task analysis that can be used to prepare a patient for a needle stick. Visuals can be incorporated in order to allow the patient to see what is expected of him [21]. The patient can be gradually introduced to steps of the procedure while he is also introduced to relaxation strategies such as deep breathing or asked to utilize distraction techniques in which the parents engage him in looking at preferred activities while the qualified medical professional completes the procedure. Additionally, behavioral contingencies can be used to reinforce compliance with steps of the procedure, and attempts to remove stimuli should be blocked and redirected. These approaches have been effective in helping individuals with developmental disorders including ASD and intellectual disabilities comply with needle sticks and

Table 4.1 Example task analysis for needle stick [21]

Sit in chair and begin watching DVD
Place arm in position
Adjust clothing to expose site
Put on gloves
Touch/probe site
Tie tourniquet on the upper arm
Apply alcohol
Prepare mock needle (0/4, 1/4, 2/4, 3/4, 4/4) circle needle size
Apply mock needle (0/4, 1/4, 2/4, 3/4, 4/4) circle needle size
Apply mock needle (0/4, 1/4, 2/4, 3/4, 4/4) circle needle size
Hold in place for 5 s
Hold in place for 10 s
Hold in place for 30 s
Hold in place for 1 min
Hold in place for 1.5 min
Hold in place for 2 min
Manipulate tubing/vial with needle in place (if actual needle, qualified medical staff only)
Perform needle stick with real needle (qualified medical staff only)

blood draws despite a history of previously failed attempts [21].

Urine Sample

Successful completion of urine collection can be dependent upon the level of toilet training achieved, preferences for how the sample is obtained, and whether the individual requires discrete assistance. In practice, performance anxiety and comprehension of directions can impede noninvasive urine collection. It is important to both verbally and visually describe what is being requested, as not all toileting routines are identical. For instance, some male individuals may sit rather than stand to urinate. Offering options for mode of collection (e.g., specimen collector pan, urinal, or cup) can make the discussion more comfortable. Younger children who use diapers may be more successful when using a urine collection bag that is adhered to the skin. Timing of collection can be facilitated by asking the caregiver about the patient's toileting patterns and when the best chance to get a full sample may occur (e.g., applying a urine bag just prior to the first void of the day or waking the individual up 30 min before the normal waking time and escorting him to the bathroom). Finally, it is important to consider that gross or fine motor skills may interfere with a patient's ability to hold a receptacle for urine collection; this should be taken into account when deciding the best method for collection. Visual materials may be helpful in allowing the patient to understand what is expected of him.

Pill Swallowing

Individuals with ASD may be prescribed medications to address a number of psychiatric or medical problems. While many individuals do not have the prerequisite skills for swallowing pills, including sustained attention or oral motor abilities, others may have developed conditioned anxiety associated with repeated negative experiences (e.g., aversive taste, gagging) when trying to swallow pills [2]. Systematic desensitization paired with behavioral contingencies, including reinforcement of desired behavior and ignoring undesired behaviors, is a particularly useful approach when teaching the skill of pill swallowing. Task analyses can also be used to teach individuals with ASD steps of the process (e.g., "open mouth," "stick out your tongue," say "Ahh"). Parents or psychologists can work with patients to introduce them to "mock pills," which may include cake toppings (e.g., sugar specks, sprinkles), small candies such as tic-tacs, or empty capsules of gradually increasing sizes (see Fig. 4.3). Once a patient completes approximately 3–5 successful trials swallowing each size, the next biggest size can be introduced. Additionally, preferred drinks may be incorporated when asking a child to swallow medications that may have an aversive taste.

A routine around pill swallowing should be established in which a patient is expected to sit at a table and comply with the demand by swallowing a pill within 30–60 s of its presentation by increasing presentation of mock pills from the smallest pill to the size of pill that is equal to the

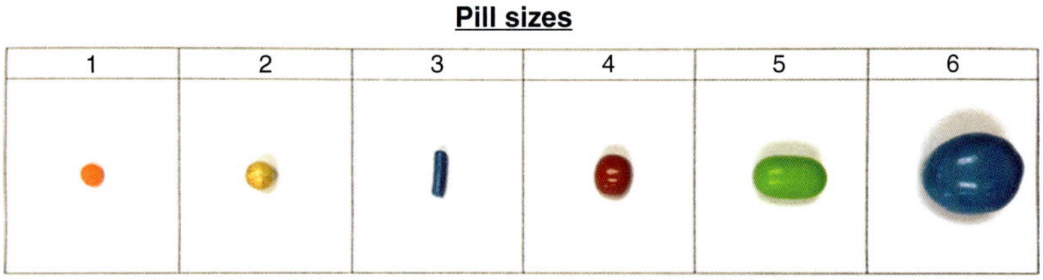

Fig. 4.3 Mock pills (candy/cake decorations) of increasing size

target medication. A parent or provider can model pill swallowing to ensure the patient understands the expectations. Any negative vocalizations or avoidance behaviors should be ignored and redirected immediately, and a patient's success should be reinforced with a preferred activity selected at the outset of the treatment.

Audiology Services

While there has been little research on systematic desensitization to hearing aids in individuals with ASD, the same procedures and approaches described in the literature have been successfully used by the authors for preparation for audiology outpatient services such as hearing aid fittings. A visual task analysis can be used to present the patient with pictures of each step of the process, from sitting in a chair to allowing a provider to touch his ears and place hearing aid molds within the ear. Multiple exposures to stimuli beginning with the least invasive procedures can be helpful in preparing the patient for the sensation of having hearing aids placed in his ears; this may include first wearing headphones and then progressing to wearing soft ear plugs and eventually hearing aid molds. By using a task analysis and shaping procedures, a patient's compliance with the procedure can be increased, and he can be taught to insert hearing aids independently. A case example is presented in the adult clinical vignette at the end of this chapter to help demonstrate this process.

Dental Visits

Like many other outpatient procedures, dental care may contribute to a high level of distress or behavioral avoidance in individuals with ASD, but behavioral contingencies and teaching trials have been effective in helping individuals complete dental procedures [5, 16]. In particular, the use of systematic desensitization, video modeling, and reinforcement has been effective in facilitating dental examination and treatments of patients with ASD [4, 11]. Cagetti et al. [4] used visual supports to help 83 children with ASD ages 6–12 years and a range of intellectual functioning tolerate oral examination, oral hygiene sessions, fissure sealant procedures, and restorative treatments. Visual supports included each step of the process from sitting in the exam chair, introducing a mirror in the mouth, and applying a fissure sealant. These visuals were reviewed with the patient for eight 1-h sessions with a psychologist (two sessions/week) and 15 min a day with parents before undergoing procedures. The patients were also shown the same visual supports throughout the dental care visit. Additionally, the amount of sensory stimuli was reduced by dimming the light, introducing the suction device at a low setting to minimize noise, and un-packaging dental instruments before the procedure in order to minimize the time and noise created by opening the packages. Use of visual supports helped over 90% of the sample complete a hygiene procedure, and fissure sealant was successfully applied in more than 80% of the sample. Children with a higher level of verbal fluency had more success in completing the procedures, although many children who were nonverbal were also able to complete the procedures.

Visual supports such as "first-then" boards can also be utilized to show the patient the expected behavior they will need to perform before accessing a preferred activity. In addition to visual supports, it is important to provide positive reinforcement for compliance while ignoring or reducing attention to noncompliance by remaining calm and redirecting the patient by providing a neutral directive (e.g., "open your mouth"). Finally, appointments should be well planned, and wait times should be kept short, preferably not exceeding 10–15 min, in order to reduce anticipatory anxiety [8]. Dental care for patients with ASD is discussed in more detail in Chap. 7.

Approaches to Procedures in Emergency and Inpatient Settings

The following section provides strategies for preparing for procedures that may be commonly conducted in inpatient or emergency settings, including electroencephalogram (EEG), electromyogram (EMG), and imaging procedures. Again, the procedures reviewed are not exhaustive, but can offer strategies and approaches that can be applied to almost any medical procedure.

Electroencephalogram (EEG) and Electromyogram (EMG) Procedures

The prevalence of epilepsy is higher in children with disabilities, including intellectual disabilities, brain injury, cerebral palsy, and ASD [7]. In fact, some estimates suggest that up to 30% of individuals with ASD experience seizures by adolescence [13]. Thus, many individuals with ASD will require an EEG at some point in their lives to monitor possible seizure activity. The EEG can be a particularly challenging procedure for many individuals with ASD given the unfamiliar sensory stimuli related to the equipment and the need to cooperative and remain still for an extended period of time. Noncompliance is sometimes met with the use of restraints, sedation, or anesthesia, which can alter test results and cause unnecessary stress for the patient [18]. Slifer et al. [18] demonstrated that behavioral training using shaping, differential reinforcement for cooperation, and blocking removal of equipment (escape extinction) has been effective in helping individuals with ASD, and developmental disabilities successfully complete EEG procedures which were previously not possible. Shaping refers to using differential reinforcement to teach successive approximations of a target behavior [18].

Shaping in preparation for an EEG includes carefully planned, gradual exposure to the procedure room, bed, equipment, and placement of electrodes on the patient's head. Specifically, patients are asked to enter the room, get into a bed, and allow the provider to touch their heads, apply gel, and begin placing electrodes one at a time. Additionally, any attempts to remove equipment are blocked and redirected, while cooperation and increased approximations to tolerating equipment are reinforced through activities such as playing a preferred video on a television in the room. Any time the patient reaches to remove the electrodes, the preferred video is paused until he cooperates; this procedure establishes a routine and expectations that the patient will not have access to preferred activities if he attempts to remove equipment. While the Slifer et al. [18] study was done in an outpatient setting where patients learned to tolerate the procedure through the course of 3–10 sessions lasting 30–60 min in duration, the same procedures can be attempted in an emergent setting through gradual exposure and behavioral reinforcement. It may be helpful to consult qualified professionals, such as psychologists or child life staff, who have experience in helping prepare individuals with ASD for medical procedures. The same process and approaches can be utilized to prepare patients for EMGs and similar procedures.

Imaging: Magnetic Resonance Imaging and X-Rays

Environmental modifications and behavioral contingencies can be used to help individuals with ASD prepare and cooperate with imaging studies such as MRI and X-rays. As with many other procedures, it is important to make the process as predictable as possible for the patient. This can be done by reviewing a social story or visual task analysis with steps of the procedure that will be completed ("I will lay down on the table," "I will wear a helmet"), expectations during the procedure (e.g., "I will try to stay very still"), and environmental stimuli he may expect to hear or see (e.g., "I may hear loud noises").

The loud noises that occur during an MRI may be particularly overwhelming for many individuals with ASD. It can be helpful to prepare them for this in several ways. One useful approach is to obtain a sample of the sound they will hear and gradually introduce them to the sound at increasing durations and volumes so that they become more familiar with what to expect. Medical professionals can supply patients and their families with a "MRI toolkit" several weeks before the procedure will take place. The toolkit could include a description of what to expect and what they will be asked to do with pictures or videos of the steps, as well as audio clips of the sounds they can be expected to hear.

It is important to thoroughly review all parts of the procedure while also using language that is simple and easy to understand. For individuals with age-appropriate receptive language skills, it can be helpful to talk to them about the noises they may hear and incorporate familiar or preferred interests. For example, a patient could be encouraged to imagine she is on a "spaceship" when listening to the sounds during the MRI scan. While familiarizing the patient with the steps of the procedure, it is also important to incorporate behavioral contingencies in the form of verbal praise and tangible reinforcement for completion of a successful procedure. During the procedure, it can be helpful to provide the patient with declarative and encouraging statements such as "You are doing well," "The scan will be done in 10-minutes," and "You are doing a great job staying still."

If possible, it is helpful to incorporate distraction in the form of preferred music or a video while the procedure is taking place. It may be especially important for caregivers to set up a behavioral contingency in which the patient is able to choose a preferred activity that he can engage in following the successful completion of the procedure. This could include earning a desired toy, going out for a favorite meal, or making a trip to a special place when the process is over. Including the patient in choosing what he would like to earn can increase his motivation and compliance with the procedure. The most important thing to remember when preparing patients for medical procedures is to consider their perspective when thinking through all steps of the procedure that it will be important to familiarize them with (e.g., what they will see, hear, and feel).

Additional Considerations for Adults and Elderly Patients

While most of the techniques and approaches for children described above can be adapted for adult patients as well, there are several considerations that the clinician should keep in mind in working with adults or elderly patients with ASD. First, it is critical to be respectful and communicate to the patient as an adult, regardless of whether or not the individual has an intellectual disability or uses a different mode of communication. If a patient is minimally verbal, do not presume that he has an intellectual impairment or cannot understand. Many patients with ASD simply need to be given additional time to process information or to have information communicated to them in a different way in order to fully understand.

It is also important to address adult patients directly, even when they are accompanied by a family member or caregiver, and to provide patients the opportunity to speak privately without family members present. Adults and elderly patients may not want to share some information in front of their caregivers.

When necessary, provide directions and information in a simple, concrete, and straightforward manner in the patient's preferred communication modality (e.g., spoken language or communication device). Providing demonstrations or visual supports can help many patients with ASD understand the components of a procedure. It is important to assume competence and check for understanding in order to guide your communication approach (e.g., ask the patient to tell you or show you what they think will happen). While it is important to initially assume competence, consider that a scripted response may not be reflective of an individual's receptive comprehension in regard to understanding the explanation of or agreement to a procedure. For example, an individual's scripting of fact-based information related to a preferred interest may not be reflective of his ability to understand details and information being provided to him. Therefore, it is important to assess understanding by asking the patient to state his understanding of what is expected of him during a procedure and what may happen. Finally, allow the patient to express his opinion and ask questions. Adults or elderly patients may demonstrate a delay in responding or need extra time to process information before responding to prompts or questions. Be patient and allow time for a response.

Knowing When to Terminate a Procedure/Interaction

Finally, it is critical to assess when terminating a procedure may be in the best interest of the patient. If care is not urgent and is contributing to significant behavioral distress, requires a high level of restraint, or raises concerns for safety, it may be best to terminate a procedure until safer methods and approaches are identified. When it is not possible to implement a procedure due to safety concerns, it may be appropriate to enlist the supports of a psychologist, behavioral therapist, or other qualified professional. Some patients may benefit from brief outpatient therapy to prepare for medical procedures, including use of behavioral contingencies and mock trials that can be designed and implemented to help ensure compliance with the procedure in the future. It can be helpful to notice caregiver cues to determine whether the patient may become increasingly dysregulated if the procedure continues. It is best to terminate a procedure when a patient is still compliant in order to increase the likelihood that he will be willing to engage in the procedure in the future rather than pushing too far and creating a traumatic experience for the patient and caregiver.

Clinical Vignette #1: A Pediatric Patient

Bradley is a 12-year-old boy with a diagnosis of ASD. He is minimally verbal and typically communicates by pointing at objects in close proximity or pulling a caregiver to the object. When he is very anxious, he may use some words to express his needs with scripted language. Bradley is participating in a clinical trial that requires an electrocardiogram (ECG), vital signs, anthropometric measures, DEXA scan (to measure bone density), and sample collection (blood, saliva, urine) at multiple time points over the course of 12 months. When a new task is presented in the medical office setting, Bradley has historically presented challenging behavior including yelling, bolting from the office, and lunging at objects and staff.

At the first visit, Bradley was visibly anxious with clammy palms and pacing, and he scripted softly under his breath with sporadic verbal outbursts, saying "one more time... all done...bookstore." This comment is a known script for him to communicate to others that he is done and wants to leave the current environment. He tolerated sitting quietly in the room for some time during the visit with several shouts to his mother to confirm what his schedule was for the day. His mother would reply, "First, Mom and doctor talk, then Bradley checks his height, then we get the medicine, then we go home." He often said "Ok, then we go book?" His mother would respond yes. This dialogue would go on every 5–7 min as a means for Bradley to confirm what was next on his schedule since the visit deviated from his typical routine of going to school.

When it was time to proceed to the vital signs room, Bradley ran three hallways down and hid in an office with his fingers in his ears, scripting and pacing. Staff and his mother were able to coax him back to the room and allowed him time to cross the door threshold with a promise that once he had his height, weight, vital signs, ECG, and samples collected, he was done for the day. He was resistant to the approach of staff but allowed his mother to help facilitate each task. At times, he would say in a very loud pressured voice "no talking, no talking." If the room was quiet, he tolerated each task by closing his eyes and scripting under his breath. He refused distractors including spinning lights, a hand-held fan, and a koosh ball, as well as reinforcements in the form of stickers.

Bradley was offered time between tasks, and staff approached him with whispers to describe what was next. At times his mother would provide reassurance that we were close to being done and that they would go get a new book when they left the clinic. The entire process for completing all procedures took over 1 h. Bradley's second visit was slightly improved with the understanding that there would be "no shots" at this visit.

Two months later, Bradley had a study visit at the clinic in which a blood draw was required. In preparation for the visit, his mother provided a visual schedule and verbal reassurance. Upon meeting with staff, Bradley was offered options to get his blood drawn first or last. He promptly told staff "shot then book?" Taking his verbal lead, staff were able to transition him to the blood collection room with slight hesitation at the door threshold at which time he said "What next, Bradley home?" Staff provided the next steps in the order they were to be completed. The entire process took only 30 min.

Six months of routine vital sign assessment and three blood draws proved to be less anxiety-provoking with each visit, and the time needed dramatically decreased to less than 15 min. At the 6-month time point, Bradley was introduced to a new environment where he would participate in a DEXA scan and wrist X-ray at the main hospital. Both his mother and study staff implemented the same strategies previously employed at each study visit, including allowing his mother to facilitate tasks by interfacing between Bradley and staff, minimal talking by staff, whispering to him to communicate next steps, whispering or gesturing between staff when needed, offering choices for the order of tasks, identifying rewards prior to study visits upon completion of the visit tasks, and informing radiology staff of Bradley's preference for minimal talking during procedures. With the assistance and cooperation of the health-care team, Bradley was able to complete both imaging studies without any behavioral outbursts, bolting, or raised voice.

Subsequent visits to the clinic proved that Bradley had developed an understanding of the expectations as he complied with requests and made few verbal commands to study staff. In months 9 through 12, he spontaneously and independently initiated interaction with staff by leading them to the vital sign room to get "his work done" and then calmly returned to the exam room where his mother waited to provide his reward in the form of a sticker and granola bar. At his final study visit, Bradley approached the staff member that administered the procedures. He stood next to her and gave her a hug while stating "Good job Bradley, bookstore."

In this case example, the family and staff worked together to develop strategies to gain Bradley's cooperation in the completion of procedures in a systematic manner which allowed for realistic expectations for return office visits. A key component to Bradley's ability to tolerate unexpected and non-preferred activities was listening to Bradley's requests and assessing his response to different approaches to complete tasks. Throughout the year, it was clear that Bradley understood that he was expected to complete non-preferred activities, and when given the option to choose the order of completion, it fostered independence and a sense of control and accomplishment on his part.

Clinical Vignette #2: An Adult Patient

Samantha is a 21-year-old young woman with ASD and bilateral sensorineural hearing loss who presents to a multidisciplinary clinic for medical care. She is nonverbal and communicates primarily through using single signs and the Picture Exchange Communication System (PECS). Samantha's mother is seeking support from the clinic staff and medical providers and reported significant difficulties with dental cleanings. Samantha is also expected to begin wearing hearing aids in order to improve awareness of her surroundings for safety purposes. The barriers to accessing consistent and comprehensive care have been Samantha's limited communication, a high level of anxiety about unfamiliar procedures, and sensitivities to touch.

First, her dental team and audiologist worked in collaboration with her mother and a psychologist to determine the best method in which to begin approaching her dental cleanings and hearing aid fittings. They began by providing Samantha pictures of the dentist's and audiologist's offices and a visual task analysis with each step of a dental cleaning and hearing aid fitting so that she could become familiar with what to expect. Samantha was asked to look at pictures of each step of the procedures and comply with each step of the process, beginning with the least anxiety-provoking tasks (e.g., sitting in a chair and then allowing the dentist to approach her). This was a useful communication tool to help Samantha understand what she would be expected to do. Additionally, Samantha's providers consulted with her mother to determine how Samantha could most clearly request a break or ask for help as needed using a combination of sign language and picture exchange, including a picture with a stop sign that Samantha used in school. This was comforting to Samantha, as she was able to understand that it was okay to ask for a break when she was feeling overwhelmed.

Related to dental cleanings, exposure to stimuli was increased until Samantha could tolerate someone approaching her mouth with tools, prompting her to open her mouth, and cleaning her teeth with a toothbrush and other more invasive tools, such as a scaler, for a longer duration of time. Providers showed her all of the items before approaching and allowed her to become more familiar with the items before beginning the dental cleaning. Additionally, pictures of each step were shown to her before beginning a new step in order to reduce her fear and anxiety.

Regarding hearing aid fittings, Samantha was introduced to stimuli, beginning with the least-restrictive items (e.g., headphones on her ears) and working toward tolerating longer periods of time with ear buds in her ears. While working to increase exposure, Samantha was provided with positive reinforcement for each step of the process, allowing her to participate in preferred activities after completion of each step, such as looking at magazines. Eventually, Samantha was able to tolerate her hearing aids and learned to independently place them in her ears and remove them when needed. In addition to systematic desensitization and exposure to stimuli, behavioral strategies were utilized to increase compliance, including blocking removal of hearing aids or dental tools and using distraction techniques to help sustain her compliance with the procedures.

In this case example, Samantha's providers worked collaboratively and were able to use her mother as a resource to learn strategies that were effective in working with Samantha. Additionally, they prioritized communication in their care, using visual tools and her primary modes of communication in the form of signs and pictures to help with communication. Finally, the providers treated Samantha with respect and dignity, remaining sensitive to her needs and comfort level throughout the process. By using these tools, they provided Samantha with patient-centered care and successfully completed multiple outpatient procedures to facilitate her health.

Clinical Pearls

Pediatric pearls

- Assess the patient's communication capabilities and preferences.
- Be patient and allow more time for procedures when possible.
- Provide visual and auditory supports.
- Consider the patient's sensitivities and triggers when completing medical procedures.
- Utilize rewards and reinforcements in order to motivate the child to complete non-preferred procedures.
- Involve the child's parents as a resource.
- Work as a team – multidisciplinary collaboration is essential to effective treatment of children with ASD.

Adult pearls

- Treat patients with dignity and communicate with them directly.
- Check for the patient's understanding of procedures (e.g., by asking them to repeat or demonstrate what they expect will occur).
- Allow adult patients the opportunity for privacy if family or caregivers are present.
- Ask caregivers and family members about the patient's past experiences and successes to help inform useful tools or strategies for medical procedures.

Survey for Preparation of Medical Procedures

Communication

- What is the patient's preferred method of communication (e.g., verbal, gestures, signs, writing, AAC device)?
- Does the patient prefer to know the details of what to expect or is it better to provide the patient with less details?

Visual Supports

- Does the patient prefer to see the steps that they will be expected to follow? Is it helpful for the patient to see a demonstration of what they will be expected to do?
- Is it helpful for the patient to see how much time is left in a procedure in order to sustain their compliance with a task (e.g., use of visual timers)?

Behavioral Contingencies and Positive Reinforcement

- Does the patient have interests or preferred activities that can be incorporated into the procedure or used as effective distraction techniques during the procedure? Does the patient benefit from receiving praise, physical touch, or access to a preferred item (e.g., toy, magazine, snack) to help motivate them to comply with difficult tasks?
- Does the patient have any behaviors or fears that may make certain steps of the procedure more difficult? If so, what has been effective in minimizing or reacting to these behaviors?

Relaxation Strategies

- What are strategies that the patient, caregivers, or family members can use to help the patient remain calm or relaxed during the procedure?
- How can the environment be set up in a way that the patient is most comfortable (e.g., minimizing distractions, loud noises)?

Collaboration with Other Providers or Individuals Familiar with the Patient

- Reflect with the patient, family, or familiar providers about what past procedures have been more difficult. What about these procedures was most challenging?
- What past procedures have been successful with other providers and what tools did they use to help the patient remain comfortable and compliant?
- Are there other providers that I can speak with who know the patient or can inform any strategies or approaches that may be helpful in completing a successful procedure?

References

1. American Speech-Language-Hearing Association. http://www.asha.org (2015). Accessed 1 May 2016.
2. Beck MH, Cataldo M, Slifer KJ, Pulbrook V, Guhman JK. Teaching children with attention deficit hyperactivity disorder (ADHD) and autistic disorder (AD) how to swallow pills. Clin Pediatr. 2005;44:515–26.
3. Braff M, Nealon L. Sedation of autistic dental patient for dental procedures. ASDC J Dent Child. 1979;46(5):404–7.
4. Cagetti MG, Mastroberardino, Campus S, Olivari B, Faggioli R, Lenti C, Strohmenger L. Dental care protocol based on visual supports for children with autism spectrum disorders. Med Oral Patol Oral Cir Bucal. 2015;20(5):e598–604.

5. Davit CJ, Hundley RJ, Bacic JD, Hanson EM. A pilot study to improve venipuncture compliance in children and adolescents with autism spectrum disorders. J Dev Behav Pediatr. 2011;32(7):521–5.
6. HANDS in Autism. Toolkit for medical professionals: tips and supports for working with individuals with autism spectrum disorders. Indianapolis: Christian Sarkine Autism Treatment Center, Riley Child & Adolescent Psychiatry Clinic, Indiana University School of Medicine – Department of Psychiatry; 2008. https://handsinautism.iupui.edu/toolkit.html#.VyZknTFWWMN. Accessed 1 May 2016.
7. Heller KW, Alberto PA, Forney P, Schwartzman MN. Learning and behavioral characteristics. In: Heller KW, Alberto PA, Forney P, Schwartzman MN, editors. Understanding physical, sensory and health impairments. Pacific Grove: Brookes/Cole; 1996. p. 35–42.
8. Kamen S, Skier J. Dental management of the autistic child. Spec Care Dentist. 1985;5(1):20–3.
9. Keck J, Gerkensmeyer J, Joyce B, Schade J. Reliability and validity of the faces and word descriptor scales to measure procedural pain. J Pediatr Nurs. 1996;11(6):368–74.
10. Love SR, Matson JL, West D. Mothers as effective therapists for autistic children's phobias. J of Appl Behav Anal. 1990;23(3):379–85.
11. Luscre DM, Center DB. Procedures for reducing dental fear in children with autism. J Autism Dev Disord. 1996;26(5):547–56.
12. McDowell RH, Scher CS, Barst SM. Total intravenous anesthesia for children undergoing brief diagnostic or therapeutic procedures. J Clin Anesth. 1995;7(4):273–80.
13. Mehta UC, Patel I, Castello FV. EEG sedation for children with autism. J Dev Behav Pediatr. 2004;25(2):102–4.
14. Merkel SJ, Voepel-Lewis T, Shayevitz JR, Malviya S. The FLACC: a behavioural scale for scoring postoperative pain in young children. Pediatr Nurs. 1997;23(3):293–7.
15. National Institute on Deafness and Other Communication Disorders. https://www.nidcd.nih.gov 2015. Accessed 1 May 2016.
16. Pilebro C, Backman B. Teaching oral hygiene to children with autism. Int J Paediatr Dent. 2005;15(1):1–9.
17. Shabani DB, Fisher WW. Stimulus fading and differential reinforcement for the treatment of needle phobia in a youth with autism. J Appl Behav Anal. 2006;39(4):449–52.
18. Slifer KJ, Avis KT, Frutchey RA. Behavioral intervention to increase compliance with electroencephalographic procedures in children with developmental disabilities. Epilepsy Behav. 2008;13(1):189–95.
19. Slifer KJ, Babbitt RL, Cataldo MD. Simulation and counterconditioning as adjuncts to pharmacotherapy for invasive pediatric procedures. J Dev Behav Pediatr. 1995;16(3):133–41.
20. Slifer KJ, Eischen SE, Busby S. Using counterconditioning to treat behavioural distress during subcutaneous injections in a paediatric rehabilitation patient. Brain Inj. 2002;16(10):901–16.
21. Slifer KJ, Hankinson JC, Zettler MA, Frutchey RA, Hendricks MC, Ward CM, Reesman J. Management during needle sticks in children with intellectual and developmental disabilities. Clin Pediatr. 2011;50:688–97. https://doi.org/10.1177/0009922811398959.
22. Solodiuk JC, Scott-Sutherland J, Meyers M, Myette B, Shusterman C, Karian VE, Harris SK, Curley MAQ. Validation of the individualized numeric rating scale (INRS): a pain assessment tool for nonverbal children with intellectual disability. Pain. 2010;150(2):231–6. https://doi.org/10.1016/j.pain.2010.03.016.
23. Switkin MC, Gelfand KM, Amari A, Dahlquist LM, Slifer K, Eskenazi AE. The impact of types of distractors on child-critical statements by a caregiver during chemotherapy injections: a case study. Child Health Care. 2002;31(4):311–9.

5 Quality Improvement

Jocelyn Carter and Christiana Iyasere

Introduction

There is a clear and demonstrated need to improve the quality of medical care delivered to individuals with autism spectrum disorder (ASD), but efforts in this area face many challenges. While over $400 million dollars a year is spent on autism research focused on pathophysiology, early diagnosis, and treatment [32], there are ongoing gaps in knowledge of ASD among healthcare providers both in community and medical settings [19, 43]. Furthermore, although there are a number of well-founded guidelines on best practices in autism, these guidelines focus primarily on the treatment of this disorder itself, and there is little in the way of cross-sectional validated best practices in healthcare delivery for this patient population. Here we describe the ongoing gaps in the medical care of patients with ASD and recommendations for designing systemic improvements in healthcare quality for patients with ASD. Finally, we present a case study for quality improvement in this area based upon our experience at Massachusetts General Hospital (MGH).

Evidence for Unmet Needs

The evidence for improved outcomes for those accurately diagnosed with ASD prior to the age of 3 years is well established [9, 10]. However, current literature suggests that a number of patients are diagnosed after the age of 3 years old and even into adulthood [17, 15, 42]. Following diagnosis, individuals with ASD face significant barriers in their access to healthcare. In a recent survey of 54 pediatricians and 59 parents of children with ASD, providers reported inability to complete examinations, patient fears about the encounter, and difficulty communicating as barriers to providing care, whereas parents reported child behavior, sensory issues, and feelings of a disconnect with the healthcare provider as barriers [5]. With regard to the inpatient setting, adolescents and families of adolescents with ASD were surveyed and identified factors including addressing communication and sensory challenges and inflexible protocols, processes, and providers as barriers to adequate care [27].

Limited access to care in the outpatient setting is another major problem. Studies have shown that limited access is a problem across the age

J. Carter (✉)
Department of Medicine, Massachusetts General Hospital, Boston, MA, USA
e-mail: jcarter0@mgh.harvard.edu

C. Iyasere
Department of Medicine, Massachusetts General Hospital, Boston, MA, USA
e-mail: ciyasere@mgh.partners.org

E. P. Hazen, C. J. McDougle (eds.), *The Massachusetts General Hospital Guide to Medical Care in Patients with Autism Spectrum Disorder*, Current Clinical Psychiatry,
https://doi.org/10.1007/978-3-319-94458-6_5

spectrum, affecting youth, those transitioning to adult care [20, 33, 37], and adults [16]. A study by Liptak and associates found particularly large disparities in access to healthcare in children with ASD in traditionally underserved populations [22].

Healthcare experience and patient satisfaction have also been studied. Parents of children with ASD surveyed with regard to their healthcare experiences have reported consistent themes that include concern with medications, frustrations with healthcare services, problems recognizing secondary health issues, and the need for more resources and services [35]. In a compelling study conducted by Nicolaidis and colleagues, perceptions of healthcare experiences were obtained by surveying 209 individuals with ASD and 228 individuals without ASD [30]. They found that adults with ASD reported lower satisfaction with patient-provider communication and were more than twice as likely to have unmet healthcare needs and to use the emergency department (ED) for services. Furthermore, individuals with ASD were twice as likely to have unaddressed mental health needs.

In another study performed by Fortuna and colleagues, comorbid conditions including intellectual disability and functional status were explored in adults with ASD [11]. This cross-sectional evaluation demonstrated higher rates of seizure disorders and depression among 18–29-year-olds with ASD. Among those 40 years of age or older, 55% of the participants had a documented IQ score. Of those, 91% had intellectual disability with an IQ<70. Only 54% could independently perform their activities of daily living in this cohort.

Quality Improvement Research: Areas for Intervention

While there are no universal, validated quality improvement approaches for the delivery of healthcare to patients with ASD, there are several systemic interventions that have shown promise, including education for hospital staff about ASD. McGonigle and partners developed and implemented educational materials for ED providers to improve care of patients with ASD in the ED [24]. Similar tools to help address agitation in the crisis or emergency setting were developed for patients with ASD [25]. One of the most promising leads in this area is the development of an interactive toolkit for both patients and providers as an evidence-based intervention funded by the National Institute of Mental Health (NIMH) to improve healthcare quality [31].

Environmental modifications such as decreasing unwanted stimulation, background noise, and light brightness have been shown to reduce stress among patients with ASD [36]. One study examining visual and auditory stimuli as obstacles to care delivery found that noise levels in the ED of an urban teaching hospital setting were in excess of both WHO and EPA recommended maximums for public health and welfare [36]. This kind of environment clearly poses a challenge in the care of patients with ASD with sensory sensitivities.

Implementation of an inclusive care plan that patients with ASD and their families can complete prior to or during clinical encounters has also been shown to improve the quality of healthcare experiences [3]. Routine use of visual aids such as social stories and visual schedules has also been shown to help reduce anxiety induced by new or unfamiliar healthcare settings and improve patients' experiences [26, 38]. Similarly, in inpatient settings, minimizing nonessential blood draws and batching diagnostic tests have been shown to improve outcomes [14]. Gabriels and associates showed that a systemic intervention that included minimizing sensory stimuli, reducing noncritical diagnostic procedures, and partnering with patients and families to create patient-centered care plans was effective in decreasing 30-day hospital readmissions as well as the length of hospitalization for psychiatric patients with ASD [13]. Problems with discharge planning and case management services have been identified as two of the largest barriers to the delivery of quality healthcare in ASD. Specialized units structured to address these barriers have shown improved outcomes [34].

Nicoloidis and associates (2014) shared a number of interventions that they implemented in order to augment healthcare for patients with ASD seen in the outpatient setting. These interventions included decreasing stimulation in waiting rooms, allowing patients to utilize preferred modes of communication, allowing patients to reconcile unfamiliar information in their own time, creating step by step instructions for making appointments and obtaining prescriptions, and providing a fact sheet to notify patients about who they can contact for questions or additional support services [29]. The utility of these types of interventions is supported by similar findings from Bultas and colleagues highlighting specific resources described by parents surveyed to identify which interventions would help improve care. Identified resources included provider adaptations to the patient, such as slowing down the delivery of care and implementing environmental adaptations, to make the office more comfortable for those with ASD [5].

Another important focus of quality improvement initiatives is the transition from pediatric to adult medical care. A study by Kuhlthau and associates demonstrated effective interventions in this area, such as providing families with written medical summaries to give to adult providers as patients transition from pediatric to adult healthcare settings, compiling lists of available adult providers or community resources, coordinating care and communication between individual pediatric and adult providers, making transition-specific appointments, and using checklists to track transition progress [18]. Informational workshops to train families and youth about healthcare transitions as well as training adult providers and medical students on care of the ASD population were also suggested as another potentially helpful intervention.

The Quality Improvement Journey: Creating Change

As reviewed above, the current evidence base may serve as an initial guide for quality improvement and innovation. The approach to quality improvement in the healthcare of individuals with ASD should include certain critical steps that will maximize the chances of success. These steps include identifying the target population, defining the problem, building a case for improvement with preliminary data, identifying key stakeholders, implementing the intervention, and measuring improvement. These processes are described in detail below and should also include education of providers and support staff and resource development for both providers and patients/families.

Describing the Target Population

For institutions that deliver healthcare to patients with ASD, the very first step toward improving care for this population may be to understand and describe the patient population they serve. While this may seem like a rudimentary task, often times identifying patients within healthcare systems that either carry a diagnosis of ASD or display characteristics or behaviors suggestive of ASD can be quite challenging [1, 15]. Clearly, the challenge of identifying patients for quality improvement efforts is part of the broader issue in ASD treatment of making early and accurate diagnoses of those with ASD and avoiding misdiagnosis in those without the condition. Despite best efforts, a number of individuals with ASD are not correctly diagnosed until later in life and thus do not benefit from the resources and services that they need most early in life [4].

Furthermore, identifying patients with ASD for quality improvement purposes can be confounded by how clinical providers bill for their encounters as well as the way that providers construct problem lists within clinical documentation. For example, a provider seeing a patient with ASD for a specific medical problem, such as asthma, may not always include ASD as a billing diagnosis or include ASD in the problem list. This can result in limited ability to capture those with ASD via review of billing data or the electronic medical record. This can lead to an underestimation of the numbers of patients with ASD in a clinical sample.

For these reasons, those seeking to quantify the number of patients with ASD within a specific healthcare setting should be cautioned to consider variation in billing and diagnostic code use if this is to be the relied-upon method for data collection. Chart review can be more reliable but is a more resource-laden and time-consuming approach. There are a number of examples of capturing patients with ASD via providers or services that come in contact with them outside of the healthcare system. These may include caseworkers, social workers, and governmental agencies providing financial support services. While there is no single approach to quantifying the number of individuals with this condition, those approaching or seeking to embark on an initiative to improve the quality of care for individuals with ASD should consider methods for identifying the target population as well as potential barriers to accurate identification.

Defining the Problem: Measuring Unmet Care Needs and Gaps in Care Quality

While there is no set pre-existing panel of recommendations for metrics to use in measuring the performance of healthcare delivery specific to individuals with ASD, there are a number of variables that may be considered for analysis. From a quantitative perspective, one approach is to use performance metrics such as those established by the Centers for Medicare and Medicaid Services (CMS) based on patient and caregiver experience, care coordination, patient safety, and preventative health interventions [7]. CMS recommends 33 different quality metrics with regard to process and outcome measures for which healthcare institutions are responsible. While this mission requires significant effort for any healthcare institution, patients with ASD could certainly benefit from a number of the metrics as described, and this is information that institutions are likely to be gathering already. Alternatively, institutions that are just beginning to embark upon the quality journey may consider simplifying metrics to focus only on the following: patient and family experience or satisfaction, ED visit rates, hospital admission rates, rates of hospital readmission within 30 days, and access to care.

Patient and family healthcare experience and satisfaction were measured by Nicoloidis and associates, who successfully developed a survey to assess the quality of care being delivered for patients with ASD [30]. In doing so they were able to identify key quality gaps that existed in their specific healthcare system and begin to strategize in terms of interventions. While ED visit rates are not considered to be a CMS recommended metric for process performance, current data suggests that patients with ASD are more than twice as likely to receive healthcare in ED settings compared to those without ASD [11]. Thus, use of ED visit data as a metric may benefit populations by highlighting an underlying lack of care in ambulatory settings.

Another potential key metric includes the percentage of ASD patients that are supported by primary care providers as compared to non-ASD patients within a particular healthcare system. Although access to ambulatory care for all patients continues to be an area in need of improvement, a survey of primary care providers demonstrated that only a fraction of those caring for patients with ASD have appropriate training and comfort in caring for these patients [41]. For this reason, improving access to primary care providers for patients with ASD and providing education about ASD to existing providers can be a critical quality improvement intervention.

Assessing admission or readmission rates to inpatient hospital settings within a particular healthcare system can also be helpful in guiding and understanding healthcare needs for patients with ASD that are being served in a particular catchment area. Given the high rates of comorbid medical diagnoses, including gastrointestinal disorders, sleep difficulties, food allergies, and epilepsy [8], patients with ASD are likely to present to acute care settings. Having an awareness of utilization of acute care services both from the perspective of diagnoses associated with inpatient hospitalizations and frequency of usage may identify underlying needs for pathway-specific or disease-specific improvement protocols for ASD populations in order to address common issues leading to hospitalization. Alternatively, many hospitals may serve as a safety net for individuals with ASD that have unmet needs in areas of social support systems, financial resources, and nonclinical outpatient services or programming. As such, the inpatient setting may serve not only to treat patients with ASD medically but also to serve patients with unmet financial and social support needs. Ultimately, the objectives and priorities of individual institutions or care centers should drive the chosen quality metrics. While the metrics that are pursued may vary from setting to setting, one of the first steps in quality improvement is identifying some measurable metrics to guide the intervention and determine its impact.

Building a Case for Improvement with Preliminary Data

Without measurement, it's impossible to know where care gaps arise or where the opportunities for healthcare improvement exist [2, 28]. Often a case must be made to hospital administrators and other stakeholders that there is a need for a quality improvement initiative before the resources for a detailed analysis are made available. Depending upon what measures are chosen, there may be a variety of ways to obtain initial data supporting the case for an improvement initiative.

After developing a way to identify patients with ASD (e.g., through billing, coding, chart review, or some other internal tracking process), preliminary data can be generated either through qualitative or quantitative means. In terms of qualitative data, disseminating surveys to providers or patients may generate a deeper understanding of issues with regard to access to care, patient and family experience with the healthcare system, and general quality of care. Partnering with other local institutions or tapping formal or informal data stores may allow for the creation of a database of individuals with ASD tracking admission and readmission rates, ED visits, or unfilled medication prescriptions. Utilizing providers that routinely connect with patients with ASD (e.g., primary care physician practices, nurse practitioners, case managers, or social workers in the community) may also allow for development of a reliable data source.

Alternatively, using narratives or testimony from patient or patient-family stories about healthcare experiences can sometimes present a strong case for a quality improvement initiative. While it's important that whatever patient experiences are highlighted are factual and representative of core issues, there are times that even one or two egregious events can merit an impetus for transformational change. In this way, use of safety reporting can be valuable in discovering issues in processes of care that need to be addressed. Having a system for review of safety reports can generate a meaningful platform for creating quality improvement initiatives.

The quality of the preliminary data used to establish the need for improvement is critical since the more flawed the data is, the less likely any correct and meaningful conclusions can be made from it. In some respects, any initiative is only as good as the preliminary data it is based upon. Ensuring the integrity of the chosen data source as well as data collection is critical. While no dataset is perfect, knowing where the potential weaknesses are as well as having alternative sources to cross reference the data can be very helpful.

Identifying Stakeholders and Champions

The success of quality initiatives depends upon the involvement of key stakeholders, defined as individuals who are concerned with the processes being addressed. Key stakeholders may include patients and families affected by ASD, administrative leaders, and clinical providers who work directly with patients with ASD, such as nurses, occupational therapists, speech therapists, physicians, case workers, and social workers [23]. While the organizational map will look different at every institution or care setting, identifying those that are the work (e.g., individuals that have ASD and are supportive of those that have ASD), those that do the work (e.g., individuals that provide clinical care to ASD populations), those that will be affected by the work (including administrative and clinical support staff), and those that are needed to approve or endorse the work (e.g., administrative or clinical leaders) should all be involved.

Engaging these individuals by presenting the preliminary data and establishing a platform for change can ignite a working group or sometimes multiple groups. Bringing these individuals together and presenting the data may peak interest, generate meaningful questions, and create forward momentum for change. The first step in this process is identifying those that may be primed for a working group or task force as well as delegating those that can help lead specific working groups or subcommittees based on their background, expertise, and historical involvement with issues or the specific population at hand. Making individuals and groups accountable by working together to create an agreed-upon consensus for mission, vision, and global and specific aims as well as a strategic plan to meet those objectives is the next step. Once this is in place, additional stakeholders, resources, and support may be identified in order to execute the described strategic plan for intervention in moving forward.

Implementing Interventions

In identifying the mission, vision, and global and specific aims, the strategic plan for improvement should begin to take shape. The plan may be based on a number of different quality improvement initiatives described in the literature or may be entirely novel [6]. Regardless, a strategic plan for quality improvement should generally include one or more of a variety of characteristics, such as education for clinical and administrative providers, additional support via electronic medical record resources specific to ASD care, improvements in processes of care to better support patient communication within clinical settings, or informational resources for patients and families. For example, interventions might include finding ways to educate clinical providers and support staff on ASD, developing and implementing a patient-centered care plan for patients with ASD, creating patient- and family-friendly resources to help educate patients and families on what to expect in the clinical environment, or augmenting social support for patients and families with ASD.

Depending upon the setting, the strategic plan may simply involve completion of a formal survey of providers and patients to better identify how to meet the needs of ASD patients that are cared for within a setting so that any discovered care gaps may be used to direct future plans for improvement or intervention.

Measuring Improvement/Transformational Change

Each improvement journey will be uniquely punctuated by the iterative ebb and flow of discovery, challenges, reassessment, learning, and implementation [12, 40]. Models such as the "plan, do, study, act (PDSA) cycle" have been invoked as a guide to the improvement process [21]. The PDSA cycle is an iterative four-step method used to understand and drive process improvement in a continuous way. In this model, trends in the qualitative or quantitative data can be used to assess progress toward outcomes. Measures like readmission rates, ED visits, access to care, physician confidence in taking care of ASD patients, and patient satisfaction, or other measures of interest may be employed.

While movement forward may not always be in a straight line from start to finish, adapting to emerging results of ongoing data collection or responses to interventions from providers or patient stakeholders is key. Although ongoing robust data collection may not be possible in some clinical settings, real-time feedback from those helping design or experiencing the strategic plan and interventions drive the pathway forward to change.

Summary

There is a clear, demonstrable need for systemic quality improvement initiatives related to the medical care of patients with ASD. Research in this area is beginning to help define best practices in ASD care. Improving quality in ASD care delivery involves several critical steps, including definition of the target population, identification of a problem or quality gap, collaboration with key stakeholders, determination of useful performance metrics, careful data collection, and implementation of interventions via iterative cycles of change to generate continuous improvement. Some of the specific initiatives that have been shown to be effective in improving care in ASD include the following:

- Increasing patient participatory research to assess and address current gaps in healthcare delivery in ASD
- Formal efforts to educate clinicians on the care of patients with ASD
- Provider adaptations to the patient, including slowing down the delivery of care and environmental adaptations geared toward reducing stimulation [5, 39]
- Use of care plans can improve the patient experience in inpatient settings [3]
- Use of care plans and reduced stimulation in clinical environments to help reduce readmissions and length of stay in inpatient settings [13]
- Reducing sensory stimuli in healthcare settings to reduce anxiety in individuals with ASD and improve care [14]
- Use of visual symbols to assist communication for individuals with ASD in healthcare settings [38]
- Specialized units for patients with ASD to enhance care delivery [34]
- Positive behavioral support with individualized schedules for patients with ASD [26]

Massachusetts General Hospital Autism Care Collaborative: A Case Study

The MGH Autism Care Collaborative (ACC) was initiated in the fall of 2013 as a result of the collaboration between a group of patients, families, and MGH clinicians with the shared goal of improving the patient care experience of individuals with ASD at MGH. An inpatient hospital admission is challenging and disorienting for most, but for a patient with ASD, the new sounds, changes to routine, and exposure to multiple unfamiliar providers can be overwhelming and lead to behavioral changes that negatively impact care. The concerns of the collaborative group were grounded in these challenges, as well as those associated with the transition from pediatric to adult medical care experienced by many of the patients, families, and providers. To begin to address these issues, three guiding objectives of the ACC were defined: (1) to educate inpatient providers and staff on the distinct needs of hospitalized adults with ASD, (2) to develop resources for inpatient providers to help facilitate optimal decision-making in the care of patients with ASD, and (3) to augment the inpatient care experience for adults with ASD.

Resource Development

The MGH ACC sought to develop a "toolkit" of resources available to inpatient providers at the point of interaction with adult patients with ASD. The Collaborative was comprised of a leadership team of physician experts in the care of both adult and pediatric patients with ASD, adult and pediatric nursing directors, internal medicine physicians, pediatric hospitalists, occupational therapists, speech therapists, and parents of individuals with ASD.

From this group, four smaller working groups were identified to work on specific issues. These workgroups were defined as follows:

- Medical management of adults with ASD on inpatient units
- Education of staff and providers about ASD
- Flow of patients with ASD through the healthcare system
- Communication/information transfer between hospital units

Each of the groups worked to create both a patient and provider toolkit that contained actionable resources to help educate staff about the optimal care for patients with ASD. Specific details of work groups are listed below.

Medical Management of Adults with ASD on Inpatient Units

This subcommittee worked to identify the distinct needs of adult patients with ASD when hospitalized, critical knowledge gaps between best practices and what was known by existing staff, and tangible resources that staff could quickly access when a patient with ASD was admitted. They then worked to develop a flexible plan for appropriate care through:

- Seamless coordination with outpatient providers and families for anticipatory planning through the utilization of an accessible, individualized "Acute Care Plan" that can provide guidance about how to support a particular patient in outpatient, ED, or inpatient settings
- Clear, concise educational tools for all providers that offer both basic information on ASD and an algorithm for involvement of resources based on ASD disease severity
- Useful order sets for the electronic medical record system that prompt providers to consider available resources during an inpatient stay, such as an occupational therapy consult or involvement of social work
- Development of an autism consultant role, or "Autism Patient Navigator," available on call to the medical team for additional support and expertise in helping patients with ASD and their families by guiding them through an inpatient admission

Education of Providers and Staff

The educational workgroup created educational resources for hospital staff about the unique challenges of caring for patients with ASD. Of note, the goal was to provide educational outreach and materials for *all* hospital staff that could encounter a patient with ASD when admitted to a medical unit. This included not only clinical staff such as nurses, physicians, and medical assistants but also nonclinical employees, such as custodial staff, front desk staff, and food service workers, who are also likely to interact with patients with ASD in the hospital. The emphasis was to anticipate and respond appropriately to the needs of patients with ASD. In particular the workgroup emphasized the following principles:

- Preparedness – A variety of "just-in-time" tools, resources, and other supports are available and easily accessible for use by clinicians at all times
- Inclusiveness – Patients with ASD and their families feel cared for: moving beyond patient-family-centered care to establish a culture of higher quality, safety, and satisfaction
- Standardization – Consistency in the care provided from clinicians who are all prepared and have the right resources available at the right time

In addition to reaching out to hospital staff, the group also highlighted the importance of providing families with key facts about what to expect from an inpatient medical stay. As a result, a "What to Expect Guide" for patients and families was created for use at the time of or prior to a hospital admission.

Patient Flow

The goal of the patient flow work group was to help optimize the hospital admissions process for patients with ASD. Guiding principles of the patient flow workgroup included:

- Minimizing patient wait times in crowded, sensory stimulating environments
- Working to outline and develop a seamless process for preadmission and admission via each entry point to the inpatient clinical setting that is interdisciplinary, effective, and patient-family centered
- Identifying opportunities to ensure single patient rooms with the capacity for caregivers to stay overnight

Communication and Information Transfer

The communication and information transfer workgroup focused on efforts to improve communication systems throughout the hospital with the goals of optimizing the patient experience for all patients with ASD and supporting staff in their commitment to provide outstanding patient care effectively and efficiently. Specific goals of this workgroup included:

- Evaluating existing materials available for patients with ASD and their families to ensure that they are accurate and up to date
- Utilizing the Autism Care Questionnaire, a survey tool for providers that helps guide them through a series of important questions to ask patients with ASD and their families to help identify patient preferences (e.g., about preferred methods of communication, behavioral triggers, and calming strategies) to improve the patient experience
- Developing a new position, an Autism Patient Navigator, who has familiarity with ASD, appropriate resources, and how to attain them and can act as a resource available to patients and their families prior to, during, and after an inpatient admission
- Identifying basic communication systems related to medical issues that should be widely available throughout the hospital (i.e., Mayer-Johnson picture board) to help patients with ASD communicate if needed
- Creating decision support tools that can help clinicians provide adequate resources for patients with ASD, such as reasons for considering occupational therapy consults for patients with ASD and checklists of considerations for patients with ASD being discharged from the hospital

Final Results

The ACC worked collaboratively over the course of the following year to execute the goals that had been defined. All materials were developed via consensus and group feedback. At the conclusion of the ACC, final deliverables included:

- Creation of three 10-min videos for hospital staff on optimal care for ASD patients, which were viewed by 80% of all nursing and support staff throughout the hospital
- Identification of two to three floors within the hospital that could serve as educational reference points for other medical floors in the hospital. These "autism knowledge units" were given more intensive orientation and training and presentations to nursing staff about existing hospital resources for providers caring for patients with ASD
- A toolkit for providers to be made available at in-person presentations and virtually for

download at any time by any provider in the hospital. This toolkit included:

- *Autism Admission Basics Checklist* (see Chap. 3): things to think about when admitting a patient with ASD regarding orders, frequency of testing, sensory environment, consults, etc.
- *Autism Clinical Care Algorithm* (see Chap. 3): a clear and concise decision tree to help providers decide appropriate resources for patients admitted to the hospital with ASD based on severity of symptoms and behavioral triggers.
- *Autism Care Questionnaire* (see Chap. 3): a survey administered either by outpatient providers prior to admission or by providers at the time of admission to identify patient communication and sensory needs. This was designed to become part of the medical record for future provider reference.
- *Patient and Family Guide: What to Expect* (see Chap. 3) – descriptive document that outlines care team membership, times to anticipate when providers will see you, and in-hospital resources.
- *Case Management Guide* (see Chap. 3): a list of available community resources to assist in the transition from the hospital to home or alternative care environment. Example information included location of facilities familiar with the care of patients with ASD and relevant disability resources.

Next Steps

The MGH ACC continues to seek opportunities to improve the care provided to adults with ASD when admitted to the hospital. To that end, next steps include program evaluation, funding for the proposed Autism Patient Navigator role, and ongoing dissemination of developed materials.

Summary

As discussed in detail above, converging evidence from many studies has demonstrated that there are significant problems with the accessibility and quality of medical care for individuals with ASD under our current healthcare system. These problems may result in greater healthcare expenditures, inefficient resource utilization in the form of frequent ED visits and hospital readmissions, significant unmet medical need, and lower patient and family satisfaction with care for this patient population. Thus, there is a clear need for initiatives to improve the quality of care delivered to patients with ASD not only at the level of the individual healthcare provider but at the systems level across entire hospitals, clinics, and healthcare networks. This chapter is intended to provide guidance about how to initiate and effect change at this level, and provides detailed information about an initiative at our hospital, MGH, as a case study. Key principles that can optimize a quality improvement initiative's chance of success include clearly defining the target population and specific goals for the intervention, gathering preliminary data to help support the need for intervention, engaging key stakeholders and champions who will carry the initiative forward, efficiently and effectively implementing concrete changes, and measuring the impact of interventions in a quantifiable way. Ideally, quality improvement should continue to progress in a cyclical way, with the identification of new targets for intervention as well as areas that were not adequately impacted in previous interventions. Only through the dedicated efforts of providers and administrators can we move toward providing the quality of healthcare that our patients with ASD deserve.

Acknowledgments The authors would like to acknowledge all members of the MGH Autism Care Committee, without whom the work described would not have been possible. These members include Zary Amirhosseini, Sarabeth Broder-Fingert, Kathleen P. Buckley, Debra Burke, Roger Gino Chisari, Amanda B. Coakley, Eve

Megargel, Mary O. Cramer, Richard H. Evans, Theresa M. Gallivan, Ann M. Giauque, Peter T. Greenspan, Eric P. Hazen, Ann Kao, Robin Lipkis-Orlando, Denise Jordan Lozowski, Christopher J. McDougle, Brenda Miller, Helen O'Carroll, Kristen Solemina, Michael Sullivan, Carmen D. Vega-Barachowitz, Pamela E. Wrigley, Sheila Golden-Baker, Tristan Gorrindo, Carole Mackenzie, Karen E. Morse-Gallagher, Janet S. Rico, Jamie Lee Rossi, Pamela E. Wrigley, Ann Martha Neumeyer, Karen A. Turner, Kerstin Zanger, Ann Fonseca, Rachel Toran Tobin, Amy Mcguire, and Victoria Peake.

References

1. Agarwal S, Angus B. Misdiagnosis versus missed diagnosis: diagnosing autism spectrum disorder in adolescents. Australas Psychiatry. 2015;23(2):120–3.
2. Batalden P. Making improvement interventions happen--the work before the work: four leaders speak. BMJ Qual Saf. 2014;23(1):4–7.
3. Broder-Fingert S, Shui A, Ferrone C, Iannuzzi D, Cheng ER, Giauque A, Connors S, McDougle CJ, Donelan K, Neumeyer A, Kuhlthau KA. Pilot study of autism-specific care plans during hospital admission. Pediatrics. 2016;137(Suppl 2):S196–204.
4. Brugha TS, McManus S, Bankart J, Scott F, Purdon S, Smith J, Bebbington P, Jenkins R, Meltzer H. Epidemiology of autism spectrum disorders in adults in the community in England. Arch Gen Psychiatry. 2011;68(5):459–65.
5. Bultas MW, McMillin SE, Zand DH. Reducing barriers to care in the office-based health care setting for children with autism. J Pediatr Health Care. 2016;30(1):5–14.
6. Calderwood AH, Mahoney EM, Jacobson BC. A plan-do-study-act approach to improving bowel preparation quality. Am J Med Qual. 2016;32:194–200. pii: 1062860616628642. [Epub ahead of print].
7. Centers for Medicare & Medicaid Services. Accountable care organization 2015 program analysis quality performance standards narrative measure specifications. 2015.: Available at https://www.cms.gov/medicare/medicare-fee-for-service-payment/sharedsavingsprogram/downloads/ry2015-narrative-specifications.pdf.
8. Croen LA, Zerbo O, Qian Y, Massolo ML, Rich S, Sidney S, Kripke C. The health status of adults on the autism spectrum. Autism. 2015;19(7):814–23.
9. Eaves LC, Ho HH. The very early identification of autism: outcome to age 4 1/2-5. J Autism Dev Disord. 2004;34:367–78.
10. Filipek PA, Accardo PJ, Ashwal S, et al. Practice parameter: screening and diagnosis of autism: report of the quality standards subcommittee of the American academy of neurology and the child neurology society. Neurology. 2000;55:468–79.
11. Fortuna RJ, Robinson L, Smith TH, Meccarello J, Bullen B, Nobis K, Davidson PW. Health conditions and functional status in adults with autism: a cross-sectional evaluation. J Gen Intern Med. 2016;31(1):77–84.
12. Foster T, Ogrinc G, Hamby L, Weeks WB. Improving the effectiveness of physician participation in local quality improvement efforts. Qual Manag Health Care. 2002 Spring;10(3):25–30.
13. Gabriels RL, Agnew JA, Beresford C, Morrow MA, Mesibov G, Wamboldt M. Improving psychiatric hospital care for pediatric patients with autism spectrum disorders and intellectual disabilities. Autism Res Treat. 2012;2012:6850–3.
14. Giarelli E, Nocera R, Turchi R, Hardie TL, Pagano R, Yuan C. Sensory stimuli as obstacles to emergency care for children with autism spectrum disorder. Adv Emerg Nurs J. 2014.; 36(2), 145–163.
15. Gould J. Autism and mental health: your guide to today's mental health issues. Ment Health Today. 2010;2009(suppl):1–2.
16. Gotham K, Marvin AR, Taylor JL, Warren Z, Anderson CM, Law PA, Law JK, Lipkin PH. Characterizing the daily life, needs, and priorities of adults with autism spectrum disorder from interactive autism network data. Autism. 2015;19(7):794–804.
17. Howlin P, Asgharian A. The diagnosis of autism and Asperger syndrome: findings from a survey of 770 families. Dev Med Child Neurol. 1999;41:834–9.
18. Kuhlthau KA, Warfield ME, Hurson J, Delahaye J, Crossman MK. Pediatric provider's perspectives on the transition to adult health care for youth with autism spectrum disorder: current strategies and promising new directions. Autism. 2015;19(3):262–71.
19. Kinnear SH, Link BG, Ballan MS, Fischbach RL. Understanding the experience of stigma for parents of children with autism spectrum disorder and the role stigma plays in Families' lives. J Autism Dev Disord. 2016;46(3):942–53.
20. Kogan MD, Strickland BB, Blumberg SJ, Singh GK, Perrin JM, van Dyck PC. A national profile of the health care experiences and family impact of autism spectrum disorder among children in the United States, 2005–2006. Pediatrics. 2008;122(6):e1149–58.
21. Langley GJ, Moen R, Nolan K, Nolan T, Norman C, Provost LP. The improvement guide: a practical approach to enhancing organizational performance. 2nd ed. San Francisco: Jossey-Bass Pub; 2009.
22. Liptak GS, Benzoni LB, Mruzek DW, Nolan KW, Thingvoll MA, Wade CM, Fryer GE. Disparities in diagnosis and access to health services for children with autism: data from the national survey of children's health. J Dev Behav Pediatr. 2008;29(3):152–60.

23. Lukas CV, Holmes SK, Cohen AB, Restuccia J, Cramer IE, Shwartz M, Charns MP. Transformational change in health care systems: an organizational model. Health Care Manag Rev. 2007;32(4):309–20.
24. McGonigle JJ, Migyanka JM, Glor-Scheib SJ, Cramer R, Fratangeli JJ, Hegde GG, Shang J, Venkat A. Development and evaluation of educational materials for pre-hospital and emergency department personnel on the care of patients with autism spectrum disorder. J Autism Dev Disord. 2014a;44(5):1252–9.
25. McGonigle JJ, Venkat A, Beresford C, Campbell TP, Gabriels RL. Management of agitation in individuals with autism spectrum disorders in the emergency department. Child Adolesc Psychiatr Clin N Am. 2014b;23(1):83–95.
26. Mesibov G, Browder D, Kirkland C. Using individualized schedules as a component of positive behavior support for students with developmental disabilities. J Posit Behav Interv. 2002;25:58–72.
27. Muskat B, Burnham Riosa P, Nicholas DB, Roberts W, Stoddart KP, Zwaigenbaum L. Autism comes to the hospital: the experiences of patients with autism spectrum disorder, their parents and health-care providers at two Canadian paediatric hospitals. Autism. 2015;19(4):482–90.
28. Nelson EC, Splaine ME, Plume SK, Batalden P. Good measurement for good improvement work. Qual Manag Health Care. 2004;13(1):1–16.
29. Nicolaidis C, Kripke CC, Raymaker D. Primary care for adults on the autism spectrum. Med Clin North Am. 2014;98(5):1169–91. https://doi.org/10.1016/j.mcna.2014.06.011.
30. Nicolaidis C, Raymaker D, McDonald K, Dern S, Boisclair WC, Ashkenazy E, Baggs A. Comparison of healthcare experiences in autistic and non-autistic adults: a cross-sectional online survey facilitated by an academic-community partnership. J Gen Intern Med. 2013;28(6):761–9.
31. Nicolaidis C, Raymaker D, McDonald K, Kapp S, Weiner M, Ashkenazy E, Gerrity M, Kripke C, Platt L, Baggs A. The development and evaluation of an online healthcare toolkit for autistic adults and their primary care providers. J Gen Intern Med. 2016;31(10):1180–9.
32. Office of Autism Research Coordination, National Institute of Mental Health, on behalf of the Interagency Autism Coordinating Committee. 2010 IACC autism spectrum disorder research portfolio analysis report. Washington, DC July 2012.
33. Roth BM, Kralovic S, Roizen NJ, Spannagel SC, Minich N, Knapp J. Impact of autism navigator on access to services. J Dev Behav Pediatr. 2016;37:188–95. [Epub ahead of print]
34. Siegel M, Doyle K, Chemelski B, Payne D, Ellsworth B, Harmon J, Robbins D, Milligan B, Lubetsky M. Specialized inpatient psychiatry units for children with autism and developmental disorders: a United States survey. J Autism Dev Disord. 2012;42(9):1863–9.
35. Strunk JA, Pickler R, McCain NL, Ameringer S, Myers BJ. Managing the health care needs of adolescents with autism spectrum disorder: the parents' experience. Fam Syst Health. 2014;32(3):328–37.
36. Suarez M. Sensory processing in children with autism spectrum disorders and impact on functioning. Pediatr Clin N Am. 2012;59(1):203–14.
37. Thomas KC, Parish SL, Rose RA, Kilany M. Access to care for children with autism in the context of state Medicaid reimbursement. Matern Child Health J. 2012;16(8):1636–44.
38. Vaz I. Visual symbols in health care settings for children with learning disabilities and autism spectrum disorder. Br J Nurs. 2013;22(3):156–9.
39. Venkat A, Jauch E, Russell WS, Crist CR, Farrell R. Care of the patient with an autism spectrum disorder by the general physician. Postgrad Med J. 2012;88(1042):472–81.
40. Wang MC, Hyun JK, Harrison M, Shortell SM, Fraser I. Redesigning health systems for quality: lessons from emerging practices. Jt Comm J Qual Patient Saf. 2006;32(11):599–611.
41. Warfield ME, Crossman MK, Delahaye J, Der Weerd E, Kuhlthau KA. Physician perspectives on providing primary medical care to adults with autism Spectrum disorders (ASD). J Autism Dev Disord. 2015;45(7):2209–17.
42. Yeargin-Allsopp M, Rice C, Karapurkar T, Doernberg N, Boyle C, Murphy C. Prevalence of autism in a US metropolitan area. JAMA. 2003;289:49–55.
43. Zerbo O, Massolo ML, Qian Y, Croen LAA. Study of physician knowledge and experience with autism in adults in a large integrated healthcare system. J Autism Dev Disord. 2015;45(12):4002–14.

Part II

Care of Specific Disorders

Neurology

6

Susanna Mierau and Ann Neumeyer

Introduction

Neurological conditions are very common in individuals with autism spectrum disorder (ASD). Both epilepsy and motor impairments have long been described in ASD. In fact, in Kanner's original description of 11 children with ASD, one child had epilepsy [9] and another developed seizures in early adult life [10]. Since then, there have been many studies focused on the frequency and types of epilepsy, the etiology of seizures, the diagnosis and treatment of seizures, and the effects of seizures in individuals with ASD. We now have better knowledge of who is at highest risk for seizures within the ASD population and when the seizures are most likely to develop. Furthermore, specific genetic syndromes have been found which predispose children to seizures and epilepsy.

Motor dysfunction in ASD has been less studied until recently, although the impairments have been noted from early on. In Kanner's original description of 11 children, there were a number of children with motor impairments: stereotypies, delays in motor development, and apraxia were noted. Motor function is crucial for the development of communication, both verbal and nonverbal. Delays in fine and gross motor skills can impair a child's ability to learn. In addition, repetitive motor behaviors often impair a child's ability to focus and engage, thus affecting overall functioning. In this chapter, the motor impairments of stereotypies or repetitive movements, motor delay, and abnormalities of gait, coordination, and praxis (dyspraxia or apraxia) will be reviewed.

A Pediatric Approach to Common Neurological Conditions

Epilepsy

Clinical Evaluation

History Epilepsy occurs in 9–22% of children with ASD [22] and has two peaks of onset, one in early childhood and one in adolescence [21]. Seizure types vary in ASD, as ASD is a heterogenous group of disorders. In children with ASD with seizure onset between 0 and 5 years old, epilepsy may present as infantile spasms or may be multifocal, focal in central regions, or present in multiple lobes. With onset in adolescence (the peak is between 10 and 15 years old), frontal and central foci may be more commonly seen.

S. Mierau
Department of Physiology, Development and Neuroscience, University of Cambridge, Cambridge, UK

A. Neumeyer (✉)
Department of Neurology, Massachusetts General Hospital, Boston, MA, USA

Lurie Center for Autism, Lexington, MA, USA
e-mail: aneumeyer@mgh.harvard.edu

E. P. Hazen, C. J. McDougle (eds.), *The Massachusetts General Hospital Guide to Medical Care in Patients with Autism Spectrum Disorder*, Current Clinical Psychiatry,
https://doi.org/10.1007/978-3-319-94458-6_6

If there is a question about whether new events observed by caregivers are seizures, it can be helpful to have the caregiver take a video to share with the provider. Children with ASD can adopt new repetitive behaviors or stereotypies that may resemble epileptic automatisms [18]. They are often unresponsive to voice and can hyper-attend to stimuli in the environment making it difficult to judge whether awareness is compromised in nonconvulsive seizures. Associated symptoms of bowel or bladder loss can be helpful in identifying seizures in children with ASD who are toilet-trained. It is also helpful to note whether suspected events are followed by periods sleep or behavioral changes, which would also favor a diagnosis of seizures. Any associated triggers (e.g., loss of sleep, fever or other illness, missed meal, menstrual cycle) should be reviewed. Caretakers can be asked to keep a seizure diary of suspected events where these factors are noted.

Physical Examination Signs of known genetic syndromes associated with ASD and epilepsy should be sought as the identification may change not only seizure management but alert providers to other non-neurological complications as well. For example, in patients with tuberous sclerosis, skin and Wood's lamp examination may reveal hypomelanotic macules ("ash leaf spots"), facial angiofibromas, thickened connective tissue hamartoma (or shagreen patch, most often found in the lower back), and periungual fibromas. Hypotonia is associated with multiple genetic disorders including Angelman syndrome (UBE3A deletion), 15q11.2–13.1 duplication, Phelan McDermid syndrome (22q13.3 deletion), or Rett syndrome (*MECP2* loss-of-function mutation). The characteristic facial features may be observed in fragile X syndrome, macrocephaly in PTEN-related disorders, or microcephaly in Rett syndrome.

Studies Electroencephalogram (EEG) is useful for diagnosis and for determining seizure type and treatment options. However, there is some controversy over the prevalence and significance of EEG abnormalities in patients with ASD but no clinical history of epilepsy. Care should be taken when interpreting the EEG, and if possible, video monitoring with EEG should be used, to distinguish whether abnormal behaviors suspected to be seizures are associated with epileptiform activity [8, 18]. The choice of a spot EEG versus 24-h monitoring is affected by the frequency and timing of the suspected seizure events. After a single event or for infrequent events, spot EEG is often used to look for subclinical epileptiform discharges or features associated with epilepsy; sleep deprivation and hyperventilation can be used to attempt to evoke seizures but can be challenging in patients with ASD who are nonverbal or who have an intellectual disability. Spot EEG is often unrevealing and requires further testing. Twenty-four hour EEG monitoring can be particularly informative for revealing whether a frequent stereotypic movement is associated with epileptic activity, especially if the behavior is occurring multiple times per day, or for increasing the likelihood of detecting epileptic or associated phenomenon during sleep or sleep-wake transitions. Obtaining EEGs in children with ASD can be particularly challenging due to language delays and hypersensitivity to touch. EEG facilities at children's hospitals are typically equipped to help pediatric patients tolerate the procedure. Children with ASD may need additional explanation and coaching ahead of time about the sequence of events, including the use of visual stories. It may also be helpful to visit the facility prior to the study and/or to acclimate the child wearing the gauze on his head (without the EEG electrodes). To help educate parents and EEG technicians about the EEG for people with ASD, a guide has been created by Autism Speaks and is available online at https://www.autismspeaks.org/science/resources-programs/autism-treatment-network/atn-air-p-eeg-guides. Additional discussion about helping children with ASD tolerate procedures such as EEGs is provided in Chap. 4 "Procedures."

Genetic screening for known mutations related to ASD and seizures can be helpful to identify the etiology for diagnostic, prognostic, and treatment purposes. Magnetic resonance imaging (MRI) can be revealing in cases of tuberous sclerosis, showing characteristic cortical hamartomas (or "tubers"), or in the evaluation of children with growth asymmetries, spasticity, or unilateral weakness.

Treatment

There may be a significant treatment benefit with regard to cognitive and language development in treating children with ASD for seizures after the first unprovoked, afebrile seizure. In a recent study of 153 children with ASD, the risk of a second seizure was estimated to be 92%, compared to previous reports of 46–66% in children without ASD [18]. More controversial is whether children with ASD and epileptiform abnormalities on EEG but no clinically apparent seizures should be treated with antiepileptics [23]. Epileptiform abnormalities have been found in 8–60% of children with ASD and no history of seizures. Small open-label studies have suggested that there may be cognitive or behavioral benefits to treatment with antiepileptics in these children, but these results have not been born out in larger, double-blind studies. Some of these studies also may have been confounded by mood stabilizing or other effects of the antiepileptic medications tried.

The choice of an antiepileptic treatment will be determined by the seizure type as well as the identification of any known underlying genetic cause of seizures in the patient. The diagnosis of ASD doesn't affect antiepileptic medication choice. Ketogenic or low glycemic diets may be particularly successful for some seizure types and syndromes, such as infantile spasms, myoclonic astatic epilepsy, GLUT-1 deficiency, Dravet syndrome, Rett syndrome, and tuberous sclerosis. Surgical interventions to resect seizure foci may also be warranted in refractory cases.

Clinical Vignette # 1

A 12-year-old female with nonverbal ASD presents for evaluation of intermittent staring spells. She comes with her mother who is an excellent historian. Recently, her therapists have noticed changes in her attention. For the past couple of months, she sometimes stares when she is doing her schoolwork with her behavioral therapist and, on occasion, as she is eating or engaging in repetitive behaviors. Her mother reports that these events seem different in that she occasionally drools during the staring spells, which typically last less than 20 s. She has never been responsive when her name is called, and she is not responsive during these new spells either.

The exam shows a well-developed Tanner stage 4 female with self-directed behaviors, hand flapping and other stereotypies. She follows simple commands. She is cooperative during the evaluation but initially fearful of the examiner. Her general exam showed a head circumference which was average for age, no neurocutaneous stigmata, and symmetric extremities. There were no focal findings on neurological examination. She was not cooperative with fundoscopy. Her tone, reflexes, and movements were symmetric. She was not cooperative with hyperventilation, which was done in an attempt to elicit an absence seizure. However, during the evaluation, she had a brief 10 s episode characterized by an arrest of hand flapping, turning her head, staring off to the right, and unresponsiveness to voice and touch.

Outcome A: Because the spells have changed in their quality with unresponsiveness to touch and drooling, there is more concern of a seizure disorder. For this reason, an EEG was ordered. An MRI is not requested because of the nonfocal examination, and an MRI in this child would require general anesthesia. As expected, there were bursts of spike and wave activity captured during the EEG. The patient was started on levetiracetam, which resulted in decreased frequency of the episodes.

Outcome B: The EEG was normal. However, because the spells also involve drooling (which can be a manifestation of gastroesophageal reflux pain) and head turning (a slight dystonic reaction), an endoscopy was performed. This study showed that there was evidence of gastroesophageal reflux. This child was diagnosed with a late onset form of Sandifer syndrome, a form of spasmodic torsional dystonia that involves arching of the back and rigid posturing, often in response to the pain associated with gastroesophageal reflux or esophagitis. It is important to be aware that seizure-like spells can be caused by medical problems or pain in addition to epileptic events.

Motor Abnormalities

Clinical Evaluation

History Motor abnormalities are common in ASD and may contribute to the core feature of delay in, or absence of, expressive language development. The most common types of motor abnormalities include stereotypies, fine and gross motor delays, praxis, and gait and coordination abnormalities [15]. Tics also occur at a higher rate in ASD [3, 20]. Stereotypies take the form of repetitive movements, often in the hands, that can be quite disabling (e.g., rubbing fingers to the extent the skin is damaged) or distracting such that activities of daily living cannot be completed. The etiology of stereotypies is not well understood; they are usually voluntary movements and often self-stimulatory. It is important to understand that these repetitive behaviors may be reinforcing or soothing for some individuals.

Fine and gross motor delays are common in children with ASD and often are the trigger for an assessment for ASD. Difficulty with praxis in hands is commonly reported by parents. This can be manifested in children with ASD holding a writing or eating utensil in their fist rather than between the forefingers. Fine motor delays in the hand are often accompanied by increased difficulty with expressive language. Difficulty with praxis for speech and writing production only compounds delays in language development as less language use results in less reinforcement of the motor patterns necessary for the rapid speech and writing demands as the child progresses through school. Gait abnormalities include toe walking as young children (often helpful in the diagnosis of ASD in children) and may take the form of a more general lack of coordination as development progresses. Toe walking in ASD is discussed in more detail in Chap. 16 "Musculoskeletal Disorders."

Physical Examination Multiple forms of ASD with known gene mutations are accompanied by motor abnormalities that may aid in the diagnosis or trigger genetic testing. Hypotonia is associated with multiple genetic disorders including Angelman syndrome (UBE3A deletion), 15q11.2–13.1 duplication, Phelan McDermid syndrome (22q13.3 deletion), or Rett syndrome (*MECP2* loss-of-function mutation).

Studies Genetic testing for syndromic forms of ASD

Treatment

The treatment of interfering or self-injurious repetitive behaviors is quite challenging as few, if any, of the psychiatric medications for reducing these undesirable behaviors have been found to be effective in placebo-controlled trials [6, 16]. Antipsychotics and selective serotonin reuptake inhibitors have been studied extensively; however, they do not show efficacy, and treatment is often limited by side effects. Replacement therapy can prove successful for some patients with ASD (e.g., wearing a rubber band around the wrist that the patient can snap on him- or herself instead of rubbing the skin); however, these approaches must be tailored to the individual with ASD. In children or adults with sufficient communication skills, cognitive behavioral therapy may provide some symptom improvement [16].

Clinical Vignette # 2

A 15-year-old boy with a history of ASD presents to his pediatrician because he is no longer continent of urine. For the past several months, his mother has noted that he wets his bed, and occasionally he is incontinent during the day. The urinalysis has been normal twice. He has not had any fevers. Upon further questioning, his mother reports that the patient has been napping occasionally during the day, which is unusual for him. He has also been doing slightly worse in school and is not sleeping well. The physical and neurological examination are unremarkable except for some stereotypic behaviors. An EEG study revealed spike and wave activity suggestive of epileptiform activity. He was diagnosed with focal aware onset epilepsy and started on valproate. When at a therapeutic level, his incontinence and napping resolved.

This vignette demonstrates the fact that seizures may not always have a typical, clearly neurological presentation. Sometimes they present instead with medical or behavioral complaints, such as incontinence and sleep disruptions. The key points in the history of this patient suggestive of possible seizure disorder are that the incontinence is secondary (he was previously continent of urine), there is no evidence of a urinary tract infection, and increased napping and poor sleep during the night are frequent problems in children with new onset or a recurrent seizure disorders.

An Adult Approach to Common Neurological Conditions

Nonverbal and limited-verbal adults with ASD face particular challenges with access to care in our current healthcare system. In contrast to pediatrics, many internists and adult-trained medical and surgical subspecialists may be unfamiliar or uncomfortable treating adult patients who cannot endorse symptoms, or these providers may be reluctant to perform invasive procedures necessary for diagnosing even common medical conditions. Care of adults with ASD is also complicated by the presence of sensory hypersensitivities, which make it difficult to perform tests and procedures. While in pediatric facilities accommodations are frequently made to acquire necessary testing without patient cooperation, in adult clinics there are few ancillary staff members willing or trained to make similar accommodations for nonverbal adults with ASD. Diagnostic testing requires planning, flexibility, sensitivity, and generally extra time by ancillary staff.

Neurologists can play an important role in the care of adults with ASD, especially those with limited communication skills. In addition to a higher comorbidity of neurologic and psychiatric disorders (e.g., epilepsy, anxiety, sleep disturbances), adults with ASD also share a similar risk with the general population for common neurological illnesses including headaches and, later in life, neurodegenerative conditions. Many signs and symptoms of these disorders may be expressed differently in nonverbal adults, typically presenting as an increase in self-injurious behavior (SIB), aggression, or social withdrawal. Pain or other uncomfortable sensations from medical or neurological illnesses may also present as an increase in repetitive behaviors. Often these symptoms are addressed first by caretakers with behavioral interventions before an underlying medical condition is considered.

The approach to nonverbal or limited-verbal adults with ASD in the neurology clinic is similar to pediatric care in that extra time is typically required in order to address the chief complaint. At the Massachusetts General Hospital Lurie Center for Autism, we typically schedule 1.5 h for a new neurology consultation and 45 min for follow-up appointments. Individuals with ASD typically have difficulty transitioning, and it often takes 10–20 min for the patient to calm down behaviorally in an office visit to the point that the neurologist can observe the baseline behavior and perform a neurological exam. The patient history, as in pediatrics, is typically provided by an accompanying adult. However, in contrast to pediatrics, it is often the case that the person who brings the patient to the appointment is not the one who has observed the chief complaint. Most nonverbal or limited-verbal adults with ASD either live with their parents or in a group home or institution. Adults with ASD living in group homes or institutions are often accompanied by staff members, family members, or state-appointed guardians who have not directly observed any of the behaviors that triggered the appointment.

The purpose of the visit is almost always motivated by a caretaker's concern over a change in behavior or new sign. Even in adults with ASD who are able to communicate basic wants, there is typically difficulty reporting emotions, internal mood states, or pain. Thus, there is an additional onus on the neurologist during the history and neurological exam to be on the lookout for conditions that might be affecting the patient's quality of life or risk for future decline in health.

It is not uncommon that an experimental approach is required for diagnosis and treatment as any change in health in the patient may present with the same symptom. For example, after collecting the history and exam for an increase in SIB, the differential may still span multiple organ systems and include common conditions such as headaches, sinus congestion, or gastroesophageal reflux disease. To differentiate these conditions, we may start by treating the most likely condition—based on observed signs, family history, age, or season of the year—for a set period of time and have the caregiver report back to us whether there is any improvement. If not, we treat the second most likely condition and see if there is any improvement. This approach requires a high degree of cooperation and observation on the part of the caregiver, but gives the patient a chance at receiving effective treatment.

Seizures and Epilepsy in Adults with ASD

Clinical Evaluation

History Epilepsy associated with ASD and related neurodevelopmental disorders typically presents in childhood or, more often, during adolescence and often continues into adulthood. Bolton and colleagues did a follow-up study with 150 individuals with a childhood diagnosis of ASD and found that 22% of them had been diagnosed with epilepsy [2]. The majority of patients developed epilepsy after age 10 years. A new presentation of seizures or seizure-like behaviors in adults with ASD after the age of 30 years should be investigated thoroughly as it would in an adult without ASD. Adults with ASD are also at the same risk as the general population for new brain lesions that would trigger seizures; however, adults with ASD are unlikely to have the studies performed to identify new lesions [2].

Adults with ASD and comorbid epilepsy should also have their antiepileptic medications thoroughly reviewed. It is not uncommon for adults with ASD in the third to sixth decade of life to be on older generation antiepileptics such as valproate, phenytoin, or phenobarbital. Years to decades of exposure to these drugs may lead to many manifestations of the side effects of chronic use (e.g., gingival hyperplasia with phenytoin, gait instability and hyperammonemia with valproate) that may go unnoticed by caregivers and primary care doctors but are causing significant harm or discomfort to the patients. In some cases, the patient may not have had any seizures in decades, and consideration may be given to gradually weaning off of antiepileptic medications. The weaning process can be spread over months, and EEG would not typically be necessary to begin the taper.

Physical Examination For adults with a long history of epilepsy, evaluate for signs of side effects from antiepileptic medications including nystagmus, gingival hyperplasia, tremor, gait instability, and sensory neuropathies. For adults with ASD presenting with new onset of seizures, look for focal neurologic signs that may represent a new brain lesion, unrelated to ASD.

Studies If seizures are well-controlled and there is no concern for toxicity, we do not generally monitor medication levels in adults with ASD as blood draws can prove difficult, particularly in individuals with hypersensitivity to touch and/or limited communication.

For adults with ASD and a new presentation of suspected seizures, EEG is recommended. To accommodate adults with a high degree of sensory sensitivity, the preparation can be done in stages prior to the procedure. First, the caregivers can wrap the head in gauze at home for short periods of time to acclimate the patient to having his or her head wrapped. The adult with ASD may need more than one visit to the facility where the EEG technicians will apply the EEG leads prior to the procedure. (See Chap. 4 for more information on how to help patients with ASD tolerate procedures.) Sleep-deprived EEGs are preferred for increasing the sensitivity in detecting epileptiform activity; however, sleep deprivation can cause behavioral issues that may decrease the chance of cooperation for many adults with ASD. In these cases, it may be useful to have the EEG applied at the clinic and then have the patient return home for monitoring overnight.

If there are signs or symptoms suspicious for a new brain lesion, neuroimaging with an MRI is recommended, as it would be in adults without ASD. However, nonverbal or limited-verbal patients or patients with hypersensitivities to sound or touch may require general sedation in order to tolerate an MRI. This requires significant coordination of care, but other testing, such as blood draws, can also be done at the same time. Many adults with severe ASD are given general anesthesia once per year to have their teeth cleaned and to get any blood draws that are needed.

Treatment

Medication should be tailored to seizure type and the treatment of comorbid conditions (e.g., migraine). In neurotypical adults, levetiracetam (Keppra) is commonly used because of the ability to start and stop the drug with a short taper, or with no taper at all, and the low side effect profile. However, levetiracetam is generally avoided in patients with ASD because the side effect of irritability can lead to an increase in self-injurious or aggressive behaviors.

Clinical Vignette # 3

A 54-year-old man with ASD and a distant history of seizures presents for neurological evaluation. He was brought to the appointment by his adult sibling and elderly parent who exclaimed that they had been "waiting for decades for care for adults with autism." The patient is nonverbal and lives in a group home with frequent visits to his family's home. He had been on the same dose of primidone for many years, but his last seizure was so long ago that they could not remember how many decades he had been seizure-free. Over the last few years, he had developed hypertension and other signs of vascular disease, and there was the possibility he may need anticoagulation in the future. The decision was made to very slowly taper the primidone over the next 4–6 months and observe for any sign of seizure recurrence. The medication was successfully discontinued without any signs of seizure activity.

Headaches in Adults with ASD

Clinical Evaluation

Headaches occur with the same prevalence in adults with ASD as in the general population. Yet headaches are very likely to be missed in patients with communication impairments because of difficulties conveying the nature of their pain or distress.

History Adults with ASD and limited ability to communicate emotion or pain due to headache will most often present with an increase in SIB, aggression, or irritability. Sometimes the SIB is directed at the location of the pain. Thus, patients who have recently begun to hit their heads or bang their heads into the wall or other objects should raise the suspicion of headaches. Observers may report that the patient often goes to bed or withdraws to another room after the behavioral episodes or that the patient appears to be less aggressive if he has slept after an episode. This pattern may indicate migraine disorder, even if the patient is unable to report photo- or phonophobia. Observers can often accurately estimate the length of time the episodes last and any temporal relation to fatigue, hunger, or menstrual cycle. If they have not observed these symptoms, a "suspected-headache" diary can be quite helpful for recording observations around the time of the behaviors that might lead to headache cause (e.g., concurrent nasal discharge). Considering factors specific to season of the year or the patient's developmental age can also be revealing. In one case of a nonverbal teenager with ASD, the cause of his behavioral change was discovered to be the emergence of his wisdom teeth.

Family history is one of the most helpful diagnostic tools for headache in nonverbal adults with ASD. A family history of migraines increases the likelihood of a patient having this condition, and we have had considerable success improving the behaviors in young adults with ASD by treating with the same preventative medications that have controlled migraines in their family members. Likewise, for seasonal allergies that lead to sinus congestion as the cause for head pain, family history can be very instructive for both diagnosis and treatment. When questioned about signs of allergic rhinitis, the caregivers often have noticed the symptoms but did not think to treat the adult with ASD with over-the-counter allergy medications.

Physical Examination As in adults without ASD, any new focal neurological signs on exam may raise possibility of headaches due to a new brain lesion and can prompt neuroimaging.

Studies No neuroimaging is recommended, unless a new brain lesion is suspected.

Treatment

The clinician should treat based on suspected headache etiology as in patients without ASD. For migraine, sumatriptan nasal spray can be very effective if the caregiver is able to give it within 30 min of symptom onset (e.g., rocking, moaning, SIB) as it does not require the patient to swallow a pill, which is challenging for many patients with ASD. For migraine behaviors happening more than a few times per month, preventative medications should be tried. Many of the preventative medications for migraine are also seizure medications and thus can be titrated if the patient also has epilepsy to treat both conditions with one medication (e.g., topiramate). For behaviors suspicious for headache that are also accompanied by signs of nasal congestion, loratadine or fexofenadine can be effective at reducing allergic rhinitis and sinus discomfort. Due to the limited reporting ability of some adults with ASD, many conditions typically diagnosed by primary care providers go undiagnosed and untreated in nonverbal adults with ASD.

Clinical Vignette # 4

A 19-year-old nonverbal man presents with his parents to establish care for ASD. Despite no history of seizures, he is on three antiepileptic medications from a previous provider, and the plan is arranged to slowly wean him off of these medications. As the topiramate is weaned, an increase in episodes of aggressive behavior is observed along with occasions where he will hit himself in the head or hit his head on the wall. His mother has a history of migraines. It is suspected that the topiramate was actually treating undiagnosed migraines. The topiramate dose was adjusted to therapeutic levels typical for migraine, rather than seizure, for which higher doses are typically prescribed, and the frequency of episodes of aggressive behavior and hitting his head decreased.

Movement Disorders in Adults with ASD

Clinical Evaluation

History Movement disorders are more common in adults with ASD than in the general population and are primarily related to medication side effects. Antipsychotic medications are used frequently to treat aggression or SIB; however, both the use and the withdrawal of antipsychotic medications increase the risk of developing or unmasking tardive dyskinesia, involuntary stereotypic movements or sense of restlessness that can be very distressing and in some cases disabling for the patient. Multiple commonly prescribed antiepileptic medications also can affect gait and balance over time.

Physical Examination Many adults with ASD make repetitive movements, especially with their hands (i.e., stereotypies), that should not be confused with a movement disorder. Signs of non-physiologic tremor in the arms, head, or legs are not typical in patients with ASD and warrant further investigation. Some adults with ASD have lifelong difficulties with gait or balance; however, new or worsening changes in gait or balance suggest non-ASD-related etiologies.

Studies For concerns about toxicity from supratherapeutic levels of antiepileptics leading to gait imbalance, blood levels can be drawn.

Treatment

The treatment of a movement disorder should be tailored to its cause. If the patient has developed tardive dyskinesia, the causative antipsychotic medication should be *gradually* reduced and discontinued. If this medication had been used to treat aggression and/or SIB, the challenge will be to identify a medication from a different class of drugs that is effective for this purpose. Naltrexone, SSRIs (e.g., fluvoxamine, fluoxetine), and buspirone have been found to be effective for stereotypies and other repetitive movements in some adults with ASD [6, 14]; however, buspirone is generally avoided in patients with ASD and comorbid epilepsy as it may decrease seizure threshold.

Clinical Vignette # 5

A 35-year-old nonverbal man with ASD, severe intellectual disability, and a history of epilepsy is brought to the clinic by the staff at his group home for difficulty walking and imbalance. Until a few months ago, he was able to walk independently, but he then started to have frequent falls such that one staff member started walking beside him to assist with balance. Over the last few months, his balance has worsened such that he now requires two-person assist anytime he is out of bed. His balance and walking are worst in the morning when he gets out of bed, and his walking is at its best in the late afternoon. He has been on the long-acting formulation of valproate for many years, and he gets the entire dose at night right before he goes to bed. On exam, he appears drowsy, although he does respond with a smile when stimulated with voice or light touch. He requires assistance to stand and has very poor balance. His ammonia levels are very high, and the decision is made to start a new antiepileptic medication in order to wean off the valproate. Unfortunately, the care home does not follow the medication plan, and new seizures occur after he misses multiple doses of the valproate. The patient is transferred to a specialized unit for adults with intellectual disability at a local rehabilitation hospital where his medication is adjusted under more specialized supervision. On a new antiepileptic medication, his ammonia levels return to the normal range, and his problems with balance improve considerably. The difficulty walking due to gait instability was caused, at least in part, by the metabolic disturbances from long-term valproate use. Because the valproate was given as single dose at night, the patient was experiencing toxic levels in the morning causing the gait instability that improved as the medication levels dropped over the course of the day. Adults with ASD, severe intellectual disability, and epilepsy can remain on the same antiepileptics for years and accrue significant morbidity from the side effects, such as the metabolic impairment caused by the valproate. Close monitoring is necessary during the transition to new antiepileptic medications to achieve good seizure control.

Cognitive Decline in Adults with ASD

Clinical Evaluation

History Complaints of decreased speech production, apathy, and skill loss are often brought by caretakers of patients with ASD who are in their early twenties. In many cases, the decreased speech and motivation coincides with both physical and environmental changes in the young adult's life, such as relief from the hormonal changes of adolescence, improved frontal control of impulsivity with age, and decreased demands as young adults attend day programs rather than formal schooling. As in typically developing adults, sleep disorders such as obstructive sleep apnea should also be investigated if there is a behavioral or other functional decline. Review of medications may also be useful, as decline in daily functioning may be the first sign that a dose of a medication is too high.

In contrast, individuals with genetic disorders such as Down syndrome (trisomy 21) are known to already have amyloid deposition in the brain by their early twenties, similar to Alzheimer's disease (AD), as the APP gene is located on chromosome 21 [7]. Early signs of AD are different in Down syndrome than the general population and may lead to a delay in diagnosis [12]. People with

Down syndrome and AD are more likely to show "frontal" signs early including apathy, stubbornness, lack of concern for others, sadness, self-injury, and other behavioral changes that may predate memory, language use, and comprehension loss [12]. One of the best indicators of AD is loss of function in the activities of daily living with a decline in their concern for personal hygiene often being the first noticeable change [12].

Physical Examination The cognitive exam modified for the individual's baseline abilities can be very useful. Even if the patient is not able to complete the bedside cognitive testing with standardized scores for dementia (e.g., the Montreal Cognitive Assessment (MoCA) or the Mini-Mental Status Exam (MMSE)), the patient's performance can be tracked with repetitions of the modified exam at subsequent visits. New exams to screen for dementia in persons with intellectual disability are being developed [11]; however, they will need to be validated for patients with Down syndrome and ASD.

Studies Lumbar puncture, MRI of the brain, and positron emission tomography (PET) scan for beta-amyloid can be useful for diagnosis in AD in Down syndrome [4]. These tests have become standard for diagnosis of AD and should especially be considered in patients with Down syndrome who show a decline in daily function [5, 13, 17]. Abnormal Pittsburgh Compound B (PiB) binding [1] or tau accumulation [19] on PET scans correlates with dementia and cognitive decline in Down syndrome patients. Volume loss on MRI on repeat scan also correlated with the onset of dementia, as the volumetric differences between Down syndrome and neurotypical patients are stable over time in Down syndrome individuals without cognitive decline [19].

A sleep study can be helpful for looking for obstructive sleep apnea in patients, although a sleep specialist may need to make modifications to their testing procedures to accommodate adults with ASD based on the individual's needs.

Treatment

Treatment will be based upon etiology. If continuous positive airway pressure (CPAP) is required for sleep apnea, considerable patience may be required by ancillary staff and caretakers to gradually acclimate the patient to a mask and the sound of the machine. Once the patient begins to experience the benefits of better sleep, the CPAP machine may become more desirable.

Clinical Pearls

- Medical conditions should be explored when children or adults with ASD show increased behavioral aggression or self-injurious behavior.
- Staring spells or developmental regression can be the first sign of seizures.
- Children with ASD are sometimes not verbally responsive, so calling a child's name is not a good way to see if a child is responsive. It may be preferable to gently touch the child on the arm or say a word which typically alerts the child.
- Medical conditions can be the first presentation of a neurological disorder. Seizures can be subtle in their presentation and should be considered when there are episodic behavioral changes or new repetitive movements that cannot be interrupted or are accompanied by impaired awareness.
- Repetitive behaviors can be soothing in ASD, so treating the underlying cause for the behavior may improve or lessen repetitive behaviors. There is no medication with a primary benefit for repetitive behaviors.
- Family history can be very helpful in diagnosing common conditions (e.g., headaches, allergies) in adults with ASD.
- Nonverbal or limited-verbal adults with ASD often need similar accommodations provided to the pediatric population for studies such as imaging and blood draws.

References

1. Annus T, Wilson LR, Hong YT, Acosta-Cabronero J, Fryer TD, Cardenas-Blanco A, et al. The pattern of amyloid accumulation in the brains of adults with Down syndrome. Alzheimers Dement. 2016;12(5):538–45.
2. Bolton PF, Carcani-Rathwell I, Hutton J, Goode S, Howlin P, Rutter M. Epilepsy in autism: features and correlates. Br J Psychiatry. 2011;198(4):289–94.
3. Canitano R, Vivanti G. Tics and Tourette syndrome in autism spectrum disorders. Autism. 2007;11(1):19–28.
4. Castro P, Zaman S, Holland A. Alzheimer's disease in people with Down's syndrome: the prospects for and the challenges of developing preventative treatments. J Neurol. 2017;264(4):804–13.
5. Dekker AD, Fortea J, Blesa R, De Deyn PP. Cerebrospinal fluid biomarkers for Alzheimer's disease in Down syndrome. Alzheimers Dement (Amst). 2017;8:1–10.
6. Doyle CA, McDougle CJ. Pharmacotherapy to control behavioral symptoms in children with autism. Expert Opin Pharmacother. 2012;13(11):1615–29.
7. Grieco J, Pulsifer M, Seligsohn K, Skotko B, Schwartz A. Down syndrome: cognitive and behavioral functioning across the lifespan. Am J Med Genet C: Semin Med Genet. 2015;169(2):135–49.
8. Jeste SS, Tuchman R. Autism spectrum disorder and epilepsy: two sides of the same coin? J Child Neurol. 2015;30(14):1963–71.
9. Kanner L. Autistic disturbances of affective contact. Nerv Child. 1943;2:217–50.
10. Kanner L. Follow-up study of eleven autistic children originally reported in 1943. J Autism Child Schizophr. 1971;1(2):119–45.
11. Kuske B, Wolff C, Gövert U, Müller SV. Early detection of dementia in people with an intellectual disability – A German pilot study. J Appl Res Intellect Disabil. 2017;30(Suppl 1):49–57. 28332285.
12. Lautarescu BA, Holland AJ, Zaman SH. The early presentation of dementia in people with Down syndrome: a systematic review of longitudinal studies. Neuropsychol Rev. 2017;27(1):31–45.
13. LeVine H, Spielmann HP, Matveev S, Cauvi FM, Murphy MP, Beckett TL, et al. Down syndrome: age-dependence of PiB binding in postmortem frontal cortex across the lifespan. Neurobiol Aging. 2017;54:163–9.
14. Maltête D. Adult-onset stereotypical motor behaviors. Rev Neurol (Paris). 2016;172(8–9):477–82.
15. Maski KP, Jeste SS, Spence SJ. Common neurological co-morbidities in autism spectrum disorders. Curr Opin Pediatr. 2011;23(6):609–15.
16. Péter Z, Oliphant ME, Fernandez TV. Motor stereotypies: a pathophysiological review. Front Neurosci. 2017;11:171.
17. Portelius E, Soininen H, Andreasson U, Zetterberg H, Persson R, Karlsson G, et al. Exploring Alzheimer molecular pathology in Down's syndrome cerebrospinal fluid. Neurodegener Dis. 2014;14(2):98–106.
18. Qadir AA, Obringer E, Hageman J, Marcuccilli C. Risk of second seizure in pediatric patients with idiopathic autism. J Child Neurol. 2017;32(10):876–9.
19. Rafii MS, Lukic AS, Andrews RD, Brewer J, Rissman RA, Strother SC, et al. PET imaging of tau pathology and relationship to amyloid, longitudinal MRI, and cognitive change in Down syndrome: results from the Down Syndrome Biomarker Initiative (DSBI). J Alzheimers Dis. 2017;60(2):439–50.
20. Ringman JM, Jankovic J. Occurrence of tics in Asperger's syndrome and autistic disorder. J Child Neurol. 2000;15(6):394–400.
21. Scott RC, Tuchman R. Epilepsy and autism spectrum disorders: relatively related. Neurology. 2016;87(2):130–1.
22. Srivastava S, Sahin M. Autism spectrum disorder and epileptic encephalopathy: common causes, many questions. J Neurodev Disord. 2017;9:23.
23. Trauner DA. Behavioral correlates of epileptiform abnormalities in autism. Epilepsy Behav. 2015;47:163–6.

Oral Health

7

Anne-Frederique Chouinard
and Jennifer A. Magee

Introduction

The dental office environment poses a challenge for individuals with autism spectrum disorder (ASD), as it presents a unique variety of sights, sounds, and smells. Dental anxiety is common in the general public and can develop either in response to a bad experience or out of concern about the unfamiliar environment that the dental office presents. Dental anxiety is more prominent in the ASD population [4], and the dental exam can be more distressing to individuals with ASD compared with typically developing individuals [37].

One may assume that routine dental care is most often neglected because medical and behavioral issues take precedence over the need for dental care, but that is not the case [17]. More commonly the primary barrier is a family's inability to find a willing dental provider, especially for patients with behavioral difficulties [6]. Although dental education aims to address diagnosis and treatment of patients with special needs, instruction and experience are typically limited, resulting in low comfort levels in treating these patients [11]. This leads to an increase in unmet dental needs for patients with ASD compared to typically developing individuals [18].

Identifying a dental provider and establishing a dental home are a key step for a lifetime of good oral health. To this end, the American Academy of Pediatric Dentistry (AAPD) recommends the first dental visit by age 1 year and the establishment of a "dental home," in recognition of the importance of routine dental exams and building a relationship of trust between the dentist and patient. Additionally a person with ASD may have a high pain threshold or difficulty expressing their pain and therefore may be unable to describe the type and location of the pain he is experiencing [13]. This makes routine dental examinations important. The dental profession must continue to work toward increasing training opportunities for providers to feel competent serving the ASD population [10].

A successful visit begins before the patient with ASD arrives, when the office staff helps to create an environment with minimal distractions by turning off loud machinery and keeping background noise low. Prior to the appointment, the

A.-F. Chouinard (✉)
Department of Oral Maxillofacial Surgery, Massachusetts General Hospital, Boston, MA, USA

J. A. Magee
Department of Oral Maxillofacial Surgery, Massachusetts General Hospital, Boston, MA, USA
e-mail: jamagee@partners.org

E. P. Hazen, C. J. McDougle (eds.), *The Massachusetts General Hospital Guide to Medical Care in Patients with Autism Spectrum Disorder*, Current Clinical Psychiatry,
https://doi.org/10.1007/978-3-319-94458-6_7

dental provider should speak to the patient's caretaker to discuss concerns and potential triggers for agitation or behavioral difficulties. This can be accomplished by interviewing the caretaker by phone or sending a questionnaire to be completed prior to the appointment. The patient's difficulty in verbal communication while experiencing distress, which a dental visit may cause, can lead to undesirable or uncooperative behavior [37], which may sidetrack the visit.

Careful evaluation may be challenging with a patient with ASD, but recognition and diagnosis are important for the development of a treatment plan. Dental and oral surgical concerns in children and adults with ASD are similar with the potential for more severe ramifications over time if the condition is allowed to persist. Therefore, a problem may be more severe in an adult patient because it has had more time to develop. Anticipation of common issues helps to create an individualized care plan for children and adults (see Table 7.1).

Common Pediatric and Adult Conditions in ASD

Bruxism

Bruxism (Fig. 7.1) is characterized by a movement of the lower jaw that is not related to normal function. This parafunctional condition involves grinding of teeth against teeth during the night or day secondary to masticatory muscle hyperactivity, and it is more common in patients with ASD than in the general population [29]. Bruxism can be a reaction to psychological stress or simply a habit to increase sensory feedback. It can cause significant attrition (tooth wear) and in more extreme cases

Table 7.1 Common dental and oral surgery concerns in patients with ASD

Dental issue	Cause	Concern if left untreated	Treatment options
Dental decay	Poor home care, dietary issues, pouching food, trouble with mastication	Infection, pain	Dental fillings
			Diet changes
			High concentration fluoride
Gingival and periodontal disease	Poor home care leads to gingival inflammation secondary to persistent plaque and calculus accumulations	Pain, bleeding gums, tooth mobility or loss, bad breath	Oral hygiene instructions, more frequent office visits
Bruxism	Parafunctional habit, may be stress induced	Attrition, loss of vertical dimension of occlusion space, pain, fractured teeth	Occlusal splint if tolerated
			Botulinum toxin injections
Erosion	Acidity from GERD, vomiting, or diet	Loss of enamel	Adjust medications and diet
Malocclusion	Variety of genetic and parafunctional habits	Difficulty chewing, esthetics	Functional appliances if tolerated
Dental and facial trauma	Falls or other injuries, including SIB	Pain, tooth loss, malocclusion, infection, dental ankylosis, growth disturbance	Depending on nature of trauma
Dental anxiety	History of bad experience or fear of the unknown	Difficulty tolerating dental care, especially during emergencies	Desensitization
			Establish dental home

GERD gastroesophageal reflux disease, *SIB* self-injurious behavior

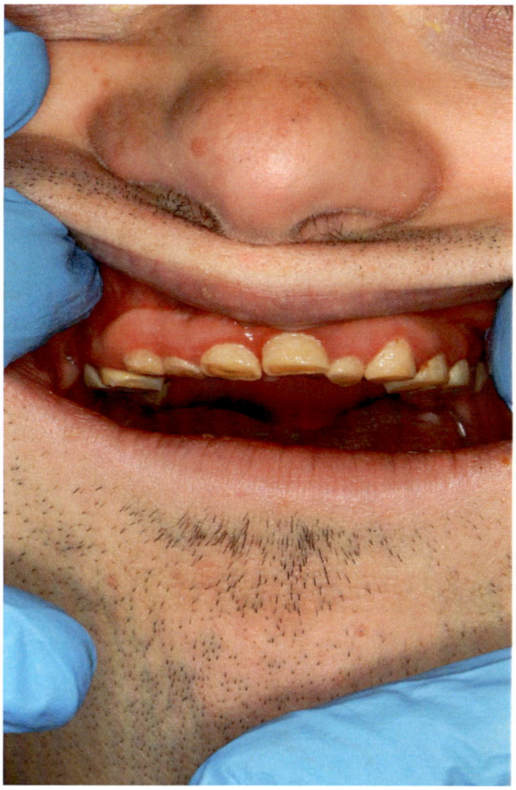

Fig. 7.1 Severe attrition due to bruxism. Note the loss of tooth structure and flattened biting surfaces due to grinding over time. This patient also has moderate marginal gingivits due to the buildup of plaque along the gumline and inability to cooperate with daily oral hygiene home care

lead to tooth fracture, pulp exposure, or myofascial pain.

Dental Decay

The incidence of dental decay in individuals with ASD is thought to be similar to that of the general public [5]. Though there are some studies that report higher or lower rates of decay, there are few well-controlled studies [10]. A predilection for sticky, sugary foods, pouching of food, and poor home care may increase the risk of dental decay in this population [29]. Additionally, the eating of non-edible substances (pica) may increase risk of decay or fracture of the teeth, depending on the item selected and the frequency of this behavior.

Dental decay occurs when oral bacteria are provided with a refined carbohydrate in the presence of a susceptible substrate (the tooth). The bacteria create an acidic environment which leads to tooth decay. If allowed to progress, the decay must be removed and a restoration placed. In order to prevent this from occurring, sugar in the diet should be limited, the patient must have adequate saliva to buffer against the acid, and the sugar and bacteria must be manually removed by brushing and flossing. In addition to limiting sugary food, one must be mindful of food textures, as soft or sticky foods are harder to remove and remain attached to the tooth for longer periods of time, making decay more likely.

Prevention is key, and brushing teeth twice a day with a fluoride-containing toothpaste should be reinforced at every appointment. For patients with high decay risk, a 1.1% fluoride toothpaste can be prescribed. However, in order to use this toothpaste, the patient should be able to spit to avoid fluoride toxicity by swallowing. If texture is a problem, the patient can use fluoride rinses or gels. It is important to work with the patient and caretaker to individualize the home care plan. If the patient does not have the coordination or muscle strength to brush independently, the caretaker must accomplish this task. This can be challenging if the patient is unable or unwilling to cooperate; many people with ASD are not able to adequately perform oral hygiene independently [29]. Oral hygiene support relies on the caretaker's understanding of oral home care and ability to perform it properly. Studies have shown differing techniques to help with home care, including repetition, routine, and consistency. Video or pictures of toothbrushing and flossing can be helpful in developing an oral hygiene routine by explaining and demonstrating the desired behavior [31]. It is important that oral care at home becomes a part of the daily routine for individuals with ASD.

Gingival and Periodontal Disease

Poor dental care at home is commonly reported among people with ASD [18] and will result in buildup of plaque and calculus leading to marginal inflammation (gingivitis) (Fig. 7.1) or loss of the supporting bone (periodontitis). In time, without improvement of home care, gingival inflammation will worsen and progress to periodontitis. Periodontitis is a nonreversible disease which, if not controlled, will result in tooth mobility and loss.

Gingival hyperplasia is a common side effect of a few antiepileptic drugs, especially phenytoin [9]. Overgrowth can be significant enough to cover the crowns of the teeth completely (Fig. 7.2a, b) which may cause delayed eruption of the teeth [39]. Gingival inflammation, pain, difficulty chewing, and difficulty maintaining good oral hygiene are consequences of gingival hyperplasia.

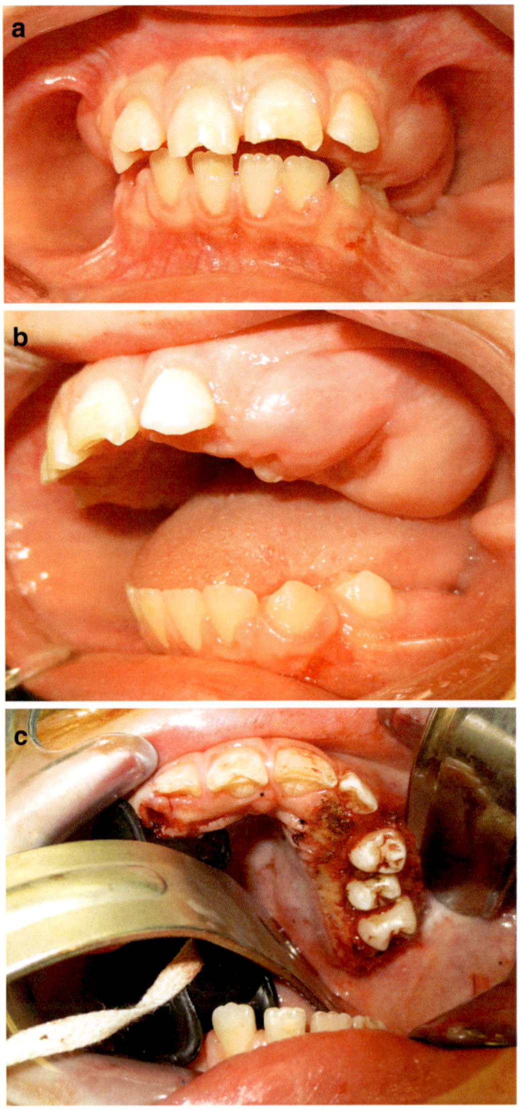

Fig. 7.2 Drug-induced gingival hyperplasia. (**a**) Frontal view showing the lower teeth are impinging on the gingival overgrowth. Enamel fractures also present on upper anterior teeth; (**b**) lateral view of the same overgrowth; (**c**) immediate result after gingivectomy. Upper posterior teeth are fully exposed after surgery

Bad Breath

Poor home care or pouching of food can also lead to impaction of food and bad breath. In addition, medical conditions, including side effects from medications, can lead to changes in breath and unpleasant odor.

Xerostomia

Xerostomia or "dry mouth" can be a side effect of many medications commonly prescribed to patients with ASD (Table 7.2) or salivary gland dysfunction. Lower salivary rates in patients with ASD [5] have been found and can have serious consequences for the patient's oral health. The lack of adequate saliva can lead to an increase in dental decay due to the absence of saliva's buffering capacity, especially in combination with poor home dental care and diet. Dry mouth can also contribute to bad breath from decreased oral clearing with the lack of secretions.

Table 7.2 Medications associated with xerostomia

Class of drug	Example
Alpha agonists	Clonidine
Antidepressants	Fluoxetine
Antiepileptics	Clonazepam
Antipsychotics	Risperidone
Anxiolytics	Alprazolam
Mood stabilizers	Lithium
Stimulants	Methylphenidate

Excessive Drooling

Excessive drooling (sialorrhea) can develop due to poor muscle control or difficulty with swallowing. This can lead to an increase in calculus buildup, resulting in marginal gingival inflammation and periodontal disease. Angular cheilitis (fungal infection at the oral commissure) and perioral irritated chapped skin are also signs of sialorrhea. Another important aspect of excessive drooling is that it can cause constant damp, soiled clothing, and can come with an unpleasant odor and poor hygienic considerations, which may contribute to social rejection.

Erosion

Long-term exposure to acids, such as with gastric reflux or excessive vomiting, can lead to erosion of the teeth. It results in the wearing away of the enamel of the tooth, making the tooth more susceptible to dental decay or sensitivity.

Malocclusion

Several conditions contribute to an increase in the observation of an unideal relationship of the teeth in the upper and lower jaw (malocclusion) in the ASD population [29]. Tongue thrust, a condition where the tongue pushes forward on the front teeth during speaking and swallowing, and other non-nutritive habits, like thumb or finger sucking, can lead to or cause persistence of an anterior open bite or dental crowding (Fig. 7.3). Malocclusion can cause problems with the ability to chew and speak as well as with esthetics and makes hygiene more difficult.

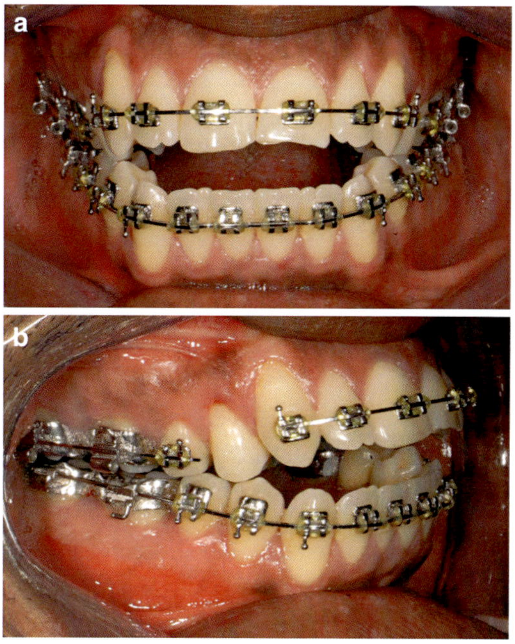

Fig. 7.3 Tongue thrust habit can lead to severe malocclusion with anterior open bite which requires combined orthodontic and surgical treatments. (**a**) Frontal view; (**b**) right lateral view

Self-Injurious Behavior

Self-injurious behavior (SIB) is a deliberate harm to the body without suicidal intent. Injuries can be superimposed upon a pre-existing lesion, secondary to an established habit, or the result of an unknown or complex etiology. SIB may rise from a stressful situation or can be an escape or attention-seeking behavior. Persons with intellectual disabilities are more prone to SIB [26]. Abnormal sensory processing leading to altered pain perception is one of the main factors contributing to SIB in children with ASD [15]. Children with ASD have been shown to sustain 7.6 times more self-inflected injuries compared to typically developing peers [24].

Dentists play an important role in identifying facial and oral habits that can lead to SIB, such as digit sucking, fingernail and lip biting, bruxism, scratching, and head banging. In fact, 70% of pediatric patients with ASD show SIB at one point during their life, and 75% of these injuries are head and neck related. Females under the age of 5 years are more frequently affected [25]. The most common self-induced oral lesions are gingivitis, periodontitis, and ulcers. The most serious self-inflected injuries from a dental perspective are self-extractions. When recently erupted, permanent teeth are more vulnerable to autoextraction. Missing teeth should not be assumed to be congenitally missing [34, 41]. Finally, a foreign body can also be lodged in the gum causing gingival irritation or infection. In order to be properly addressed, SIB has to be identified and not mistaken for a biological response or pathology from a different etiology.

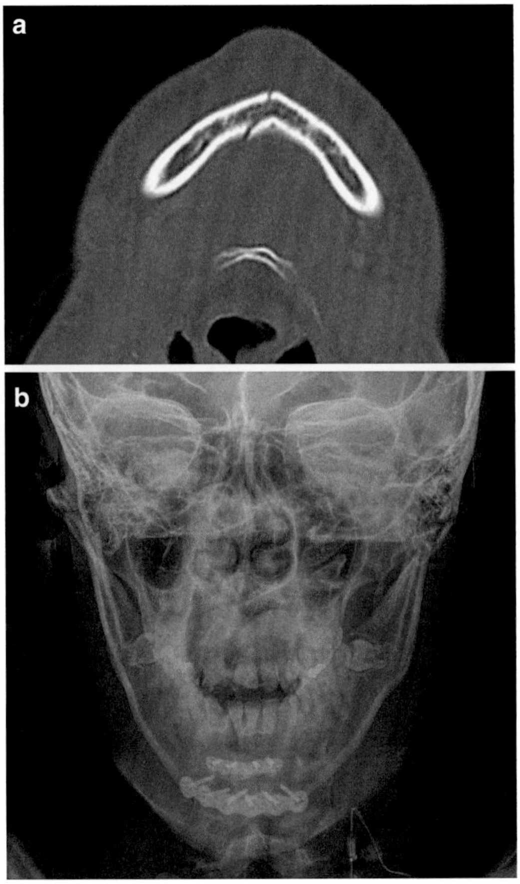

Fig. 7.4 A 16-year-old nonverbal boy sustained an unwitnessed fall. (**a**) Axial cut CT scan showing mandibular symphysis fracture; (**b**) postoperative frontal skull radiography demonstrating two osteosynthesis plates following open reduction with internal fixation (ORIF) of mandibular symphysis fracture

Trauma

According to the literature, no statistically significant differences in rates of traumatic dental injury have been identified between children with ASD and children without ASD [1, 14]. Risk factors between those two groups are different. Children with ASD sustain more injuries during routine activities, from falling while walking and secondary to SIB [14]. Girls with ASD are more prone to dental trauma than boys with ASD [14]. The types of injuries are the same for patients with and without ASD. The most frequent injury is enamel fracture (Fig. 7.2) [1, 14]. Finally, children with ASD are significantly more prone to head, face, and neck injuries compared to normal developing peers (Fig. 7.4) [24].

Clinical Evaluation

History

The examination should start with a thorough medical history, including a consultation with the primary care physician if indicated, to determine if the patient can safely be treated in the dental office. This will also allow the provider to predict potential dental issues arising from medical conditions (Tables 7.3 and 7.4). Many medications have dental side effects, and a complete list of all medications should be obtained from the caretaker or the primary care doctor prior to the appointment.

A complete dental history is also necessary, including what has been completed and how it was tolerated. Understanding the patient's triggers will help to avoid behavioral difficulties that can lead to a negative situation, including possible injury to the patient or staff. The caretaker should be interviewed to find out how the patient

Table 7.3 Dental issues arising from medical conditions

Medical condition	Dental ramifications	Treatment considerations
GERD	Dental erosion	Adjust medications to minimize reflux
		High fluoride toothpaste[a]
Seizure disorder	Increased risk of dental and facial trauma	Optimize medical control, wear a helmet
	Drug-induced xerostomia	Modify drug therapy, salivary substitutes, salivary stimulants, water
	Drug-induced gingival hyperplasia	Gingivectomy
Pica	Decay	Improved home care and high fluoride toothpaste
	Fractured teeth	
ADHD	Difficulty with dental exams	Minimize distractions
Behavioral issues	Increased risk for facial and dental trauma	Reinforcement interventions
Anxiety/ depression	Drug-induced xerostomia	Modify drug therapy
		Salivary substitutes, salivary stimulants, water

GERD gastroesophageal reflux disease, *ADHD* attention-deficit/hyperactivity disorder

[a]Use of high fluoride toothpaste assumes use of appropriate amount and that patient does not swallow toothpaste

Table 7.4 Resources

Helpful resources for families
Autism Speaks Family Services Community Connections Dental Guide (https://www.autismspeaks.org/sites/default/files/documents/dentalguide.pdf)
Practical Oral Care for People with Autism – NIH (https://www.nidcr.nih.gov/sites/default/files/2017-09/practical-oral-care-autism.pdf)

reacts in other situations, such as doctor's appointments, blood draws, haircuts, and shaving. Discussion with the patient and/or caretaker about any concerns prior to the appointment may illuminate potential difficulties related to procedures or products [33], avoiding conflict during the visit. Encourage the caretaker to book the appointment at a time when the patient is most likely to cooperate and discuss what motivates the patient so it can be used as an incentive to cooperate during the appointment. For example, if the patient enjoys showing family pictures to others, save them in an envelope on the counter until the end of the appointment. Lack of a motivating factor for cooperation has been shown to negatively impact behavior during the dental visit.

Finally, it is important to determine if the patient is legally competent to consent to care and if not who the legal guardian is. The guardian should be present at the first appointment and any future appointments that require additional consent to be signed (e.g., for extractions) and should be easily reached by phone when not present.

Physical Examination

Consistency and predictability are keys to a successful exam with a patient with ASD. All instruments should be out of sight when the patient is seated. Background noise should be kept to a minimum. Use of "tell, show, do" is a fundamental approach in pediatric dentistry and has been shown to be helpful in the ASD population, with the caveat that the patient may not respond that they understand the procedure. "Tell, show, do" starts prior to initiating the exam, by discussing with the patient and caretaker what the procedure is, using simple, concrete words and, if possible, showing pictures. Then the procedure is demonstrated, and finally the procedure is performed as described.

Examination should start with the hands only to gauge the patient's level of cooperation and then use a mirror and explorer if allowed. For patients unwilling to open their mouth, starting with toothbrushing may be a way to motivate the patient to open, as it is part of a familiar routine.

After brushing one can reattempt to examine the patient with a mirror and explorer. Examination should be directed and as quick as possible. Expect frequent interruptions, and stop as the patient requires.

As with a typical dental examination, it is important to start with an extraoral exam, evaluating for any swelling or asymmetry. The examination should proceed intraorally to see if there is any swelling, gross decay, or fractured teeth. Marginal gingival inflammation and plaque or calculus accumulation should be noted. If the patient is able to tolerate it, periodontal charting should be completed.

Studies

If the patient is able to cooperate, intraoral radiographs should be obtained. A goal of four dental radiographs and a panoramic radiograph should be attempted at the first appointment and repeated as age and caries history dictate [2]. Patients with sensory issues or strong gag reflexes may not be able to tolerate intraoral radiographs. For oral lesions, advanced imaging may be necessary, including MRI or CT scan.

If the patient's ability to cooperate hampers proper examination and diagnosis, various sedating agents, such as nitrous oxide, oral midazolam, or intramuscular ketamine, can be considered depending upon the clinical situation.

Treatment

General Considerations

Treatment of a patient with ASD can be more difficult for the dental provider due to great difficulty in establishing the rapport necessary for cooperation [19]. Desensitization has been shown to help some individuals with ASD better tolerate treatment. Slowly allowing the patient to become accustomed to the dental environment works well because it proceeds as the patient's comfort grows. Initially the patient may only enter the dental operatory, the next time they may sit down in the chair, and the following time teeth may be counted. This process can be time-consuming for both the dental provider and family, so in lieu of frequent visits, reenactments at home may be helpful. It has been demonstrated that it can be helpful to have the patient practice the appointment with a therapist or caregiver, including review of pictures of the planned procedure over the course of many sessions, and this may increase the patient's ability to tolerate treatment [7].

Time in the waiting room should be kept to a minimum, and the same room and staff should be used whenever possible. A welcoming environment for the patient may be fostered by minimizing office noise and outside distractions. There appears to be some benefit in sensory adaptation of the office environment for ASD patients to reduce anxiety and improve tolerance of the visit [8]. A sensory-adapted dental environment is an individualized process which can lead to a calmer environment from the patient's perspective [36]. This may involve playing videos or soothing music, use of softer lighting, or availability of weighted blankets. During treatment, good behavior should be praised and unwelcome behavior ignored. When problem behavior develops, try to quickly identify and remove the stimulus instead of focusing on the behavior itself [13]. Work with the caretaker to determine what incentive helps motivate the patient in order to encourage good behavior. At the end of the appointment, follow up with the caretaker to discuss how they feel the appointment went compared to previous experiences, and note anything that works well for the next appointment.

All methods to improve in-office cooperation should be explored, including protective stabilization, which is a physical aid for immobilizing the patient to allow safe treatment (Fig. 7.5). Some patients with ASD may find the snugness of the harness reassuring and may respond well to this tactic. If utilized, protective stabilization should be the least restrictive possible and be in accordance with state guidelines around the use of medical restraints.

In some cases communicative behavior management techniques are not enough. For these patients, pharmacological behavior management with conscious sedation may be an alternative to general anesthesia. Different agents are routinely

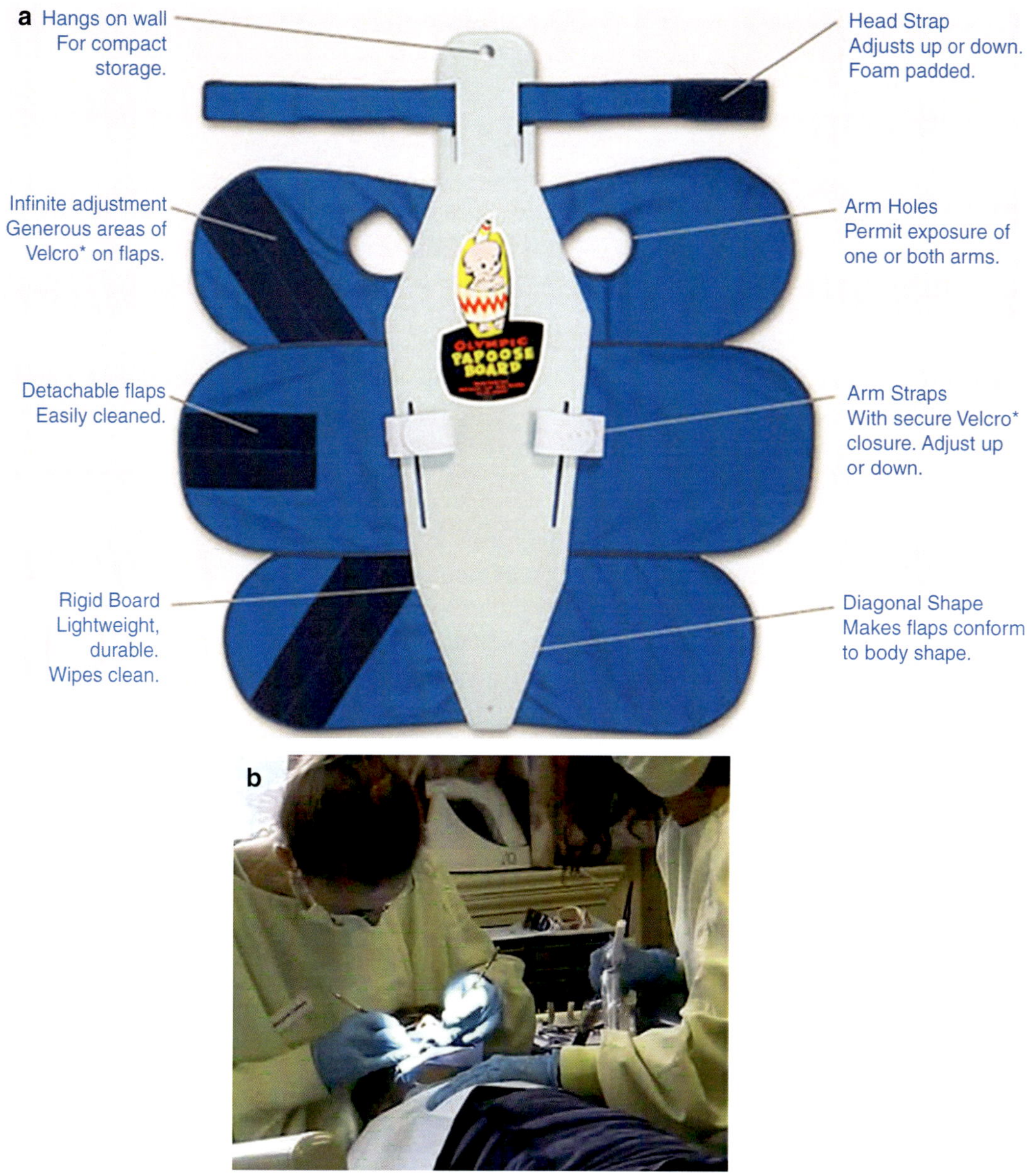

Fig. 7.5 (**a**) Example of protective stabilization device, Olympic Papoose Board by Natus Medical Incorporated, San Carlos, CA, a splint principle of binding the patient to a rigid board using three sets of opposing flaps that fold over the patient body; (**b**) Olympic Papoose Board used during dental treatment in a child (Courtesy of Dr. Vu, Montreal Children's Hospital)

used in the dental office, including diazepam, midazolam, ketamine, and nitrous oxide [32, 35, 38, 40].

Consideration of the patient's ability to process the information and cooperate is important. If other methods have failed, the ability to properly diagnose and treat the patient will be compromised. In those cases, treatment in a controlled setting under general anesthesia in the operating room (OR) must be considered. Approximately 37% of patients with ASD require dental treatment in the OR [22]. Treatment in the OR also provides the opportunity to achieve other difficult medical tasks, such as blood draws, vaccine administration, and examinations by other services, such as gynecology. Patients treated in the

OR should return for a follow-up appointment to review oral hygiene instructions and establish an in-office recall schedule to help reduce the need for treatment under general anesthesia in the future [23].

Treatment of Common Pediatric and Adult Conditions

Bruxism

If persistent, the ideal treatment for bruxism is a custom fabricated occlusal splint (nightguard) to minimize the force expressed to the teeth. Bruxism can be difficult to treat in children and persons with intellectual disability due to difficulty tolerating an oral appliance. Therefore in those populations one must watch for and treat the signs of severe bruxism, such as tooth fracture, as well as monitor and eliminate potential triggers.

Another option is botulinum toxin injections in masticatory muscles which result in muscle paralysis. The decrease in the strength of these muscles prevents bruxism. This approach is especially useful when the patient is not aware of the habit or cannot control it [28].

Finally, an anxiolytic such as buspirone has been used with success to treat anxiety-related bruxism. This treatment alternative is based on the proposition that chronic diurnal and nocturnal bruxism in patients with developmental disabilities can be a response to emotional stress [30].

Dental Decay

Treatment of established dental decay is important to prevent the development of infection and pain. Selection of restorative material depends upon a variety of factors, including the size of the cavity, mechanical forces expected to be placed on the restoration, and the ability to adequately isolate the tooth during placement. Additionally, the dentist must consider the expected life span of the restoration and the likelihood of need for additional treatment. For example, restorations on primary teeth may not need to last as long given the time until exfoliation; teeth with deep decay may require pulpal therapy now or in the future.

Given the wide variety of clinical presentations, risk factors for caries, and level of cooperation of the patient, the selection of restorative material is highly individualized. Traditionally, decay requiring removal involves local anesthesia of the tooth and placement of an amalgam or composite restoration, with amalgam being the preferred choice when there is not good moisture control during placement. For primary teeth with large restorations or pulp therapy, prefabricated stainless steel crowns have the best longevity. There is some promising data that the method of Atraumatic Restorative Technique (ART) may be comparable with traditional restoration techniques in the special needs population in short-term follow-up [27]. ART involves excavation of caries with hand instruments and placement of a glass ionomer cement; this often can be accomplished without the need for local anesthesia and therefore may be better tolerated.

The teeth with extensive decay or infection may require pulpal therapy or extraction. The final decision for treatment relates to the prognosis of the tooth, both short and long term, as well as patient cooperation. Treatment performed in the operating room under general anesthesia tends to require a more aggressive approach [22], since the patient is unable to cooperate in the clinic if a dental issue develops between OR visits.

After treatment it is important to review home care to ensure that the patient has adequate fluoride exposure and oral hygiene assistance and is seen in the office for regular cleanings and examinations. A healthy diet with limited exposure to sugar should be encouraged to help prevent further decay.

Gingival and Periodontal Disease

Gingival inflammation must be managed by manual removal of plaque and calculus. More advanced disease may require a deep cleaning with hand instruments or periodontal surgery.

Excellent home care is necessary to prevent progression of disease. This may be challenging depending upon the patient's cooperation at home or manual dexterity. The use of a power toothbrush has been shown to decrease the presence of gingival plaque [3]. The standard office visit schedule for cleanings is every 6 months, but many patients require more frequent visits in order to remove plaque and calculus accumulations. Some patients may also benefit from the use of daily chlorhexidine antibacterial rinse.

Drug-induced gingival hyperplasia, which is a side effect of some antiepileptic medications, can be managed by gingivectomies (recontouring of the gumline) (Fig. 7.2c). The possibility of discontinuation of the offending agent and substitution with another medication should be discussed with the prescribing clinician.

Xerostomia

There are some agents available that have shown limited efficacy to increase saliva production, including pilocarpine. Other options, such as salivary substitutes, are also available. If the condition may be the result of a medication side effect, the possibility of a medication change should be discussed with the prescribing clinician.

Excessive Drooling

Excessive drooling can be addressed at different levels. Current medications should be evaluated for side effect profiles and adjusted if possible. Options for physical or occupational therapy should be discussed with the primary care physician to help with muscle control or swallowing. Pharmacologically, oral glycopyrrolate or scopolamine can be tried to reduce the amount of saliva production [20]. Botulinum toxin injections into the salivary glands can also be used to address excessive drooling [21]. A more drastic alternative is to remove the submandibular glands. Other surgical options are to reposition posteriorly the submandibular gland excretory canals that are located on the floor of the mouth or to ligate them [12].

Erosion

To help prevent erosion, the caretaker should evaluate the patient's diet and eliminate or limit acidic foods. After vomiting the patient should rinse the mouth with water to remove residual acid. The patient should be referred to a primary care doctor for evaluation and possible treatment of gastric reflux or recurrent vomiting.

Malocclusion

Treatment of malocclusion varies significantly based on the presentation and the patient's ability to tolerate intraoral appliances. There are several functional orthodontic appliances which can be used to reeducate the tongue into its proper position. Speech therapy with different exercises can also help to address that issue. If the patient or caretaker is concerned about malocclusion and the patient is cooperative, referral to an orthodontist (a dental specialist focused on alignment of the teeth and jaws) would be indicated.

Self-Injurious Behavior

Oral and facial injuries secondary to SIB should be treated just like any other lesion. Important emphasis has to be placed on working with the patient's care team to address the behavior leading to the injury. Once identified, different reinforcement- or extinction-based interventions, such as alternative forms of stimulation, physical restraint, and crisis and stress management, can be applied to reduce SIB [16, 26].

Trauma

Management of dental and facial trauma depends on the type of injury and on the patient's behavior. Some injuries necessitate long-term treatment, which can be a great ordeal for some patients. Close follow-up is important, particularly when treating patients with communication impairments or altered pain perception.

Clinical Vignette #1

A 23-year-old patient presented with his parents to establish dental care for the first time. He has the diagnosis of ASD and is nonverbal. He exhibited repetitive behaviors and has significant anxiety about the visit. He lives at home with his parents, who are his legal guardians and primary caretakers. He goes to a day program, which he enjoys.

He has never seen a dentist, but the staff at his day program noticed some skin irritation on his face and recent changes in his behavior, and they worry that he is having tooth pain. His father had not noticed any changes at home and believed that the skin irritation may be from shaving, which the patient allows his father to do for him.

Examination is attempted, but the patient paced the room and would not sit in the chair. There was no facial asymmetry or swelling noted. The patient would not open his mouth for examination but did allow for a toothbrush cleaning while he stood. A brief exam revealed no gross decay or swelling but moderate gingival inflammation. He could not tolerate any radiographs. Options were discussed with his parents, and treatment in the OR under general anesthesia for radiographs and a full assessment were recommended.

In the OR (Fig. 7.6), it was revealed that he had moderate gingivitis but no decay or infection. He received a thorough cleaning and application of fluoride varnish. Once a full assessment was completed and his decay risk was determined to be low, a customized plan was formulated for future care in the dental clinic. He has been seen every 6 months for the past several years; his father has declined more frequent visits to attempt desensitization. For the follow-up appointments, he has continued to pace the room but will sit in the dental chair for increasing amounts of time. He will now allow examination with a mirror and explorer and toothbrush cleaning in small bursts of up to a minute, followed by more pacing and sitting again for treatment. He continues to be unable to tolerate radiographs or a thorough cleaning with scaling of the teeth. The plan will be to return to the OR as needed or for comprehensive exam, radiographs, and a cleaning every few years given his low decay rate.

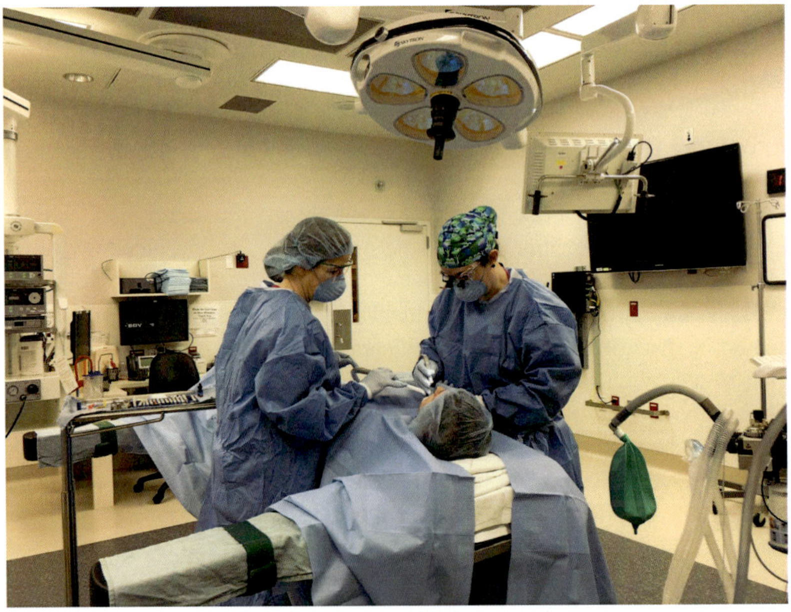

Fig. 7.6 Full mouth rehabilitation in the operating room allows for examination, diagnosis, and treatment of patients with special needs in a controlled environment

Clinical Vignette #2

A 16-year-old nonverbal boy with ASD and a seizure disorder presented to the emergency department following an unwitnessed fall. His fall was thought to be related to recent changes in his antiepileptic medication. On presentation, the patient was unable to cooperate with a clinical exam. Bilateral preauricular swelling was noted. His anterior-inferior mandibular contour and preauricular areas bilaterally were tender to palpation. After the use of a visual storyboard and the promise of a reward, the patient was able to cooperate for a facial CT scan. Imaging revealed bilateral mandibular intracapsular condylar head fractures (minimally displaced) and mandibular symphysis fracture (slightly displaced) (Fig. 7.4a).

These kinds of mandibular fractures can be treated with maxillomandibular fixation (MMF) (closed technique) and diet restriction. MMF is normally maintained for a period of 6 weeks. It is achieved most of the time under local anesthesia by placing arch bars (heavy metal bars with hooks) at the gumline level on both jaws. Occlusion is reestablished and maintained by metal loop wires going from the upper arch bar to the lower one (Fig. 7.7). By reestablishing the premorbid occlusion, the mandibular fractures are reduced and stabilized.

It was decided that the patient would be best treated differently because MMF treatment requires patient compliance to be successful and the patient's parents expressed concern about his ability to cooperate with this treatment. An alternate treatment plan was then pursued involving open reduction with internal fixation (ORIF) of his mandibular fractures under general anesthesia (Fig. 7.4b). ORIF is a more invasive treatment compared to MMF but allows more diet flexibility, and there is no restriction in jaw movement and no apparent hardware during the healing period. Also, with ORIF, unlike MMF, no other intervention after the healing period is required for hardware removal. Arch bars in MMF need to be removed once they are no longer used.

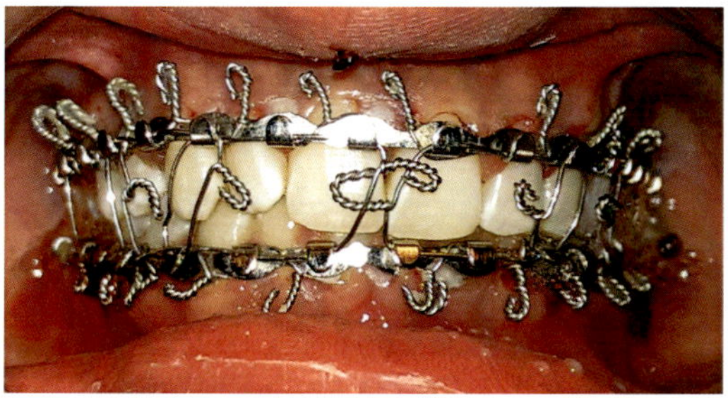

Fig. 7.7 Example of maxillomandibular fixation as closed reduction treatment of mandibular fracture

The patient's postoperative course was without any complications and resulted in a favorable outcome. Treatment choice has to be adapted for every patient, especially those with ASD. Rigidly adhering to a standard treatment approach without consideration of the patient's ability to cooperate with care and tolerate procedures may result in worse outcomes and greater distress for the patient.

Clinical Pearls

- Encourage establishment of a dental home.
- Utilize "tell, show, do" to explain procedures and improve cooperation.
- Watch body language and behavior for signs of distress or agitation.
- Identify stressful stimuli, and remove them quickly.
- Use positive reinforcement of desired behaviors and ignore negative behaviors.
- Start slow, let the patient lead, and gain trust for the next step.
- Rely on the expertise of caretakers, interviewing them to determine what motivates the patient and what areas may be challenging.
- Minimize wait time and distractions.
- Review proper home care and trauma prevention at each visit.
- Modifications of the environment in the office and the approach to care and treatment may be necessary for some individuals with ASD.

Acknowledgment We would like to thank Dr. Maria Troulis, Chief of the Department of Oral and Maxillofacial Surgery at Massachusetts General Hospital, for her support and guidance with this chapter.

References

1. Altun C, Guven G, Yorbik O, Acikel C. Dental injuries in autistic patients. Pediatr Dent. 2010;32:343–6.
2. American Academy of Pediatric Dentistry (AAPD). Guideline on prescribing dental radiographs for infants, children, adolescents and persons with special health care needs. Ref Man. 2016;38(6):355–7.
3. Awasthi P, Peshwani B, Tiwari S, Thakur R, Shashikiran N, Singla S. Evaluation and comparison of the efficacy of low fluoridated and calcium phosphate-based dentifrice formulations when used with powered and manual toothbrush in children with autism. Contemp Clin Dent. 2015;6(6):188.
4. Blomqvist M, Dahlla G, Bejerot S. Experiences of dental care and dental anxiety in adults with autism spectrum disorder. Autism Res Treat. 2014;2014:1–9.
5. Blomqvist M, Bejerot S, Dahlla G. A cross-sectional study on oral health and dental care in intellectually able adults with autism spectrum disorder. BMC Oral Health. 2015;15:81. https://doi.org/10.1186/s12903-015-0065-z.
6. Brickhouse T, Farrington F, Best A, Ellsworth C. Barriers to dental care for children in Virginia with autism spectrum disorders. J Dent Child. 2009;76(3):188–93.
7. Cagetti M, Mastroberardino S, Campus G, Olivari B, Faggioli R, Lenti C, et al. Dental care protocol based on visual supports for children with autism spectrum disorders. Med Oral. 2015;20:e598–604.
8. Cermak S, Stein Duker L, Williams M, Dawson M, Lane C, Polido J. Sensory adapted dental environments to enhance oral care for children with autism spectrum disorders: a randomized controlled pilot study. J Autism Dev Disord. 2015;45(9):2876–88.
9. Chen B, Choi H, Hirsch LJ, Moeller J, Javed A, Kato K, Legge A, Buchsbaum R, Detyniecki K. Cosmetic side effects of antiepileptic drugs in adults with epilepsy. Epilepsy Behav. 2015;42:129–37.
10. Delli K, Reichart P, Bornstein M, Livas C. Management of children with autism spectrum disorder in the dental setting: concerns, behavioural approaches and recommendations. Med Oral. 2013;18:e862–8.
11. DeLucia L, Davis E. Dental students' attitudes toward the care of individuals with intellectual disabilities: relationship between instruction and experience. J Dent Educ. 2009;73(4):445–53.
12. Formeister EJ, Dahl JP, Rose AS. Surgical management of chronic sialorrhea in pediatric patients: 10-year experience from one tertiary care institution. Int J Pediatr Otorhinolaryngol. 2014;78:1387–92.
13. Gandhi R, Klein U. Autism spectrum disorders: an update on oral health management. J Evid Based Dent Pract. 2014;14:115–26.
14. Habibe RCH, Ortega AOL, Guare RO, Diniz MB, Santos MTBR. Risks factors for anterior traumatic dental injury in children and adolescents with autism spectrum disorders: a case-control study. Eur Arch Paediatr Dent. 2015; https://doi.org/10.1007/s40368-015-0207-7.
15. Hazen EP, Stornelli JL, O'Rourke JA, Koesterer K, McDougle CJ. Sensory symptoms in autism spectrum disorders. Harv Rev Psychiatr. 2014;22:112–24.
16. Howlin P. Behavioural techniques to reduce self-injurious behaviour in children with autism. Acta Paedopsychiatr. 1993;56:75–94.
17. Huebner C, Chi D, Masterson E, Milgrom P. Preventive dental health care experiences of preschool-age children with special health care needs. Spec Care Dent. 2014;35(2):68–77.
18. Jaber M. Dental caries experience, oral health status and treatment needs of dental patients with autism. J Appl Oral Sci. 2011;19(3):212–7.
19. Kamen S, Skier J. Dental management of the autistic child. Spec Care Dent. 1985;5(1):20–3.
20. Lakraj AA, Moghimi N, Jabbari B. Sialorrhea: anatomy, pathophysiology and treatment with emphasis on the role of botulinum toxins. Toxins (Basel). 2013;5:1010–31.
21. Lim M, Mace A, Nouraei SA, Sandhu G. Botulinum toxin in the management of sialorrhoea: a systematic review. Clin Otolaryngol. 2006;31:267–72.
22. Loo C, Graham R, Hughes C. The caries experience and behavior of dental patients with autism spectrum disorder. J Am Dent Assoc. 2008;139(11):1518–24.
23. Mallineni S, Yiu C. A retrospective review of outcomes of dental treatment performed for special needs patients under general anaesthesia: 2-year follow-up. Sci World J. 2014;2014:1–6.
24. McDermott S, Zhou L, Mann J. Injuries treatment among children with autism or pervasive developmental disorder. J Autism Dev Disord. 2008;38:626–33.
25. Medina AC, Sogbe R, Gomez-Rey AM, Mata M. Factitial oral lesions in an autistic paediatric patient. Int J Paediatr Dent. 2003;13:130–7.
26. Minshawi NF, Hurwitz S, Morriss DH, McDougle CJ. Multidisciplinary assessment and treatment of self-injurious behavior in autism spectrum disorder and intellectual disability: integration of psychological and biological theory and approach. J Autism Dev Disord. 2015;45:1541–68.
27. Molina G, Faulks D, Mazzola I, Mulder J, Frencken J. One year survival of ART and conventional restorations in patients with disability. BMC Oral Health. 2014;14(1):49.
28. Monroy PG, da Fonseca MA. The use of botulinum toxin-a in the treatment of severe bruxism in a patient with autism: a case report. Spec Care Dent. 2006;26:37–9.

29. Orellana LM, Silvestre F, Martinez-Sanchis S, Martinez-Mihi V, Bautista D. Oral manifestations in a group of adults with autism spectrum disorder. Med Oral. 2012;17:e415–9.
30. Orsagh-Yentis DK, Wink LK, Stigler KA, Erickson CA, McDougle CJ. Buspirone for bruxism in a child with pervasive developmental disorder-not otherwise specified. J Child Adolesc Psychopharmacol. 2011;21:643–5.
31. Pilebro C, Backman B. Teaching oral hygiene to children with autism. Int J Paediatr Dent. 2005;15(1):1–9.
32. Pisalchaiyong T, Trairatvorakul C, Jirakijja J, Yuktarnonda W. Comparison of the effectiveness of oral diazepam and midazolam for the sedation of autistic patients during dental treatment. Pediatr Dent. 2005;27:198–206.
33. Rada R. Controversial issues in treating the dental patient with autism. J Am Dent Assoc. 2010;141(8):947–53.
34. Ross-Russell M, Sloan P. Autoextraction in a child with autistic spectrum disorder. Br Dent J. 2005;8:473–4.
35. Shah S, Shah S, Apuya J, Gopalakrishnan S, Martin T. Combination of oral ketamine and midazolam as a premedication for a severely autistic and combative patient. J Anesth. 2009;23:126–8.
36. Shapiro M, Melmed RN, Sgan-Cohen, Eli I, Parush S. Behavioural and physiological effect of dental environment sensory adaption on children's dental anxiety. Eur J Oral Sci. 2007;115:479–83.
37. Stein L, Lane C, Williams M, Dawson M, Polido J, Cermak S. Physiological and behavioral stress and anxiety in children with autism spectrum disorders during routine oral care. BioMed Res Int. 2014;2014:1–10.
38. Udhya J, Varadharaja MM, Parthiban J, Ila S. Autism disorder (AD): an updated review for paediatric dentists. J Clin Diagn Res. 2014;8:275–9.
39. US Department of Health and Human Services. Practical oral care for people with autism. Bethesda: National Institute of Dental and Craniofacial Reaseach; 2009.
40. Van der Walt JH, Moran C. An audit of perioperative management of autistic children. Pediatr Anaesth. 2001;11:401–8.
41. Williams AC. Autoextraction of twelve permanent teeth in a child with autism spectrum disorder. Int J Paediatr Dent. 2015; https://doi.org/10.1111/ipd.12161.

8 Ophthalmology

Aubrey L. Gilbert and Melanie Kazlas

Introduction

The prevalence of ophthalmic pathology is higher in individuals with autism spectrum disorder (ASD) than in the general population. Those with ASD have higher incidences of refractive error, especially astigmatism, and of strabismus and amblyopia. It has also been shown that they may have retinal pathology as well as various abnormalities in higher-order visual processing, especially for processing of biological motion and faces and for integration of complex visual information. Some of these differences in visual processing may contribute to behavioral difficulties. Problems with visual processing of faces, for example, may play a role in difficulties with social interactions.

Among autistic patients, restrictive diets may also lead to systemic vitamin deficiencies, which may manifest in a number of ways but may be appreciable on ophthalmic exam with signs such as decreased vision, xerophthalmia, or optic neuropathy. Because of the known high incidence of ophthalmic pathology in the autistic population, a comprehensive eye examination by an ophthalmologist is recommended for all children diagnosed with ASD. As some patients with ASD may have difficulty cooperating with the examination, there is a higher likelihood that such abnormalities might be missed, so follow-up examination may be needed. Each patient with ASD requires a tailored approach to maximize examination yield. It is recommended to start the examination with the most relevant testing first, in case it is not possible to complete a full exam. The approach to the patient should take into account their special needs, and consideration should be given to ways to minimize stress to reduce the chances of increased apprehension and poor cooperation with future examinations.

Common Conditions

In a retrospective review of pediatric autistic patients in an ophthalmology practice in Baltimore, Black et al. [4] found that 52% of patients had some ocular abnormality, with 41% having strabismus, 27% with significant refractive error, 7% with anisometropia, and 11% with amblyopia. The prevalence of these conditions is higher than those for the general pediatric popu-

A. L. Gilbert
Department of Ophthalmology, Boston Children's Hospital, Massachusetts Eye and Ear Infirmary, Boston, MA, USA
e-mail: audrey.gilbert@childrens.harvard.edu

M. Kazlas (✉)
Department of Ophthalmology, Boston Children's Hospital, Massachusetts Eye and Ear Infirmary, Boston, MA, USA
e-mail: melanie.kazlas@childrens.harvard.edu

E. P. Hazen, C. J. McDougle (eds.), *The Massachusetts General Hospital Guide to Medical Care in Patients with Autism Spectrum Disorder*, Current Clinical Psychiatry,
https://doi.org/10.1007/978-3-319-94458-6_8

lation. This was corroborated in a larger study by Ikeda et al. [19] who did a retrospective chart review of 478 autistic children and found ophthalmic pathology to be present in 40% of patients, with 29% having significant refractive errors, 21% demonstrating strabismus, and 10% having amblyopia. A similar study done in Turkey [22] noted ophthalmic pathology in 26.9% of autistic patients, of which 22% had significant refractive errors and 8.6% had strabismus. A small study done in Niger [13] found that astigmatism was the most common refractive error among autistic children.

A number of case reports have also detailed ocular abnormalities related to vitamin deficiencies in the setting of severe food selectivity and highly stereotyped diets, especially vitamin A and vitamin B12 in autistic children [9, 28, 32]. Such deficiencies can have serious ophthalmic and systemic consequences, and signs of them should be screened for on exam and by history. An association of ASD has also been reported in children with Möbius sequence, CHARGE syndrome, and oculo-auriculo-vertebral spectrum [21]; however this association has not been widely corroborated, and some studies suggest it is not as common as previously speculated [6].

A variety of visual tasks have been reported in which individuals with ASD actually outperform controls and the explanation for this has been a matter of some debate [30]. Some early studies showed enhanced visual acuity in autistic children [7], but these studies were found to be methodologically flawed, and we know, as discussed above, that children with ASD actually have higher incidences of refractive error and amblyopia. Later studies (e.g., [1]) showed that children with ASD did not actually demonstrate superior acuity.

Some studies have shown impaired retinal activity in patients with ASD as well. Lavoie et al. [23] provide a nice summary of many of the studies showing abnormal electroretinographic findings in some children with ASD. Early visual cortical processing has been studied in patients with ASD, and, for the most part, studies (e.g., [30]) do not show enhanced early cortical function. Finally, it has been suggested that there are differences in higher-order visual processing in pediatric patients with ASD that could account for differential performance on visual tasks. Guy et al. [17] demonstrate that the development of contrast sensitivity for spatial frequencies follows a different trajectory in autistic patients compared to controls, and Davies et al. [12] found that children with autism experience impairment in trajectory discrimination and high spatial frequency contrast. Visual recognition of biological motion was also found to be impaired in children with ASD by Blake et al. [5]. An interesting study by Happé [18] showed that children with ASD are less likely to succumb to visual illusions and suggests that this might be due to weak central coherence, i.e., inability to "see the big picture," in visual processing. In fact, within the realm of perceptual processing in children with ASD, three main themes have persisted: enhanced processing of local structure, inferior processing of global structure, and impaired perception of motion, especially of biological motion [11]. There have also been studies documenting abnormalities in eye movement, fixation, and visual behavior and attention, and we discuss some of these below.

Anomalies in fixation patterns and the ballistics of eye movements are well documented in children with ASD, with off-center fixations being very common. Some studies also suggest that patients with ASD have abnormal saccadic eye movements, but a study by Pensiero et al. [27] did not confirm the presence of saccadic movement alterations in subjects with ASD. They did however frequently observe instability of fixation in the ASD population. Furman et al. [14] examined eye movements in verbal children with ASD and did find increased saccade latency but normal saccadic velocity and accuracy. Grossman et al. [16] found that individuals with high-functioning ASD demonstrate maladaptive fixation behavior in auditory-visual processing of speech by spending less time looking at the mouth region of the face. Anderson et al. [3] also found significant decrease in visual scanning behavior in children with ASD, and whereas controls demonstrated pupillary dilation when shown faces, children with ASD had pupillary constriction. Chawarska and Shic [8] likewise found atypical visual scanning and recognition of faces in 2- and 4-year-old children with ASD. A study by Shi et al. [31] with preschool-aged children with ASD found that they had different visual preference patterns compared to typically developing children in response to simple and complex dynamic social stimuli. They found that children with ASD attended significantly less to dynamic social images showing two or more children playing than to similar images showing a single child, and they suggest that visual attention preference in young children with ASD may be modulated by the type of visual stimuli.

Some degree of physiologic variation may underlie these observed differences. One study [29] used magnetic resonance imaging (MRI) to demonstrate larger extrastriate receptive fields in high-functioning patients with ASD compared with controls and speculated that visual function in patients with ASD may be characterized by extrastriate cortical hyperexcitability or differential attentional deployment. Some studies have suggested too that there might be enhanced integration of motion information in individuals with ASD and that this might actually lead to feelings of "sensory overload" [25] and that this overload may underlie some of the social difficulties the patients' experience. Interestingly, Frey et al. [15] suggest that the differential visuospatial cortical mapping that has been observed in children with ASD may be a consequence of stereotyped visual behaviors and peculiarities in gaze that affect experiential development of retinotopic maps.

Some studies have suggested an altered balance between excitation and inhibition in cortical networks in individuals with ASD. Stroganova et al. [34] used magnetoencephalography to investigate this in processing of visual motion and found there may be reduced excitability of fast-spiking inhibitory neurons in a subset of children with ASD. Visual processing in individuals with ASD has also been investigated with electroencephalography. Cléry et al. [10] found that, compared to controls, children with ASD show an earlier visual mismatch response, suggesting a hypersensitivity to visual deviancy. They suggest that this atypical change detection processing may contribute to some individual's intolerance of change. In another electroencephalographic analysis focusing on synchrony of visual evoked potentials between homologous early visual areas, Isler et al. [20] found reduced functional connectivity in children with ASD in spite of bilaterally increased power. They suggest that the cortices of children with ASD are hypersensitive to stimulation yet have diminished interhemispheric connectivity and speculate that this may be due to increased intra-hemispheric processing or perhaps to regulation by the thalamus, a theory that might be consistent with some others regarding attention modulation effects in patients with ASD.

Interactions between the visual and other systems may also be affected in ASD. For example, evidence has suggested impaired auditory-visual integration in high-functioning individuals with ASD for verbal information but not for simple nonverbal auditory stimuli [33]. Nebel et al. [24] also point out that children with ASD exhibit what appears to be a specific bias against using visual feedback during motor learning. They used functional MRI to investigate this and found increased intrinsic asynchrony between visual and motor systems in children with ASD. Interestingly, the degree of asynchrony correlated to the severity of autistic traits in individual participants.

Clinical Evaluation

History The same basic history should be obtained for a patient with ASD as for any patient undergoing ophthalmic evaluation. It may be more difficult to obtain history directly from the patient in some cases, and so external sources of information, such as family members, teachers, and healthcare aides, should be addressed for details. Assessment should include questions about any past ophthalmic history including any history of prior eye traumas or surgeries; problems with reading or distance vision; any notice of eye misalignment or squinting; any preferred head postures when performing visual tasks; any visual changes (may be difficult to assess); any apparent ocular redness, discharge, or discomfort; and any other ocular complaints. In addition, questions should be posed about any stereotyped visual behaviors or peculiarities of gaze as well as any behavioral quirks that may affect visual functioning or represent a threat to safety of the eyes, such as frequent eye rubbing, which may lead to corneal ectasia. It is also important to inquire about diet and nutrition to ensure no vitamin deficiencies, as mentioned above. Finally, practitioners should ask about comorbid health issues, such as hypertension, that could affect the eyes or the visual system.

Physical Examination Ophthalmic examinations can be stressful for any patient but can be particularly so for those with ASD. They can also be frustrating and time-consuming for the practitioner. It is good to know in advance of any special triggers that may set off a patient. Our clinic uses a behavioral screening form for all patients that requests detailed information about any sensitivities or special needs. It is also important to remember that even though patients may appear totally normal, they may be impaired on various parts of the exam and should be given extra time to respond or participate if needed.

Given the wide spectrum of patients with ASD, the approach to ophthalmic examination must be tailored to the individual and to the complaint. Some authors recommend using a photoscreener that can obtain multiple measurements at once from a distance in order to decrease stress to the patient (e.g., [26]). To minimize invasiveness, the examination of visual behavior can also begin from afar in the waiting room and on the way to the exam room.

If a patient is presenting for a specific complaint, a prioritized mental list of examination items should be made, and the most important aspects should be performed first in case it is not possible to complete all parts of the examination. Some basic features normally included in a comprehensive visit include assessment of stereovision and binocular function, dynamic retinoscopy, convergence amplitudes, visual acuity with each eye, fixation preferences, convergence amplitudes, extraocular movements, presence of nystagmus, ocular alignment, external appearance including presence of any particular head turn or tilt or other posturing, pupillary responses, measurement of intraocular pressure in each eye, anterior segment examination with a penlight or handheld or standard slit lamp if possible, dilated fundus examination, and cycloplegic retinoscopy. It may be helpful to have the parents bring a few fixation targets favored by the patient. Based on some of the literature reviewed above, it may also be desirable to assess visual tracking and saccades in patients with ASD and, if any history of dietary restriction is present, to assess specifically for ophthalmic manifestations of vitamin deficiencies.

Studies Determination of appropriate studies to obtain is dependent on examination findings; some studies that require more cooperation to obtain may require sedation depending on the level of functioning of the patient. Some common studies that may be obtained in clinic include external and fundus photography, visual field testing (which may be very difficult given the high degree of attention and cooperation required), and optical coherence tomography of the optic nerves or macula. More complex studies such as visual evoked potentials and electroretinography may be appropriate in certain cases.

Treatment

Vision therapy and behavioral training may be helpful for some individuals with ASD with higher-order visual processing issues. Otherwise, treatment is dependent on pathology noted and generally would be similar for the same pathology in typically developing patients. Some individuals with ASD may be averse to wearing glasses, and having glasses that fit well is particularly important. For pediatric patients, it is preferable to have glasses made by an optometry shop that specializes in fitting children. In addition if there are behavioral issues that make wearing glasses additionally complicated, it may be helpful to have glasses wear incorporated into a behavioral therapy plan. If patients with ASD require surgery to treat their ophthalmic pathology, all of the considerations listed above in regard to tailoring the clinical experience to each patient based on their level of functioning would apply. Many ophthalmic issues require chronic management, and so forming a good rapport and trying to avoid trauma or any experiences that will heighten apprehension of future encounters are recommended.

Special Considerations in the Ophthalmologic Care of Adults

While most of the current medical literature related to ophthalmologic care in patients with ASD is focused on the pediatric population, good care should extend throughout the life span, including regular screening eye examinations. Asymptomatic adults with ASD should follow the same screening guidelines as the general population to look for signs of age-related eye diseases, such as cataracts, macular degeneration, glaucoma, and macular degeneration, as these conditions may begin in mid-life but may not noticeably affect vision until they have progressed. The American Academy of Ophthalmology currently recommends a comprehensive medical eye examination at 40 years of age, with repeat examinations every 2–4 years until age 54 years, when the interval should be decreased to every 1–3 years. After age 65 years, an examination should be done every 1–2 years [2]. More frequent examination may be indicated in symptomatic individuals or those with medical conditions, such as diabetes mellitus, that increase risk of certain ophthalmologic problems. As described in the evaluation section above, more time may be needed for appointments and examinations in adult patients with ASD, and a more tailored approach may be necessary.

Some adult patients with ASD may have guardians who are responsible for medical decision-making. It is important to clarify guardianship status prior to initiation of care and to communicate with the guardian. However, even when patients present for care with a parent or a guardian, it is important to address the patient directly and to consider the patient's wishes a priority.

There is a clear need for more adult ophthalmologists and optometrists with experience and comfort in treating patients with ASD and a need for more research into the prevalence and challenges of ophthalmologic care in adults with ASD.

Clinical Vignette # 1

Our ophthalmology service was consulted to see a 16-year-old boy with severe ASD with aggressive behavior for new apparent ocular pain. Earlier in the day, the patient had gone swimming as part of an outing with his group home, and he was noted to have bilateral eye redness after getting out of the pool. One of his aides rinsed the eyes with tap water and dried them with a paper towel. This was reportedly done with great difficulty due to the patient's agitation. Afterward, the patient was tearing and even more agitated, and he was brought to the Urgent Care clinic where a number of people held him down in order to instill fluorescein eye drops, further worsening his agitation. After instillation of fluorescein, examination was even more difficult, but it was felt that the patient's symptoms were possibly attributable to bilateral corneal abrasions, and he was again held down forcibly while kicking and yelling in order to put erythromycin ointment in both eyes.

His level of agitation worsened significantly, and he was at risk of harming himself and others despite efforts by staff and his family to soothe him and keep him safe. The decision was made to transfer the patient to the emergency department (ED), where he continued to be quite agitated. The patient kept his eyes squeezed tightly shut and was hitting, kicking, and yelling loudly in the ED. He was not approachable by any healthcare professional. No examination was possible in the ED, and the patient was sent home with an oxycodone prescription for pain with the plan to follow up in ophthalmology clinic the following day when it was felt the patient might be calmer after spending time at home.

When he returned to the clinic the following day, however, his parents reported that he had not slept overnight and had been inconsolable. His parents appeared completely exhausted. The patient was still yelling and punching and banging his head. He was immediately placed into a private room, and, after a brief attempt, it was determined that no examination would be safely possible. Since the underlying ophthalmic pathology was still uncertain, it was decided that an examination under general anesthesia would need to be undertaken. Consent was obtained from the parents, and they were returned to the ED for sedation but instead decided to take the patient home as it was felt time in a warm bath might calm him. The family was contacted by phone and asked to bring the patient back to the hospital for examination under anesthesia, but they reported that after going home and telling the patient they would not be returning to the hospital, the patient became more calm, opened his eyes, and seemed to resume his baseline level of functioning. In retrospect the patient's agitation may have been more attributable to healthcare interventions and attempts at examination than to actual underlying pathology. An early assessment of the patient's situation and ability to cope with examination and either opting for a "wait-and-watch" approach or more direct tract to examination under sedation might have provided a preferable course in this case, sparing the patient and his family multiple traumatic experiences with the healthcare system, as well as saving a significant amount of time for the patient, the family, and all of the healthcare practitioners involved.

Clinical Pearls

- Patients with ASD are known to have a higher incidence of several visual problems, including refractive error, strabismus, and amblyopia, than the general population. They also seem to manifest a number of abnormalities in higher-order visual processing.
- Patients with ASD can also present with any and every ophthalmic disease known in the general population.
- Every child with ASD should have a comprehensive examination by a pediatric ophthalmologist.
- Ophthalmic examination and management for ASD patients should be tailored for each individual based on their needs.
- Management of ophthalmic issues can be chronic, and so formation of a good rapport and taking steps to minimize apprehension about future examinations are advised.
- Abnormalities in the visual system and visual processing in individuals with ASD may contribute to some of their behavioral issues.
- Assessment of the degree of functioning should be made at the beginning of an encounter and used to guide patient interactions and goals for examination.
- In some special cases, examination under sedation may be preferable earlier rather than later.

References

1. Albrecht MA, Stuart GW, Falkmer M, et al. Brief report: visual acuity in children with autism spectrum disorders. J Autism Dev Disord. 2014;44(9):2369–74.
2. American Academy of Ophthalmology Preferred Practice Patterns Committee. Preferred practice pattern® guidelines. Comprehensive adult medical eye evaluation. San Francisco: American Academy of Ophthalmology; 2015. Available at: www.aao.org/ppp. Accessed 15 Dec 2017.
3. Anderson CJ, Colombo J, Jill Shaddy D. Visual scanning and pupillary responses in young children with autism spectrum disorder. J Clin Exp Neuropsychol. 2006;28(7):1238–56.
4. Black K, McCarus C, Collins ML, Jensen A. Ocular manifestations of autism in ophthalmology. Strabismus. 2013;21(2):98–102.
5. Blake R, Turner LM, Smoski MJ, Pozdol SL, Stone WL. Visual recognition of biological motion is impaired in children with autism. Psychol Sci. 2003;14(2):151–7.
6. Briegel W, Schimek M, Kamp-Becker I. Moebius sequence and autism spectrum disorders – less frequently associated than formerly thought. Res Dev Disabil. 2010;31(6):1462–6.

7. Brosnan MJ, Gwilliam LR, Walker IJ. Brief report: the relationship between visual acuity, the embedded figures test and systemizing in autism spectrum disorder. J Autism Dev Disord. 2012;42(11):2491–7.
8. Chawarska K, Shic F. Looking but not seeing: atypical visual scanning and recognition of faces in 2 and 4-year-old children with autism spectrum disorder. J Autism Dev Disord. 2009;39(12):1663–72.
9. Chiu M, Watson S. Xerophthalmia and vitamin A deficiency in an autistic child with a restricted diet. BMJ Case Rep. 2015;5:2015.
10. Cléry H, Bonnet-Brilhault F, Lenoir P, Barthelemy C, Bruneau N, Gomot M. Atypical visual change processing in children with autism: an electrophysiological study. Psychophysiology. 2013;50(3):240–52.
11. Dakin S, Frith U. Vagaries of visual perception in autism. Neuron. 2005;48(3):497–507.
12. Davis RA, Bockbrader MA, Murphy RR, Hetrick WP, O'Donnell BF. Subjective perceptual distortions and visual dysfunction in children with autism. J Autism Dev Disord. 2006;36(2):199–210.
13. Ezegwui IR, Lawrence L, Aghaji AE, et al. Refractive errors in children with autism in a developing country. Niger J Clin Pract. 2014;17(4):467–70.
14. Furman JM, Osorio MJ, Minshew NJ. Visual and vestibular induced eye movements in verbal children and adults with autism. Autism Res. 2015;8:658–67.
15. Frey HP, Molholm S, Lalor EC, Russo NN, Foxe JJ. Atypical cortical representation of peripheral visual space in children with an autism spectrum disorder. Eur J Neurosci. 2013;38(1):2125–38.
16. Grossman RB, Steinhart E, Mitchell T, McIlvane W. "Look who's talking!" Gaze patterns for implicit and explicit audio-visual speech synchrony detection in children with high-functioning autism. Autism Res. 2015;8(3):307–16.
17. Guy J, Mottron L, Berthiaume C, Bertone A. The developmental trajectory of contrast sensitivity in autism spectrum disorder. Autism Res. 2015;9(8):866–78.
18. Happé FG. Studying weak central coherence at low levels: children with autism do not succumb to visual illusions. A research note. J Child Psychol Psychiatry. 1996;37(7):873–7.
19. Ikeda J, Davitt BV, Ultmann M, Maxim R, Cruz OA. Brief report: incidence of ophthalmologic disorders in children with autism. J Autism Dev Disord. 2013;43(6):1447–51.
20. Isler JR, Martien KM, Grieve PG, Stark RI, Herbert MR. Reduced functional connectivity in visual evoked potentials in children with autism spectrum disorder. Clin Neurophysiol. 2010;121(12):2035–43.
21. Johansson M, Gillberg C, Råstam M. Autism spectrum conditions in individuals with Möbius sequence, CHARGE syndrome and oculo-auriculo-vertebral spectrum: diagnostic aspects. Res Dev Disabil. 2010;31(1):9–24.
22. Kabatas EU, Ozer PA, Ertugrul GT, Kurtul BE, Bodur S, Alan BE. Initial ophthalmic findings in Turkish children with Autism Spectrum Disorder. J Autism Dev Disord. 2015;45(8):2578–81.
23. Lavoie J, Maziade M, Hébert M. The brain through the retina: the flash electroretinogram as a tool to investigate psychiatric disorders. Prog Neuro-Psychopharmacol Biol Psychiatry. 2014;48:129–34.
24. Nebel MB, Eloyan A, Nettles CA, et al. Intrinsic visual-motor synchrony correlates with social deficits in autism. Biol Psychiatry. 2016;79(8):633–41.
25. Manning C, Tibber MS, Charman T, Dakin SC, Pellicano E. Enhanced integration of motion information in children with autism. J Neurosci. 2015;35(18):6979–86.
26. McCurry TC, Lawrence LM, Wilson ME, Mayo L. The plusoptiX S08 photoscreener as a vision screening tool for children with autism. J AAPOS. 2013;17(4):374–7.
27. Pensiero S, Fabbro F, Michieletto P, Accardo A, Brambilla P. Saccadic characteristics in autistic children. Funct Neurol. 2009;24(3):153–8.
28. Pineles SL, Avery RA, Liu GT. Vitamin B12 optic neuropathy in autism. Pediatrics. 2010;126(4):e967–70.
29. Schwarzkopf DS, Anderson EJ, de Haas B, White SJ, Rees G. Larger extrastriate population receptive fields in autism spectrum disorders. J Neurosci. 2014;34(7):2713–24.
30. Shafai F, Armstrong K, Iarocci G, Oruc I. Visual orientation processing in autism spectrum disorder: no sign of enhanced early cortical function. J Vis. 2015;15(15):18.
31. Shi L, Zhou Y, Ou J, et al. Different visual preference patterns in response to simple and complex dynamic social stimuli in preschool-aged children with autism spectrum disorders. PLoS One. 2015;10(3):e0122280.
32. Steinemann TL, Christiansen SP. Vitamin A deficiency and xerophthalmia in an autistic child. Arch Ophthalmol. 1998;116(3):392–3.
33. Stewart CR, Sanchez SS, Grenesko EL, et al. Sensory symptoms and processing of nonverbal auditory and visual stimuli in children with autism spectrum disorder. J Autism Dev Disord. 2016;46(5):1590–601.
34. Stroganova TA, Butorina AV, Sysoeva OV, et al. Altered modulation of gamma oscillation frequency by speed of visual motion in children with autism spectrum disorders. J Neurodev Disord. 2015;7(1):21.

Otolaryngology

9

John M. Dobrowski, Donald Keamy Jr, and Molly A. Dobrowski

Introduction

It is essential that any individual with autism spectrum disorder (ASD) who is referred to an otolaryngologist be thoroughly evaluated anatomically and functionally. The contribution that the otolaryngologist's examination provides is paramount in the overall context of any patient's diagnosis and health maintenance, and this is particularly true for patients with ASD.

The otolaryngologist is often consulted before other specialists, as many patients with ASD first come to clinical attention due to speech and language delays and may be referred for concerns about a possible hearing impairment [11]. Regardless of the patient's age, the otolaryngologist will do a comprehensive regional exam and order appropriate testing for the evaluation of the patient's or family's concerns and symptoms. The assessments and exams may be challenging to perform depending upon the cognitive, communicative, social, and behavioral capabilities of the individual. Additionally, sensitivities to physical and sensory stimuli are common among individuals with ASD, but can be quite variable between them. Therefore test results may be incomplete, require multiple attempts to complete, or be difficult to interpret.

Individuals with ASD often have associated conditions that may include mild to severe intellectual disability, language delay, hearing impairment, mood or anxiety disorders, behavioral issues, and sleep disorders. Individuals with disorders such as fragile X syndrome, Down syndrome, tuberous sclerosis, or Rett syndrome may also have symptoms of and thus be given the co-occurring diagnosis of ASD [1, 2, 4, 14, 16, 46, 49, 53, 55, 61, 62, 64, 66]. Genetic testing is helpful in distinguishing these syndromes from non-syndromic ASD.

A Pediatric Approach to Common Conditions of the Ear, Nose, and Throat in Children with ASD

Even before a diagnosis of ASD is established, the pediatric otolaryngologist may be consulted regarding delayed sound and speech production or potential hearing impairment. Early diagnosis and intervention is of utmost importance in

J. M. Dobrowski (✉) · D. Keamy Jr
Department of Otolaryngology, Massachusetts Eye and Ear Infirmary, Massachusetts General Hospital, Boston, MA, USA
e-mail: john_dobrowski@meei.harvard.edu; donald_keamyjr@meei.harvard.edu

M. A. Dobrowski
St. Louis University School of Nursing, and at Amego, Inc., Boston, MA, USA

E. P. Hazen, C. J. McDougle (eds.), *The Massachusetts General Hospital Guide to Medical Care in Patients with Autism Spectrum Disorder*, Current Clinical Psychiatry,
https://doi.org/10.1007/978-3-319-94458-6_9

ASD. The otolaryngologist can play an important role in identifying at-risk children, making referral for further diagnostic evaluation, and initiating supportive therapies [4, 5, 7, 25, 26, 35, 48].

Establishing a trusting relationship with a child with ASD often takes time and may take multiple follow-up visits. The child may grow more receptive and communicative after becoming familiar with the office environment, the testing facility, and overall surroundings. Office visits should be arranged early in the day, when the office may be quieter, and integrated into the child's normal routine as much as possible. Waiting room times should be kept brief and to a minimum [7]. The physician should select staff members who are experienced and have interacted with patients with ASD or those with similar difficulties in the past. When communicating with patients with ASD, it is important to use direct, short, and simple explanations and to prepare the patient in advance for any casual contact, loud noises, or bright lights during the exam. Use of the verbiage "first we will do_______ and then_______" can be helpful. A calm, supportive atmosphere and constant positive reinforcement during the exam and any procedures will help decrease anxiety in the patient [7, 19, 67].

Even with all of the above measures, it can be very challenging to complete all that the physician, medical professional, or technician desires to accomplish during the scheduled visit time. It may be preferable to reschedule a visit promptly when fatigue is identified or resistance is encountered and to follow the lead of the patient's parents or caregivers, as they generally know their child best.

Symptoms associated with acute or chronic medical conditions are not always clearly verbalized in the pediatric ASD population, but may manifest as anxiety, agitation, aggression, self-injury, temper tantrums, or other changes in behavior. Parents and caregivers must be mindful of this and seek help from the patient's doctors when they observe changes in behavior or emotions and subtle symptoms of illness.

Compliance with recommended regimens and medication administration are often best incorporated into routine schedules. Open access and communication between the physician's office and the parents or caregivers can allay fears that emerge and can provide reassurance, allow for a check on progress and recovery, or prompt quick action when uncertainty persists.

History

A history should be gathered from parents, grandparents, siblings, other physicians, teachers, caregivers, and allied health professionals involved in the initial and continued evaluation of the child. It can be helpful to send a questionnaire prior to the appointment so that caregivers can concentrate and answer pertinent questions at a time when they are not distracted, as may occur during the child's actual visit.

Overall, an important goal of the history is to establish a baseline of function and anatomy from which to monitor an individual's development in speech and sound production, receptive and expressive language development, auditory functioning, and reciprocal communication skills. Oral motor structures, swallowing, sleep issues, and notation of any dysmorphic facial features should be examined, discussed, and noted. Observations by parents, caregivers, primary care physicians, and therapists should be included as part of a comprehensive and detailed medical history. Focus is given to the history regarding developmental milestones with emphasis on speech and sound production, history of ear infections, oral motor difficulties, sleep disturbances, and concerns about possible hearing difficulties. Information regarding social interaction, avoidance and withdrawal from these situations, and behavioral concerns should be included in the discussion.

A history of sleep disturbances, snoring, apnea, insomnia, parasomnias, leg movement, and quality of sleep should be reviewed with the patient and the caregivers.

Physical Examination

Exams can be challenging as the level of disability and presentation of symptoms vary widely among individuals with ASD. The office environment can cause anxiety and agitation for many patients who are accustomed to their daily regimens, schedules, and environments. Patients' tolerance to even a casual touch, much less the ability of the patient to withstand mild to moderate invasive exams, will affect the level of cooperation during their visit. Below is an outline of the important features of a thorough ear, nose, and throat examination.

General Appearance

Note gross structural abnormalities, syndromic features, and general facial features.

Ears

Note appearance and development of the auricle and ear position. Examine and note the condition of the external ear canal, tympanic membrane, middle ear, and ossicular chain.

Hearing

An auditory evaluation may include infant screening with otoacoustic emissions (OAE), auditory brainstem response (ABR), audiogram, pure tone averages, speech reception thresholds, reflex testing, and tympanometry. Sound production and speech development may be noted, but a detailed assessment should be performed by a speech pathologist. With the advent and use of infant screening, the identification of children with hearing loss is discovered much earlier in their lives. Of course this has had the dramatic and beneficial effect of initiating treatment and therapy at a much earlier age.

An accurate assessment of hearing is of paramount importance, and repeated attempts to complete the exam by the audiologist may be necessary to achieve accurate testing results. Unfortunately, many patients with ASD experience hyperresponsiveness to auditory stimuli. If cooperation or reliable results are not achieved, then sedated, noninteractive testing may be required. The otolaryngologist will focus on hearing issues, sound production, patterns of speech, and social communication skills, including the ability and willingness of the patient to interact with others. The pediatrician is dependent upon the otolaryngologist's exam and testing results when formulating the differential diagnosis of speech and language delays. When conclusive test results indicate a sensorineural hearing impairment, early intervention in the form of hearing aids or cochlear implants have been found to be beneficial [17].

Establishing normal peripheral hearing through pure tone audiological testing does not prove normal central auditory processing [5, 15]. A peripheral audiological assessment which measures the function of the ear and primary ascending auditory pathways is limited to testing the integrity of the peripheral auditory system [60]. It does not confirm normal central auditory processing and system function [15, 32, 65]. Audiologists will report that hearing is adequate for speech and language development once peripheral hearing has been established [12, 15]. Davis and Stieger cautioned against making this claim because central auditory deficits can exist in the presence of a normal peripheral auditory system and this can impede the acquisition of speech and language [15]. Individuals with ASD have reported difficulty in listening in the presence of background noise as well as maintaining focus on auditory stimuli. Evidence of this is seen in adult patients with ASD who have normal peripheral hearing thresholds yet report that the way in which they process auditory stimuli is inconsistent and that their ability to utilize auditory information declines under conditions of sensory stress.

There is no consensus in the literature regarding the prevalence of hearing impairment among children with ASD [5]. Rosenhall and colleagues reported that individuals with ASD have a tenfold greater prevalence of hearing loss than the general population [52]. More recently, Meinzen-Derr reported in a study of 24 children with a dual diagnosis of ASD and hearing impairment that there is a 1.7–4% increase in possibility of hearing loss in those diagnosed with ASD [38]. However, on detailed examination of the literature, the variation in prevalence estimates of hearing impairment may be attributed to differences between study methodologies, sample size, and inconsistencies in subject inclusion criteria [8, 32, 48, 50, 52, 60].

Nose

The appearance and structure of the nose, patency, septal deviation, turbinate hypertrophy, nasal congestion from allergies, chronic rhinitis, or the inability to coordinate the act of blowing one's nose should be examined and documented. Because the sense of smell is subjective, it may be difficult to assess in a patient who has impairments in communication.

Oral Pharynx

Mouth and lip appearance, lip closure, occlusion, arch and width of the hard palate, length and competence of the soft palate, tongue size, oral strength and coordination, swallowing function, and management of saliva should be assessed. Complications may be caused by a cleft lip or palate particularly as it relates to swallowing, voice production, Eustachian tube function, and effects on middle ear ventilation. The frenulum of the tongue and the frenulum of the upper or lower lips should be examined. If the child is still breastfeeding, coordination of sucking and swallowing should be noted.

Larynx

Alterations in voice or presence of stridor will necessitate direct inspection of vocal cord appearance and mobility and observation of nodules or lesions, as well as glottis or subglottic narrowing from obstruction or stricture.

Pharynx and Upper Esophagus

The natural coordinated action of swallowing, even swallowing normal salivary secretions, may not be present, so oral competence, pharyngeal musculature coordination, and ease of swallowing should be carefully noted. A prior history of drooling, reflux, or frequent spitting and regurgitation is likewise important, and complaints or symptoms of dysphagia, achalasia, and stricture may be more dramatic and require interventional studies to confirm.

Neck

The general appearance of the neck should be visually and manually inspected and palpated to identify findings of a webbed neck, limited mobility, cranial nerve function, and overall musculoskeletal strength with or without normal supportive structures. The presence of palpable lymph nodes, cysts, or masses needs to be identified and investigated.

Treatment of Common Conditions

Speech and Language Development

The evaluation and management of speech and language development parallels the evaluation of the patient's hearing. Coordination and collaboration between the audiologist and speech therapist is paramount, and coordinated discussions, consultations, and therapy will support the development of receptive and expressive communication to the best of the child's ability.

Hearing Impairment

Interestingly, it has been noted that when there is coexistence of hearing loss and ASD, an initial diagnosis is made of one entity, but unfortunately, it often leads to a delay in diagnosing the other [30, 48].

Behavioral audiometry can be challenging in patients with ASD and should be attempted by experienced audiologists. The testing frequently requires two audiologists working together in a coordinated effort to achieve reliable results.

Even with experience, patience, and maximum effort, it is not uncommon to arrive at inconclusive findings using behavioral audiometry. In these cases, auditory brainstem response (ABR) testing is employed to obtain audiometric data [32]. However, if a child is unable to fall asleep after feeding or sleep deprivation, this test may require the use of anesthesia. The establishment of normal or abnormal peripheral hearing has profound consequences, as patients with ASD are already at risk for speech and language delay; thus, an unrecognized hearing loss will further compromise development of language.

In patients whose results show a mild to profound conductive or sensorineural hearing loss, audiologists and physicians will jointly endorse recommendations for the most effective way to treat the problem. Treatments may include bilateral myringotomy and pressure equalization (PE) tube placement, hearing aids, and possibly cochlear implants, depending upon the cause of the hearing impairment.

The discussion should include thought on the patient's suspected tolerance of these devices, as well as ways to prevent noncompliance and destruction of the devices. Hypersensitivity to sound stimuli in some individuals has to be considered, and discussing and implementing coping strategies can mitigate failure and improve compliance. Consequently, all treatment options need to be considered for hearing impairment in a patient who also has ASD.

Ear Infections

It is a recommendation from the American Academy of Otolaryngology and Head and Neck Surgery that clinicians offer bilateral PE tube insertion to children who have persisting otitis media effusion (OME) for 3 months or longer and documented hearing difficulties. In addition, PE tubes should be considered for any child affected by recurrent acute otitis media or OME of any duration who is at increased risk for speech, language, or learning problems from the conductive loss caused by the otitis media. If a conductive hearing loss is encountered, middle ear effusions are present, and there has been a history of frequent ear infections, then removal of fluid from the middle ear by means of myringotomy and placement of PE tubes can reverse this process. In doing so, a conductive hearing loss can be reversed, and a resulting language delay may be improved. Antibiotic therapy for persisting serous otitis media, without signs of acute bacterial infection, is not generally recommended [51].

Tonsils and Adenoids

The size and shape of the tonsils and adenoids can affect the upper airway during wakefulness and sleep. Recurrent infections and nasal obstruction can affect midfacial growth and development. Removal of the tonsils and adenoids may be necessary to facilitate breathing and swallowing and to eliminate snoring or potential sleep issues. Enlarged tonsils and adenoids may obstruct the posterior nares and contribute to rhinitis. The lingual tonsils, which are positioned at the base of the tongue just above the voice box, and esophagus are not easily visualized. If inflamed, they can also cause upper airway obstruction, impede swallowing, and affect the quality of the voice. When hypertrophy of the lingual tonsils causes deleterious effects, surgical correction should be considered.

Recurrent throat infections, particularly those caused by group A beta hemolytic streptococci, are an indication for tonsillectomy when recorded at a frequency of seven episodes in 1 year, five episodes per year within 2 years, or three episodes within 3 years. Certainly, compounding clinical history such as poor oral intake or refusal of key medications due to the pharyngitis will modify these strict guidelines. However, the decision to proceed with surgical intervention needs to be weighed against the increased risk of complications reported in patients with craniofacial disorders, Down syndrome, cerebral palsy, major heart disease, and bleeding diatheses as well as in children younger than 3 years of age with proven sleep-disordered breathing as seen on polysomnogram. Approximately 1.3% of patients experience delayed discharge for fluid hydration and pain management or oxygen desaturation, and 3.9% will have secondary complications requiring readmission, including dehydration, pain management, or bleeding. The rate of primary hemorrhage after surgery has ranged from 0.2% to 2.2% and the rate of secondary hemorrhage (more than 24 h after surgery) from 0.1% to 3%. Mortality for tonsillectomy has been estimated at a rate between 1 in 16,000 and 1 in 35,000. Regardless, the decision to perform a tonsillectomy and adenoidectomy needs to be carefully weighed with meticulous attention to the risks and benefits of the procedure prior to commencement [3].

Allergic Rhinitis

Generally, repeated exposures to an allergen are necessary to initiate an allergic environmental response; thus a specific seasonal environmental allergy may not be diagnosed before the age of 2 years. Family history is often found to contribute significantly in these situations. Environmental allergies affect the nasal and pulmonary airways by causing turbinate swelling, nasal congestion, and constriction of the airway. The swelling of the upper and lower airways is manifested as upper airway stridor or lower airway pulmonary wheezing and asthma. Food allergies can be identified much earlier in life, as in the case of milk, which often manifests with gastrointestinal symptoms. Oral antihistamines and nasal steroid sprays in pediatric formulations are available and beneficial. First-generation antihistamines such as diphenhydramine can cause a paradoxical reaction in some patients. Rather than cause drowsiness as seen in adults, diphenhydramine may cause stimulation and agitated behavior in some children. Paradoxical behavioral changes occur less commonly with second- and third-generation antihistamines. Desensitization, in the form of sublingual therapy or subcutaneous injections, can be of great benefit for individuals who cannot tolerate oral or nasal medications [31].

Sinusitis

At birth the sinuses are partially developed and require further pneumatization to fully mature at approximately 13–15 years of age. Repeated episodes of nasal congestion and mucopurulent secretions may indicate inflammation and early obstruction of the sinuses. These need to be distinguished from the common and frequent nonbacterial, viral self-limiting rhinitis of childhood. Additional conditions of ciliary dysfunction magnify the frequency and complexity of sinus infections. The use of saline nasal rinses should be encouraged as they are often tremendously soothing and helpful in reducing or eliminating mucus and bacterial accumulation. Of course this may need to be done with some prompting and encouragement, but once established as a routine, it is welcome and even requested by some patients with ASD. Cultures of the nasal passages may identify colonized nasal bacteria but frequently do not correlate with true sinus pathogens within the sinus cavities. Lack of response to empiric antibiotic treatment necessitates obtaining cultures by means of surgical intervention with the intention to ventilate and irrigate the sinus cavities.

Sleep Disturbances

There is a higher rate of sleep disturbances in children with ASD compared to typically developing children, although there is no evidence of an increased prevalence of obstructive sleep apnea (OSA) [43]. Sleep issues in ASD are also discussed in more detail in Chap. 11. Pediatric otolaryngologists are instrumental in evaluating obstructive sleep disturbances in the ASD population. Sleep disturbances can be related to nasal and oral pharyngeal obstruction but can often be related to insomnia and sleep fragmentation independent of obstruction. Often other forms of sleep disruption, insomnia, and parasomnias are exacerbated by obstructive sleep apnea. Therefore, diagnosis and treatment of underlying obstructive sleep apnea is an important initial goal.

Children with ASD more commonly have problems with sleep onset and maintenance of sleep when compared to their typical peers. Irregular sleep-wake patterns, problems with sleep onset, and early waking associated with overall poor sleep and sleep routine have been found at all developmental levels, with increasing severity at lower developmental levels [33, 44].

Overnight polysomnogram (PSG) is the gold standard in the diagnosis of pediatric obstructive sleep apnea. Most but not all children with ASD tolerate the study very well, despite the potential difficulties associated with sensory concerns related to placement of monitoring leads and equipment. It is prudent to obtain PSG data prior to considering adenotonsillectomy in children with developmental delay as a means of developing baseline information, even when there is a strong history of sleep-disordered breathing.

There are many tools and techniques that will help children with ASD and their families feel informed and relaxed when undergoing a sleep study. The use of social stories, a visit to the sleep lab, and favorite books, as well as providing any items of comfort during the study, can be extremely helpful when an overnight sleep study is requested and performed. These approaches are outlined in more detail in Chap. 4.

Obstructive sleep apnea in children is most commonly caused by enlarged tonsils and adenoids; therefore the primary treatment is adenotonsillectomy. For a patient with ASD, additional discussion, preparation, and support by a team of individuals involved in preoperative preparation, postoperative recovery, and follow-up will be required. If a trial of continuous positive airway pressure (CPAP) is warranted, proper fitting by a therapist skilled in pediatric positive pressure therapy is needed; often an acclimation period at home may be helpful in acceptance of the CPAP mask. However, the tactile sensory stimulation of the mask may be too overwhelming for some patients and may interfere with the use of CPAP altogether.

Sensory Issues: Olfactory and Taste

Studies performed by Bennetto and colleagues at the University of Rochester found that participants with ASD were "significantly less accurate in identifying sour and bitter tastes" and concluded that "True differences exist in taste and olfactory identification in ASD"[6]. Others have also confirmed altered taste in patients with ASD [40, 45, 47, 58]. These alterations may contribute to limited diets in which children with ASD accept only a small number of foods.

Pica

Individuals with ASD may exhibit pica, which is characterized by the ingestion of substances that are largely nonnutritive, such as dirt, paint chips, or coffee grounds, that has persisted for greater than 1 month in circumstances where eating such objects is considered developmentally inappropriate. This behavior can lead to contamination in children, for example, through lead poisoning associated with the ingestion of paint chips, which in turn can lead to further developmental delays and other medical problems. Pica can also cause nutritional deficiencies, parasitosis, and occasional surgical emergencies due to esophageal or intestinal obstruction. Symptoms of pica should be addressed when talking to caregivers. The otolaryngologist may be called upon to treat patients who have ingested substances that are dangerous and even life-threatening. Liquids such as cleaning supplies could burn and damage the mouth, throat, or esophagus, leaving permanent stricture. Items that become lodged in the throat must be removed either in the office or more often in the controlled setting of the operating room. Treatment varies depending on the location and form of the foreign body and the need for intravenous sedation or general anesthesia. In repeated episodes, a behavioral plan must be instituted to address this dangerous and at times life-threatening disorder [36].

Pediatric Otolaryngic Surgical Procedures

Preoperative preparation and planning are imperative for surgical procedures. Procedures for patients with ASD should be scheduled early in the morning, which can reduce the likelihood that the patient may eat or drink prior to the surgery. Social stories, picture icons, favorite books, a tour of the facility, meeting staff, and demonstration of the use of a breathing mask are all strategies that may be of great benefit [54].

On the day of the procedure, all members of the operating room team should be comforting and supportive. Noise, harsh lights, and confusion should be minimized.

Weighted blankets can be very helpful and comforting for many patients with ASD. Premedication in the form of intranasal, sublingual, or intramuscular injection may be necessary and is the most reliable method to decrease anxiety and improve cooperation. Restraints are not recommended during induction, and parents may wish to be present and assist by holding and gently caressing the child until the child is asleep.

Postoperatively, there are also many considerations that will make the recovery less stressful for the patient and family. When circumstances allow, recovery in the familiar environment of the patient's home is best, provided adequate supervision is available.

Pain management requires a thorough understanding of the instruction for delivery of the prescribed scheduled medication and diligent monitoring by the caregivers because individuals with ASD are often unable to communicate their level of postoperative pain. It is important that patients receive pain medications for their discomfort in order to avoid unnecessary distress and suffering. Proper hydration is critical. Fluids need to be strongly encouraged and monitored, especially in the case of postoperative tonsillectomy or oral surgery. Postoperative emergency room visits or readmissions are occasionally necessary and unfortunately can add extra anxiety for ASD patients due to disruption of their routine and the environment in which they are most comfortable [53].

Clinical Vignette # 1

RS is a 2-year-old boy with pronounced speech delay and a diagnosis of ASD. According to his parents, he passed the newborn hearing screening, but subsequent audiograms have been inconsistent. He is receiving early childhood developmental services, but there remain questions about the status of his hearing.

On examination in the clinic, the patient is noted to have bilateral middle ear effusions. It is unclear how long the effusions have been present. By history, he has had two episodes of acute otitis media in the past 6 months. An audiogram is attempted with tympanogram. The audiologist is not able to discern hearing thresholds at any frequency and finds flat tympanograms.

Options for this child include further observation of effusions, consideration of tympanostomy tubes, and obtaining a sedated auditory brainstem response (ABR) test. From the perspective of his speech delay and ASD, this child is considered "at risk" for speech delay related to the effusions and hearing loss. In this setting, it is reasonable to place tympanostomy tubes without waiting 3 months for the middle ear fluid to resolve. Additionally, placement of tympanostomy tubes allows for a sedated ABR test during the same operative setting.

Findings during the procedure demonstrate mucoid effusions that are suctioned from both middle ears, and PE tubes are placed in the tympanic membranes bilaterally. ABR testing reveals normal hearing thresholds after the removal of the effusions.

Early speech and language delays are a hallmark of ASD, so it is imperative to determine hearing levels and any changes in hearing as quickly as possible. Therefore, myringotomy and tympanostomy tube placement may not only relieve the conductive loss but also allow for a sedated ABR to effectively test hearing levels.

Clinical Vignette # 2

PJ is a 6-year-old boy with ASD. He has significant difficulty initiating and maintaining sleep. When he does sleep, there is audible snoring, but his parents are unable to confirm respiratory pauses or true apneas. He was started on melatonin by his pediatrician with some improvement in sleep initiation, but he still wakes up frequently at night and has a difficult time falling back to sleep after awakening.

On physical exam PJ has significantly enlarged tonsils and obvious mouth breathing.

His height and weight are in the 15th percentile for his age. Based on his history and exam, there is clinical suspicion for obstructive sleep apnea (OSA).

A sleep study is ordered and demonstrates severe obstructive sleep apnea (Apnea Hypopnea Index [AHI] 15.0/h). Based on this, his history, and his physical exam, adenotonsillectomy is recommended.

The patient undergoes an uncomplicated adenotonsillectomy and is discharged to his home on postoperative day 1. He is readmitted to the hospital 3 days later for dehydration and refusal to drink fluids. After intravenous hydration and pain management, he and his parents are coached to employ techniques for adequate oral intake and pain management, such as delivering small sips of liquids frequently, providing acetaminophen suppositories for pain control, and administering small partial doses of pain medicine at frequent intervals. He is discharged 2 days later with no further postoperative difficulties.

At his postoperative visit, his parents note that his sleep has improved. He is sleeping better with less frequent awakenings although he still does not sleep as well as his siblings. His snoring has resolved, and his parents note that they feel his overall daytime mood and behavior have improved. Additionally, his oral intake is better than it had been before the surgery. A postoperative study reveals resolution of his sleep apnea with an AHI of 1.0/h. He is referred to a sleep medicine specialist to further treat his remaining sleep disruption.

This clinical vignette highlights the broad impact of OSA on growth, development, and behavior. While sleep disruption and insomnia are common in patients with ASD, these conditions are even more pronounced if there is OSA as well. This case demonstrates that treatment of OSA can improve sleep and reduce the impact of concurrent sleep disorders but also that further management may be necessary.

Approach to Common Conditions of the Ear, Nose, and Throat in Adults with ASD

History

As with pediatric ASD patients, a history is gathered from data and discussions with parents, grandparents, siblings, other physicians, teachers, caregivers, and allied health professionals and therapists involved in the initial and continued evaluation of the patient. Forms with questions about medical history, current medications, current concerns, and contact information of consulting physicians should be sent to parents or caregivers well in advance of the scheduled office visit so that they can be filled out in a tranquil, uninterrupted environment. Most often the adult patient has a preexisting diagnosis of ASD, but on rare occasions adults may be newly diagnosed [35, 37, 61, 62]. In addition, while treating adult patients, it is important to establish whether the patient has medical decision-making capacity or whether he has a legal guardian responsible for making these decisions. Consent from the legal guardian must be obtained prior to any non-emergent medical evaluation or treatment.

Physical Examination

Depending upon the cooperation and tolerance of the patient, the otolaryngology examination may be difficult to complete. Each individual tolerates touch and mild to moderate invasive stimuli and reacts to being approached by strangers or "white coats" in various ways. The examination is dependent upon the patient's oral motor strength and coordination, cognitive ability, sensory defensiveness, and overall cooperation during the exam.

General Appearance

Posture, gait, repetitive behaviors, gross structural abnormalities, syndromic features, and general facial features are assessed.

Ears

The general appearance, auricle development, and location and symmetry of the ears are documented. The size, shape, and appearance of the external ear canal and presence of cerumen accumulation are noted and removed if present. Inspection of the tympanic membrane, middle ear pneumatization, and the ossicular chain must be visualized as irregularities in these structures may be the cause of a conductive hearing impairment, which can interfere with the audiological evaluation.

Hearing

An auditory evaluation should encompass audiogram with or without behavioral audiometry techniques, pure tone averages, speech reception thresholds, speech discrimination, reflex testing, tympanometry, and ABR testing as necessary to confirm and/or monitor hearing levels.

Communication

Speech and language development and cognitive assessments are impacted by apraxia or aphasia. Apraxia is a motor disorder. It is the inability to perform motor planning. A person with apraxia cannot move their lips or tongue to the correct place to say sounds even though the muscles may not be weak. The messages from the brain to the mouth are disrupted. Aphasia on the other hand is the inability to comprehend and formulate language because of dysfunction in specific brain regions. It may range from inability to find a word to express oneself to the loss of the ability to speak, read, or write. Physical capability and cooperation by the individual during assessment and treatment are paramount for success.

Nose

General appearance, structure, and patency of passage should be documented. The patency can be compromised by septal deviation, turbinate hypertrophy, allergic congestion, mucous and chronic rhinitis, or the lack of ability to coordinate clearing one's nose. Finally, if possible and since it is a subjective sensation that often requires communication to confirm, the assessment of the sense of smell is useful.

Oral Cavity and Oropharynx

Mouth and lip appearance, muscular strength, closure of lips, occlusion and alignment of teeth, arch and width of palate, length of soft palate, tonsil size, tongue size, strength and coordination, swallowing function, drooling, presence of cleft lip, and/or palate repair should be noted. The frenulum of the tongue and the frenulum of the upper or lower lips may remain present from childhood and can interfere with tongue or lip mobility. Salivary flow and coordination of swallowing may be readily apparent. The use of anticholinergic medications such as glycopyrrolate can reduce salivary flow in cases of drooling. Lingual tonsillar hypertrophy may not be obvious due to anatomical position, but needs to be evaluated when symptoms of snoring, apnea, or dysphagia are present.

Hypopharynx and Upper Esophagus

History of drooling and swallowing difficulties may highlight a prior history of reflux, dysphagia, achalasia, or stricture. Achalasia of the esophagus is failure of the smooth muscle fibers to relax. This causes a sphincter muscle to remain closed and fails to open when needed or in the case of esophageal achalasia a dysmotility of the esophageal smooth muscle layer. New onset of symptoms needs to be evaluated for developing pathology.

Larynx

Voice quality or changes that are not attributed to maturation require inspection of the vocal cords' appearance noting mobility and presence of any nodules, lesions, or strictures. Stridor, the abnormal sounds from airflow narrowing, may indicate glottis or subglottic narrowing or obstruction.

Neck

General appearance noting scars or anatomical variance, neck and muscular mobility, the presence of a webbed neck, cranial nerve function, musculoskeletal strength, firm or cystic masses, variations of normal structure, cervical lymph nodes, and thyroid size and nodularity should be examined.

Studies

As with the pediatric studies, the capability and willingness of the patient to cooperate may determine the ability of the tester to obtain consistent and reliable results in individuals diagnosed with ASD.

Hearing and Balance and Speech Evaluation

Audiogram techniques are employed using verbal and visual reinforcement in order to engage patients to assess hearing. Auditory brainstem response (ABR), acoustic reflex, and otoacoustic emissions do not require participation but the ability to lie motionless and can be used to assess hearing levels. A tympanogram requires the ability to tolerate sensory stimulation but provides information about middle ear aeration of fluid. Vestibular testing and vestibular rehabilitation may be difficult due to sensory stimulation if imbalance is apparent.

Radiographic Evaluation of Head, Neck, and Swallowing

CT of temporal bones, CT of sinuses, and MRI of temporal bones may require sedation or IV administration of contrast material. Ultrasound of the neck and salivary glands is one of the least invasive and most patient-friendly as long as the patient can tolerate skin sensory stimulation. Barium swallow, dynamic swallowing evaluation, and gastrointestinal consult and evaluation are dependent on patient cooperation.

Sleep Evaluation

Polysomnogram and CPAP titration are dependent upon the patient's ability to be connected to electrodes for brain wave monitoring. Home sleep testing can be achieved with less invasive monitoring but will only score for respiratory events and requires the cooperation of family members.

Speech and Language Evaluation

Speech and language assessment and adaptive communication assessment are dependent on patient cooperation but are essential for baseline assessment and therapeutic planning.

Dental and Orthodontic Evaluation

Dental and orthodontia evaluations are often dependent upon tolerance of oral stimulation during an examination and mouth opening motor coordination and strength. Lifelong evaluation with coordinated oral hygiene, preventative, interventional, or restorative care may be required.

Treatment

Hearing

Hearing levels need to be monitored throughout the patient's life in all individuals with ASD. For those with significant communication impairment, the identification of slowly progressive hearing loss may only be identified through repeat testing. This may be stretched to every other to every fifth year based on stability of hearing. This is meant to identify hearing loss that may require hearing aids or cochlear implants that are not appreciated by the patient, family members, or caregivers. Repeat urgent audiological testing is warranted for sudden changes in hearing levels as reported by cooperative adult patients with ASD or their caregivers. Hearing assessments must be kept up to date in changing audiological situations. Continued support for those using amplification or cochlear implants is necessary along with scheduled yearly reassessments. Maintenance of equipment as needed along with physical exams to keep cerumen from accumulating in the external ear canal and impeding hearing aid function is recommended.

The confirmation of normal peripheral hearing does not always correlate with normal auditory speech perception. Adult patients with ASD may be limited by disruption in their central auditory processing. This may inhibit word recognition and the understanding of speech, especially in the presence of background noise. Evidence of this is seen in adult patients with ASD who have normal peripheral hearing thresholds yet report inconsistent processing of auditory stimuli and a decline in the ability to utilize auditory information under conditions of sensory stress [15].

Hearing aids are beneficial in managing sensorineural hearing loss but are dependent on the tolerance and compliance of the patient. Initially, assistance is required by caregivers. Cochlear implants are tremendously helpful in bilateral profound hearing loss, allowing for perception of sound and speech [17, 18, 22, 23, 28, 38, 41, 59]. However, maintenance and care of the implant need to be addressed with the patient and caregivers.

Communication

Patients benefit from multimodality communication techniques that include oral approximation of words, sign language, storyboards, and electronic augmentative communication devices [20, 21, 42, 56, 63].

Vestibular Function

Balance and coordination are often reduced in individuals with ASD with variability in core balance. Activity levels may also be reduced but will improve with physical therapy, therapeutic horseback riding, community activities (such as YMCA and Special Olympics), and a structured fitness schedule at the individual's school or adult day habilitation programs [63]. Changes observed by the individual or caregiver need to be reported and addressed. Vestibular testing and occasional vestibular rehabilitation for balance disturbances may be indicated.

Radiographic Evaluation

CT images of the temporal bones should be obtained when hearing loss is diagnosed to identify possible structural abnormalities. Additional information may be gleaned from MR images, which more accurately enhance soft tissue and fluid structures. Ultrasound of soft tissue masses can be less intrusive and better tolerated by patients with ASD.

Abnormal soft tissue structures within the head and neck such as cysts or masses need appropriate evaluation. Imaging studies such as ultrasound, CT, and MRI define the anatomical structures in association to surrounding normal structures.

Surgical Procedures

Needle aspiration of cystic or solid masses provides cells for cytological evaluation or culture and can often confirm a suspected diagnosis. However, excisional biopsy will provide definitive pathologic diagnosis, culture material, or tissue for specialized processing. Understandably, it is a more intrusive procedure for a patient with ASD to endure and often requires intravenous sedation or general anesthesia.

Surgical intervention should be carefully considered and the risks and benefits weighed before being undertaken. Regardless of age, special considerations and arrangements for the surgical setting and postoperative care must be considered and addressed as part of the surgical planning. This has been outlined in more detail in the pediatric surgical procedure section above and in Chap. 4 on "Medical Procedures: Challenges and Strategies."

Sinuses

Nasal congestion and blockage, recurrent upper respiratory illness, poor nasal hygiene, and inability to coordinate blowing or clearing the nose may result in chronic rhinitis or sinusitis. Sinus cysts, obstruction, internal nasal deformities such as deviated nasal septum and turbinate hypertrophy, nasal polyposis, and tumors of the paranasal sinus are identified through radiographic imaging; thus CT or MR images of the sinuses may be necessary. Plain films do not generally give reliable results. Lateral films may confirm adenoid, tonsil, and lingual tonsil hypertrophy and upper airway obstruction. Surgical interventions performed to open, ventilate, and culture obstructed sinuses are mostly performed under general anesthesia.

Sleep

Sleep disturbance may be identified in childhood or emerge later in life. Obesity increases the possibility of upper airway obstruction and consequently snoring, and sleep evaluation may be necessary. Home sleep studies give information about respiratory phases but can underestimate the index of obstruction. Sleep studies conducted in a sleep center provide more definitive information about neurologic sleep stages, epileptic activity, and simultaneous respiratory and cardiovascular parameters. In-lab attended overnight sleep studies performed in a center are necessary for the titration of a positive airway pressure (PAP) unit, especially when a diagnosis of narcolepsy or central apnea is considered, or a comorbid condition such as a neurocognitive and cardiopulmonary disorder is present [13, 29].

Oral and Dental Care

The otolaryngologist often works cooperatively and in conjunction with dentists, periodontists, endodontists, and orthodontists in the identification of inflammatory and other related conditions. Each examination can assist the next professional, because they often identify issues that might require more definitive evaluation or treatment. During an oral exam, notation is made of unusual pressure points, tenderness, deterioration in tooth enamel, or excessive wear in the location of occlusive contact due to bruxism, as these may be signs of impending problems. Since communication is often limited, an individual patient may not complain of pain, so caregiver observations may be equally as important in identifying potential problems. Varying degrees of pain tolerance by ASD patients have been reported. Any new onset of severe sharp pain may elicit strong avoidance of examination, whereas dull constant pain may be more tolerable. This may be due to a higher pain tolerance or simply the inability of a patient with ASD to describe his symptoms [8–10, 20, 21, 24, 27, 34, 39, 42, 53, 56, 57]. When abnormalities are identified, the otolaryngologist has a responsibility to direct the patient to his respective dentist or coordinate care by personally alerting the dentist of his concerns. Dental health in patients with ASD is covered in more detail in Chap. 7.

Swallowing and Reflux

Functional swallowing difficulties are generally diagnosed and addressed early in childhood. However, dyscoordination, progressive muscular deterioration, or loss of dentition can interfere with chewing and swallowing later in life. Some of the acute mucosal changes that cause pain include aphthous ulcerations; mucosal lacerations from biting or seizures; acute viral, bacterial, or fungal infections; and reflux laryngitis and pharyngitis. Examination and coordinated management of candidiasis of the oropharynx, hypopharynx, and esophagus may be needed. Healthcare coordination between otolaryngologists, speech therapists, and gastroenterologists may be required for non-resolving conditions. Persistent swallowing disorders, management of reflux, and the treatment of helicobacter pylori infection may require further evaluation and testing by a gastroenterologist. Nutritional support and guidance for maintenance of body weight in dysphagia and conversely weight control and reduction in overweight or obese patients often require multispecialty collaboration and cooperative management.

Clinical Vignette # 3

MD is a 24-year-old female diagnosed with ASD. She had a successful soft tissue cleft palate repair at 8 months of age. MD has oral motor apraxia and is nonverbal. Her anatomical differences have presented problems throughout her 24 years of life. As a child she had multiple ear infections that required placement of PE tubes. This treatment was helpful and ear infections no longer occurred. Multiple hearing tests confirmed normal hearing.

However, sinusitis continued to be problematic for her. She was unable to clear her nose unless she sneezed, and other treatment methods were necessary. Bulb syringes or sinus rinse squeeze bottles were employed to mobilize secretions. Topical decongestants such as Neo-Synephrine and oxymetazoline were also necessary at times to provide patency of the nares. This was followed by nasal saline rinses with nasal cleansing agents such as Alkalol and nasal steroids.

Orthodontic treatment for malocclusion was required due to severe misalignment. Shortened dental roots and bruxism also placed oral care at high priority to prevent tooth loss. MD was home for a holiday break from her residential program when her parents noted sensitivity during tooth brushing and flossing of her front teeth. On closer inspection of the gingiva and alveolus, a small blister was seen indicating a dental abscess above the lateral incisor. This necessitated an emergency root canal by an endodontist.

The patient was not able to cooperate for such a procedure under local anesthesia; thus general anesthesia was required. While under anesthesia and after the root canal procedure was completed, impressions for a night guard and updated x-rays were taken. A night guard was used to minimize bruxism and resulting strain on the dental roots and to protect her teeth enamel. No dental caries were identified; otherwise these would have been addressed during the procedure.

This case illustrates the importance of oral care and hygiene as well as the need for careful examination by individuals, parents, or caregivers to monitor subtle changes in behavior for those that have limited cognitive or verbal communicative capabilities. The slightest change in behavior may indicate symptoms of a significant problem. It emphasizes the benefits of having a network of available specialists willing to evaluate and accommodate individuals with special needs. Parents and caregivers need to prioritize each individual's need for assistance with good oral hygiene and care of teeth. In this case, comprehensive dental care and treatment included many dental professionals and specialties over the years. They must have the experience, patience, willingness, office staff, and extra time required for appointments with individuals with special needs.

Clinical Pearls

- Monitor and reevaluate any ENT problems for progression in diagnosed areas.
- Subtle behavior changes in patients who have communication deficits may indicate illness or disease processes.
- Maintenance of oral, nasal, throat, and ear hygiene is particularly important in adults with ASD.
- Awareness of an individual's sensitivities and triggers is important for examiners and technicians to minimize stimulation and anxiety during examination and testing.
- Definitive evaluation and diagnoses may not be achieved during an initial consultation, and repeated visits may be necessary.
- Reschedule office visits when a patient becomes overwhelmed at an appointment to avoid future anxiety and enhance cooperation.
- Allow additional time for appointments for patients with ASD.
- Never assume all is "normal" and obtain comprehensive testing as indicated.

In complex patients with unusual behaviors, it is helpful to have multiple services working together, lending their opinions and documenting normal and abnormal examination findings to help in the differential diagnosis and overall management of the individual.

Summary

Autism spectrum disorder is characterized by a range of neurodevelopmental delays and disorders in social interaction, communication, and the presence of restricted interests or repetitive behaviors. The evaluation through detailed otolaryngic assessment and examination is essential in determining a baseline status of each individual. From this evaluation, a systematic multidisciplinary approach can be implemented for continued monitoring of progress or regression from natural development or intervention. The evaluation should begin at birth and be maintained throughout the individual's life. A coordinated effort by vigilant parents, guardians, caregivers, teachers, technicians, allied health professionals, and physicians is necessary to help these individuals reach their greatest potential. Since the majority of the special senses and motor function for these neurodevelopmental disorders reside within the head and neck, the otolaryngologist must play an important role in the examination, requisition, and interpretation of appropriate studies and coordination of needed evaluation and therapeutic intervention.

References

1. American Psychiatric Association. Autism spectrum disorder. Diagnostic and Statistical Manual of Mental Disorders (DMSV). 5th ed. Arlington: American Psychiatric Association; 2013.
2. Augustyn M. Autism spectrum disorder: terminology, epidemiology, and pathogenesis UpToDate. Wolters Kluwer. 2015. [Updated April 18, 2016 April 19, 2016] Nov 18, 2015. https://www.uptodate.com/contents/autism-spectrum-disorder-terminology-epidemiology-and-pathogenesis. Accessed 29 July 2018.
3. Baugh RF, Archer SA, Mitchell RB, Rosenfeld RM, Amin R, Burns JJ, et al. Clinical practice guideline: tonsillectomy in children. Otolaryngol Head Neck Surg. 2011;144(S1):S1–S30.
4. Beals K. Early intervention in deafness and autism: one family's experiences, reflections, and recommendations. Infants Young Child. 2004;17:28490.
5. Beers AN, McBoyle M, Kakande E, Dar Santos RC, Kozak FK. Autism and peripheral hearing loss: a systematic review. Int J Pediatr Otorhinolaryngol. 2014;78(1):96101.
6. Bennetto L, Kuschner ES, Hyman SL. Olfaction and taste processing in Autism. Biol Psychiatry. 2007;62(9):101521.
7. Biyani S, Morgan PS, Hotchkiss K, Cecchini M, Derkay CS. Autism spectrum disorder 101: a primer for pediatric otolaryngologists. Int J Pediatr Otorhinolaryngol. 2015;79(6):798802.
8. Breau LM, Camfield C, McGrath PJ, Rosmus C, Finley GA. Measuring pain accurately in children with cognitive impairments: refinement of a caregiver scale. J Pediatr Psychol. 2001;138:7217.
9. Breau LM, Camfield CS, McGrath PJ, Finley GA. The incidence of pain in children with severe cognitive impairments. Arch Pediatr Adolesc Med. 2003;157(12):121926.
10. Breau LM, McGrath PJ, Camfield C, Rosmus C, Finley GA. Preliminary validation of an observational pain checklist for persons with cognitive impairment who are unable to verbally communicate. Dev Med Child Neurol. 2000;42:60916.
11. Bridgemohan C. Autism spectrum disorder: surveillance and screening in primary care UpToDate. Wolters Kluwer. 2015. [Updated April 18, 2016 April 19, 2016]. https://www.uptodate.com/contents/autism-spectrum-disorder-surveillance-and-screening-in=primary-care. Accessed 29 July 2018.
12. Cloppert P, Williams S. Evaluating an enigma: what people with autism spectrum disorders and their parents would like audiologist to know. Semin Hear. 2005;26(4):253.
13. Collop NA, Anderson WM, Boehlecke B, Claman D, Goldberg R, Gottlieb DJ, et al. Clinical guidelines for the use of unattended portable monitors in the diagnosis of obstructive sleep apnea in adult patients. J Clin Sleep Med. 2007;3(7):73747.
14. Cop E, Yurtbasi P, Oner O, Munir KM. Genetic testing in children with autism spectrum disorders. Anadolu Psikiyatri Derg. 2015;16(6):42632.
15. Davis R, Stieger L. Towards more effective audiological assessment of children with autism spectrum disorders. Semin Hear. 2005;26(4):241.
16. DiGuiseppi C, Hepburn S, Davis JM, Fidler DJ, Hartway S, Lee NR, et al. Screening for autism spectrum disorders in children with Down syndrome: population prevalence and screening test characteristics. J Dev Behav Pediatr. 2010;31(3):18191.
17. Donaldson AI, Heavner KS, Zwolan TA. Measuring progress in children with autism spectrum disorder who have cochlear implants. Arch Otolaryngol Head Neck Surg. 2004;130:66671.
18. Edwards LC. Children with cochlear implants and complex needs: a review of outcome research and psychological practice. J Deaf Stud Deaf Educ. 2007;12:25868.
19. Elwin M, Ek L, Schroder A, Kjellin L. Autobiographical accounts of sensing in Asperger syndrome and high functioning autism. Arch Psychiatr Nurs. 2012;26(5):4209.
20. Fanurik D, Koh JL, Schmitz ML, Harrison RD, Conrad TM. Children with cognitive impairment: parent report of pain and coping. J Dev Behav Pediatr. 1999a;20:22834.
21. Fanurik D, Koh JL, Schmitz ML, Harrison RD, Robertson PK, Killebrew P. Pain assessment and treatment in children with cognitive impairment: a survey of nurses' and physicians' beliefs. Clin J Pain. 1999b;15:30412.
22. Geers AE, Nicholas JG, Sedey AL. Language skills of children with early cochlear implantation. Ear Hear. 2003;24:4658.
23. Geers AE, Strube MJ, Tobey EA, Pisoni DB, Moog JS. Epilogue: factors contributing to long term outcomes of cochlear implantation in early childhood. Ear Hear. 2011;32:8492.
24. Gillberg C. Endogenous opioids and opiate antagonists in autism: brief review of empirical findings and implications for clinicians. Dev Med Child Neurol. 1995;(3):37, 23945.

25. Greenspan SJ, Brazelton TB, Cordero J, Solomon R. Guidelines for early identification, screening, and clinical management of children with autism spectrum disorders. Pediatrics. 2008;121(4):82830.
26. Guardino CA. Identification and placement for deaf students with multiple disabilities: choosing the path less followed. Am Ann Deaf. 2008;153:5564.
27. Hadden K. Pediatric pain letter: abstracts and commentaries on pain in infants, children and adolescents. Commentary. 2000;4(1):45.
28. Hamzavi J, Baumgartner WD, Egelierler B, Franz P, Schenk B, Gstoettner W. Follow up of cochlear implanted handicapped children. Int J Pediatr Otorhinolaryngol. 2000;56(3):16974.
29. Harvey MT, Kennedy CH. Polysomnographic phenotypes in developmental disabilities. Int J Dev Neurosci. 2002;20(35):4438.
30. Jure R, Rapin I, Tuchman R. Hearing impaired autistic children. Dev Med Child Neurol. 1991;33(12):106272.
31. Jyonouchi H. Autism spectrum disorders and allergy: observation from a pediatric allergy/immunology clinic. Expert Rev Clin Immunol. 2010 May;6(3):397–411.
32. Klin A. Auditory brainstem responses in autism: brainstem dysfunction or peripheral hearing loss? J Autism Dev Disord. 1993;23(1):1535.
33. Kotagal S, Broomall E. Sleep in children with autism spectrum disorder. Pediatr Neurol. 2012;47(4):242–51.
34. LaChapelle DL, Hadjistavropoulos T, Craig KD. Pain measurement in persons with intellectual disabilities. Clin J Pain. 1999;15(1):1323.
35. Lord C, Petkova E, Hus V, Gan W, Lu F, Martin DM, et al. A multisite study of the clinical diagnosis of different autism spectrum disorders. Arch Gen Psychiatry. 2012;69:30613.
36. Matson JL, Belva B, Hattier MA, Matson ML. Pica in persons with developmental disabilities: characteristics, diagnosis, and assessment. Res Autism Spectr Disord. 2011;5(4):145964.
37. Matson JL, Rivet TT. Characteristics of challenging behaviours in adults with autistic disorder, PDDNOS, and intellectual disability. J Intellect Develop Disabil. 2008;33(4):3239.
38. Meinzen-Derr J, Wiley S, Bishop S, Manning-Courtney P, Choo DI, Murray D. Autism spectrum disorders in 24 children who are deaf or hard of hearing. Int J Pediatr Otorhinolaryngol. 2014;78(1):1128.
39. Mieres AC, Smallwood V, Nicholson SK. Retrospective case report: evaluation of pain in a child with pervasive developmental disorder. Pediatr Phys Ther. 2011;23(2):194200.
40. Nieminenvon Wendt T, Paavonen JE, Ylisaukko-Oja T, Sarenius S, Kallman T, Jarvela I, et al. Subjective face recognition difficulties, aberrant sensibility, sleeping disturbances and aberrant eating habits in families with Asperger syndrome. BMC Psychiatry. 2005;5:20.
41. Niparko JK, Tobey EA, Thai DJ, Eisenberg LS, Wang NY, AL Q, et al. Spoken language development in children following cochlear implantation. J Am Med Assoc. 2010;303:1498506.
42. Oberlander TR, O'Donnell ME, Montgomery CJ. Pain in children with significant neurological impairment. J Dev Behav Pediatr. 1999;20:23543.
43. Reynolds AM, Malow BA. Sleep and autism spectrum disorders. Pediatr Clin N Am. 2011;58(3):685–98.
44. Richdale AL. Sleep problems in autism: prevalence, cause, and intervention. Dev Med Child Neurol. 1999;41:60–6.
45. Rogers SJ, Hepburn S, Wehner E. Parent reports of sensory symptoms in toddlers with autism and those with other developmental disorders. J Autism Dev Disord. 2003;33:63142.
46. Rojahn J, Wilkins J, Matson JL, Boisjoli JA. Comparison of adults with intellectual disabilities with and without ASD on parallel measures of challenging behavior: the behavior problems inventory01 (BPI01) and Autism Spectrum Disorder Behavior problems for Intellectually Disabled Adults (ASDBPA). J Appl Res Intellect Disabil. 2010;23:17985.
47. Rolls ET, Scott TR. Central taste anatomy and neurophysiology. In: Doty RL, editor. Handbook of olfaction and gustation. 2nd ed. New York: Marcel Dekker; 2003. p. 679705.
48. Roper L, Arnold P, Monteiro B. Co-occurrence of autism and deafness: diagnostic considerations. Autism. 2003;7:24553.
49. Rosenberg RE, Law JK, Yenokyan G, McGready J, Kaufmann WE, Law PA. Characteristics and concordance of autism spectrum disorders among 277 twin pairs. Arch Pediatr Adolesc Med. 2009;163(10):90714.
50. Rosenblum SM, Arick JR, Krug DA, Stubbs EG, Young NB, Pelson RO. Auditory brainstem evoke responses in autistic children. J Autism Dev Disord. 1980;10(2):21525.
51. Rosenfeld RM, Schwartz SR, Pynnonen MA, Tunkel DE, Hussey HM, Fichera JS, et al. Clinical practice guideline: tympanostomy tubes in children. Otolaryngol Head Neck Surg. 2013;149(S1):S1–S35.
52. Rosenhall U, Johansson E, Gillberg C. Oculomotor findings in autistic children. J Laryngol Otol. 1988;102(5):4359.
53. Sandman C, Spence M, Smith M. Proopiomelanocortin (POMC) dysregulation and response to opiate blockers. Ment Retard Dev Disabil Res Rev. 1999;5:31421.
54. Seid M, Sherman M, Seid AB. Perioperative psychosocial interventions for autistic children undergoing ENT surgery. Int J Pediatr Otorhinolaryngol. 1997;40(23):10713.
55. Smith KR, Matson JL. Behavior problems: differences among intellectually disabled adults with comorbid autism spectrum disorders and epilepsy. Res Dev Disabil. 2010;31(5):10629.

56. Stallard P, Williams L, Lenton S, Velleman R. Pain in cognitively impaired, non-communicating children. Arch Dis Child. 2001;85(6):4602.
57. Stallard P, Williams L, Velleman R, Lenton S, McGrath PJ. Brief report: behaviors identified by caregivers to detect pain in non-communicating children. J Pediatr Psychol. 2002;27(2):20914.
58. Suzuki Y, Critchley HD, Rowe A, Howlin P, DGM M. Impaired olfactory identification in Asperger's syndrome. J Neuropsych Clin N. 2003; 15:1057.
59. Svirsky MA, Robbins AM, Kirk KI, Pisoni DB, Miyamoto RT. Language development in profoundly deaf children with cochlear implants. Psychol Sci. 2000;11:1538.
60. Taylor MJ, Rosenblatt B, Linschoen L. Auditory brainstem response abnormalities in autistic children. Can J Neurol Sci. 1982;9:42933.
61. Volkmar F, Siegel M, Woodbury-Smith M, King B, McCracken J, State M, et al. Practice parameter for the assessment and treatment of children and adolescents with autism spectrum disorder. J Am Acad Child Adolesc Psychiatry. 2014;53(2):23757.
62. Volkmar FR, Klin A. Issues in the classification of autism and related conditions. Volkmar FR, Klin A, Paul R, Cohen DJ. Handbook of autism and pervasive developmental disorders. 3rd Hoboken: Wiley; 2005. 541.
63. Weissman L, Bridgemohan C. Autism spectrum disorder in children and adolescents: complementary and alternative therapies. Wolters Kluwer. 2015. [Updated Oct 05, 2015 April 15, 2016]. https://www.uptodate.com/contents/autism-spectrum-disorder-in-children-and-adolescents-overview. Accessed 29 July 2018.
64. Wetherby AM, Prizant BM. Autism spectrum disorders: a transactional developmental perspective. Baltimore: Paul H. Brookes Publishing; 2000.
65. Wong V, Wong SN. Brainstem auditory evoked potential study in children with autistic disorder. J Autism Dev Disord. 1991;21(3):32940.
66. World Health Organization. The ICD10 classification of mental and behavioral disorders. Clinical descriptions and diagnostic guidelines. 2016. http://www.who.int/classifications/icd/en/bluebook.pdf.
67. Zimmer M, Desch L. Sensory integration therapies for children with developmental and behavioral disorders. Pediatrics. 2012;129(6):11869.

Cardiology

10

Jason G. Ho and Ana Maria Rosales

Introduction

Cardiac evaluation and treatment of a patient with autism spectrum disorder (ASD) can be necessary for a variety of conditions and can range from simple reassurance at a single visit to serial, lifelong evaluations that may even start before birth. On one end of this continuum, providers evaluate patients with varying symptoms to determine if there is an underlying condition or if the symptoms are likely limited in clinical significance. These chief complaints include chest pain, palpitations, shortness of breath, dizziness, syncope, exercise intolerance, and pallor.

Conversely, patients undergoing cardiac evaluation may have a form of congenital heart disease (CHD) with varying timelines of diagnosis and levels of severity. Mild forms of CHD, such as bicuspid aortic valve or atrial septal defects, may go undiagnosed for years in asymptomatic individuals, whereas severe forms of CHD are diagnosed prenatally with routine obstetric ultrasounds. Some conditions may be monitored without intervention, while others require multiple open-heart surgeries.

Independent of the reason for cardiac evaluation, providers must recognize potential barriers to good care and adapt accordingly when evaluating patients with ASD. There may be concerns to focus on, such as electrocardiogram (ECG) changes with psychotropic medications, as well as the need to adjust the interaction with the child and the family to adequately evaluate the history and physical in the setting of children who have special needs.

Evaluating an individual who has both ASD and CHD would most likely occur in the context of a specific syndrome, such as trisomy 21, and its associated comorbidities. Concerning those individuals sporadically affected with both conditions, a review of the incidence of both conditions is important to determine the likelihood of this occurrence. Of note, recent research has started to uncover genetic links between the two conditions.

Congenital Heart Disease: Population Studies

CHD represents nearly one-third of all major congenital anomalies and affects an estimated 9 per 1000 live births worldwide [61]. In addition, advances in care have resulted in an improvement in survival rates. Over 90% of children born with

J. G. Ho (✉)
Department of Cardiology, University of Florida College of Medicine, Jacksonville, FL, USA
e-mail: Jason.Ho@jax.ufl.edu

A. M. Rosales
Department of Pediatrics, Massachusetts General Hospital, Boston, MA, USA

E. P. Hazen, C. J. McDougle (eds.), *The Massachusetts General Hospital Guide to Medical Care in Patients with Autism Spectrum Disorder*, Current Clinical Psychiatry,
https://doi.org/10.1007/978-3-319-94458-6_10

CHD in developed countries are now expected to live into adulthood. Furthermore, the median age of death in patients with severe CHD increased significantly from 2 years of age in 1987 to 23 years of age in 2005, reflecting a 31% decrease in overall mortality [33]. Due to prolonged longevity, there are now more adults living with CHD than children [34].

Accordingly, the prevalence of CHD has increased. Population studies from 1968 to 1997 in Atlanta report 15-year prevalence rates of 6.2 and 9.3 per 1000, respectively [7]. A study from England spanning 1985–2004 reported a prevalence of 6.4 per 1000 [66]. Most recently, a group in South Carolina evaluated data from 1996 to 2010 that showed a prevalence of 16.7 per 1000 [56]. In total, approximately two million people were estimated to be alive with CHD in the United States in 2010 [39].

The Centers for Disease Control (CDC) Autism and Developmental Disabilities Monitoring (ADDM) Network has provided insight into the prevalence of ASD. This network includes sites across the United States that conduct records-based surveillance for ASD. Population-based data has been collected on 8-year-old children every 2 years since 2000. The CDC more recently expanded the data collection to include 4-year-old children in 2010.

The 8-year-old cohort data has shown that, as with CHD, the prevalence of ASD has increased with time. The ADDM surveillance areas in 2000 reported an ASD prevalence of 6.7 per 1000. A decade later, this estimate had increased to 14.7 per 1000 [11]. At 4 years of age, the prevalence of ASD was 13.4 per 1000 [12]. The authors stated that often ASD screening does not occur until after 4 years of age, so this number may be an underestimation of the true prevalence.

Association Between Autism Spectrum Disorder and Congenital Heart Disease

There is a consistent finding that children with ASD have a higher frequency of congenital anomalies compared to healthy controls. In one study, out of 417 children with ASD, 3.1% had CHD, compared to 1.9% of healthy controls. The only organ system that was found to have higher risk with children with ASD was the gastrointestinal system [65].

Conversely, multiple studies have provided data to suggest that children with CHD have an increased risk of ASD compared to the general population, along with higher rates of communication impairments and decreased social competence [40].

Researchers reviewed data from the 1997 to 2011 National Health Interview Survey to study long-term outcomes in children with CHD aged 0–17 years to compare comorbidities—including autism/ASD—from this population against age-matched controls without CHD. The study found that 2.6% of those with CHD had autism, while 0.6% of those without CHD had autism, reflecting an approximate fivefold increase in odds of ASD in children with CHD compared to those without CHD [50].

A group of physicians in Taiwan conducted a retrospective population-based case-control study to investigate the impact of CHD on the development of both attention-deficit/hyperactivity disorder (ADHD) and ASD. The researchers used national health database statistics to evaluate children between 1997 and 2009 and compared those with CHD against age- and sex-matched controls. The researchers found that ASD occurred in 0.99 per 1000 person-years in the CHD cohort versus 0.2 per 1000 person-years in the control group. This represented a significantly higher risk for developing ASD in children with CHD. The researchers found that children with CHD and early developmental delays might additively increase risk of developing ASD later in life [59].

A large-scale longitudinal study from 2017 involving 195 children with a history of CHD noted a rate of ASD diagnosis of approximately 1 in 31 individuals compared to the national rate of 1 in 68. The authors found the following variables to be associated with an increased risk of screening positive for ASD: genetic disorder and certain genetic genotypes, postoperative length of stay after first surgery, cumulative deep hypothermic cardiac arrest time from the first surgery to 4 years of age, and delayed sternal closure after surgery. The latter three factors suggest that difficult perioperative courses become a risk for subsequent developmental delay and possible ASD diagnoses.

On the other hand, factors that decreased the chances for positive screens for ASD included maternal education, socioeconomic status class, certain genetic genotypes, the absence of genetic disorders, better language and social skills, and older gestational age [4].

Concerning timing of diagnosis, severe types of CHD are typically diagnosed in the fetal or neonatal periods. Less significant CHD often may be found years later as incidental findings in asymptomatic patients. ASD is commonly diagnosed between 2 and 4 years of age. Thus, at the time of diagnosis for CHD, ASD may not be detectable for years. If a commonly associated syndrome is also identified at birth, this could allow the family to prepare for an increased risk of ASD later in life.

Children with significant CHD are commonly screened for developmental disorders, as there is an increased risk of developmental delay including deficits in cognitive capabilities, academic achievement, language, visual construction and perception, attention, executive functioning, fine and gross motor skills, and psychosocial functioning [40]. Executive function involves the control and execution of complex behaviors such as planning, working memory, set maintenance and shifting, and inhibition of prepotent processes. Impairments in this area are considered a core feature of ASD [2].

Surgical intervention for CHD is necessary for survival but does place children at risk for developmental issues. Neurocognitive development after cardiac surgery may be affected by perioperative brain injury and hemodynamic factors [29, 43]. These cardiac-related issues can result in impaired cerebral brain flow and subsequent abnormal neurodevelopment and immunological dysregulation, which may play a role in the development of ASD [59].

Children with more domain-general neurocognitive issues at 4 years of age (i.e., cognitive, language, and attention issues) are at higher risk and need to be assessed for ASD. This is important because there are higher false-positive rates for ASD in the CHD population due to neurodevelopmental and cognitive issues that are similar but unrelated to ASD. Providers should follow the American Academy of Pediatrics (AAP) guidelines [15] recommending early developmental screening starting at 9 months and ASD-specific screening at 18 and 24 months of age. Early identification of ASD in CHD promotes better outcomes and helps identify the need for follow-up and intervention [4].

A study of 57 patients with surgically repaired CHD as infants were followed for 6–12 years postoperatively and compared to healthy controls concerning their neuropsychological assessment. Up to 25% of CHD children performed worse than expected on motor tasks. They had significantly reduced skills for imitating hand and finger positions, were slower on motor tasks, showed worse hand-eye coordination, showed less accuracy in fine visuomotor skills, and used an impulse strategy more often [42].

Children with preoperative hypoxemia in infancy are at higher risk for motor dysfunction compared to those with preoperative heart failure [27]. This process likely stems from involvement of the basal ganglia in motor deficits, as this part of the brain is most sensitive to hypoxia and ischemia. In addition, these factors are a major cause of periventricular leukomalacia, which results in neurodevelopmental delay and is present in more than 50% of neonates after cardiac surgery. Other neonatal postoperative physiologic effects likely explain other CHD-related deficits compared to controls, including in the areas of language, memory, visual attention, and impulsivity [42].

Children with comorbid attentional problems may be at risk for delayed ASD diagnosis [44], so a lower screening threshold for the CHD population may be needed to make sure that children with primary social issues are not overlooked due to their general neurocognitive delays [4].

Common Conditions/Genetic Syndromes

Although patients may sporadically have ASD and CHD together, one of the common variables is the high incidence of both as comorbidities with genetic syndromes. Thirty percent of patients with CHD have a genetic disorder [23], whereas only 5% of patients with ASD have a genetic disorder [37], commonly known by the term *syndromic ASD*. Within each genetic syndrome, there is a varying frequency of ASD, ranging from the single digits up to above 90% [70]. The following subsections will review each condition, including the related forms of CHD and the epidemiology of ASD and CHD for that syndrome.

Trisomy 21 (Down Syndrome)

Down syndrome is the result of a complete or partial trisomy of chromosome 21 and is characterized by numerous congenital defects involving multiple systems. Down syndrome is the most common chromosomal abnormality in live infants and the most frequent chromosomal cause of intellectual disability [21].

Down syndrome is estimated to occur in 1–2 per 1000 live births and at present is associated with an average life expectancy into the sixth decade. Cardiac defects occur in 45–50% of individuals with Down syndrome. Of these, the most common types involve defects in the septal wall of the chambers, including atrial (8% in isolation), ventricular (33–43%), and combined atrioventricular (39–47%) types [64].

Of the atrioventricular septal defects, the most common is the complete form, which involves a single large septal defect spanning both atria and ventricles and resulting in a common atrioventricular valve (versus the usual separated tricuspid and mitral valve). Researchers have attempted to identify the exact cause of cardiac manifestations with Down syndrome; however, this is complicated by the fact that not every patient with Down syndrome has a cardiac defect and that complete atrioventricular septal defects—the most common lesion in trisomy 21—can also occur in individuals without Down syndrome.

Patients with unrepaired complete atrioventricular septal defects may present with symptoms of increased pulmonary blood flow due to a left to right shunting of the blood across the defects to the pulmonary circulation. This increase in blood flow to the lungs can result in pulmonary hypertension, an increase in pulmonary vascular resistance, and ultimately Eisenmenger's syndrome, an irreversible condition in which the pulmonary pressures are higher than the systemic pressures, leading to a reversal of blood flow and cyanosis [64].

Corrective surgery is typically performed within the first year of life to avoid complications later. This surgery commonly involves splitting the common atrioventricular valve and placing an artificial patch in the middle of the heart to close off the systemic and the pulmonary circulations from one another.

Concerning the prevalence of ASD in individuals with Down syndrome, a study in 2013 evaluated 108 individuals using the Social Communication Questionnaire (SCQ; [53]) which consists of three subscales: communication, social interaction, and repetitive and stereotyped patterns of behaviors. They found that 19% of those with Down syndrome met criteria for broadly defined ASD and 8% for strictly defined autistic disorder [45]. Another study in 2010 evaluated 123 individuals aged 2–11 years with Down syndrome using similar screening tools and reported comparable prevalences. From this study cohort with Down syndrome, 18.2% met criteria for broadly defined ASD and 6.4% for strictly defined autistic disorder [18].

The SCQ scores for those with Down syndrome and ASD were significantly higher than those with Down syndrome alone and were similar in profile to those with ASD without genetic syndromes. Those with Down syndrome and ASD had lower levels of self-help skills, were less mobile, and had fewer verbal abilities. In addition, this group had higher rates of behavioral issues including hyperactivity, stereotyped behavior (especially relating to the hands), and inappropriate speech such as repetitive use of language. Self-injury was also more common in those with ASD. Interestingly, those with both Down syndrome and ASD were less withdrawn from their environment compared to those with ASD alone [45].

Other groups have noted that individuals with Down syndrome and ASD tend to show more social-emotional responsivity and reciprocity and possess a greater range of emotional facial expression than that seen in those with ASD without Down syndrome [51]. In addition, individuals with Down syndrome and ASD are noted to have more anxious behavior, complex and unusual stereotypies, and self-isolation or social withdrawal compared to those with Down syndrome without comorbid ASD [10].

Turner Syndrome

Turner syndrome occurs with complete or partial monosomy of the X chromosome and is the only monosomy compatible with life. Typical features include short stature, premature ovarian failure, webbed neck, impaired glucose tolerance, thyroid disease, hearing loss, and CHD. All individuals are phenotypically female. Approximately 1 in 2000 live born females have Turner syndrome [6, 32].

CHD occurs in an estimated 23–50% of individuals with Turner syndrome. The most common types are bicuspid aortic valve (BAV) (12–30%), hypoplastic left heart syndrome (10%), and coarctation of the aorta (7–18%). Septal defects (0–8%) and partial anomalous venous connection (1–13%) are rarer.

Coarctation of the aorta is the cardiac malformation classically associated with Turner syndrome. This involves a narrowing along the aortic arch that results in increased pressures prior to the obstruction and dilation of the aortic walls after the obstruction. This in turn can lead to hypertension and increased left ventricular stress and hypertrophy. Treatment involves relieving the obstruction through stenting or surgery depending on the location and severity of the narrowing and the age of the patient.

Another serious cardiac condition that commonly occurs in Turner syndrome is ascending aortic dilatation, present in 15–30% of cases. Although aortic dilation often occurs with BAV in general, the prevalence of aortic dilation is similar in Turner syndrome individuals with normal aortic valves, showing that this increase could not solely be explained by the presence of BAV in this condition. In addition, there is a higher rate of aortic dissections in Turner syndrome with ages of presentation ranging from 25 to 60 years.

There is an increased incidence of ASD in Turner syndrome compared to the general population [32]. In a study of 150 patients with Turner syndrome, 5 (3%) met diagnostic criteria for autism [16]. With the prevalence of ASD in females estimated at 4 in 10,000 individuals, this represents a 75-fold increased risk [35].

Individuals with Turner syndrome typically have normal global intellectual functioning. Verbal skills tend to be significantly higher than nonverbal skills. In fact, females with Turner syndrome have shown normal and even superior language development compared to controls, including higher reading levels, accuracy, and comprehension. They also have better receptive vocabulary skills.

However, females with Turner syndrome are more likely to have deficits in visual-spatial, visual memory, visual-perceptual, and visual-constructive abilities. Tests of these abilities include mental rotation, object assembly, and facial recognition. Individuals with Turner syndrome may have issues including right-left disorientation, problems with copying designs, and problems with planning and organization. These deficits may be explained by the fact that females with Turner syndrome often have a reduction in the volume of the parietal lobe, which is involved in these areas of cognition.

In addition, females with Turner syndrome are noted to have impairments with social functioning, including lower social activity, poor social coping skills, and increased immaturity, hyperactivity, and impulsivity [32, 35]. Females with Turner syndrome are also more likely to have fewer friends, be involved in fewer social activities, and have greater attentional and societal difficulties compared to normal peers [9].

Chromosome 22q11.2 Deletion Syndrome/DiGeorge Syndrome

The microdeletion of chromosome 22q11.2 occurs in approximately 1 in 4000 births and results in issues affecting multiple organ systems, including developmental delay, absence of the thymus and parathyroid glands, and conotruncal cardiac abnormalities. The various names given to this condition include velocardiofacial syndrome and DiGeorge syndrome.

Whereas diagnoses like Down syndrome and Turner syndrome are confirmed with karyotypes, this condition is confirmed with fluorescence in situ hybridization (FISH). FISH involves binding a fluorescent probe to a specific chromosome and then using a second probe to bind to the deleted region. If the second probe is absent, then the individual has a deletion of the targeted region, in this case chromosome 22q11.2. Often the diagnosis can be suspected prenatally as ultrasound findings of certain malformations, such as the presence of an aortic arch malformation, will result in subsequent testing.

In a cohort of 906 patients with chromosome 22q11.2 deletion, 77% had a form of CHD. This included tetralogy of Fallot in 20%, ventricular septal defect in 21%, interrupted aortic arch in 12%, truncus arteriosus in 6%, and a vascular ring in 6% [41].

Truncus arteriosus is the classic cardiac malformation associated with DiGeorge syndrome and involves a single vessel arising from the ventricles instead of the usual aorta and pulmonary artery. This is repaired by separating the branch pulmonary arteries from the truncus vessel and creating a separate pathway for the blood to flow from the ventricles to the pulmonary arteries.

Patients with deletion of 22q11.2 have a mean IQ in the borderline range of intellectual disability. They also frequently have learning disorders and speech delay. Besides ASD, other comorbidities include ADHD, anxiety disorders and depression, bipolar disorder, and schizophrenia [2]. Concerning prevalence, in 2005, researchers studied 98 individuals with 22q11.2 deletion syndrome and noted a prevalence of ASD in 14% [20]. A study from 2007 evaluated 41 children and noted a prevalence of 42% for broadly defined ASD and 20% for strictly defined autistic disorder [2]. Finally, a 2009 study evaluated 100 patients with chromosome 22q11 deletion and found that 23 individuals had broadly defined ASD and 5 had strictly defined autistic disorder [47].

Individuals with 22q11.2 deletion often have deficits in executive function and behavioral difficulties. They also may have language delays and problems with social functioning. Since patients with ASD and chromosome 22q11.2 deletion often have similar behavioral and cognitive findings, a comparison of cohorts of chromosome 22q11.2 individuals with and without ASD was performed. Those with ASD had more psychiatric comorbidities including ADHD, specific phobias, and symptoms of mania. In addition, those with both conditions were found to have a larger right amygdala, which has been associated with a variety of symptoms of ASD including socialization and communication deficits [2].

Williams Syndrome

Williams syndrome is caused by a microdeletion of 25 genes on chromosome 7q11.23 and is estimated to occur in 1 in 10,000 people. Affected individuals often have a common physical appearance featuring flat nasal bridge, long philtrum, short upturned nose, and delicate chin.

Cardiac issues include stenosis of medium and large arteries due to medial layer thickening from smooth muscle overgrowth. The deletion of the elastin gene is implicated as the cause of this issue. The location of the stenosis is commonly above the aortic valve at the sinotubular junction and is termed supravalvular aortic stenosis. This occurs in 70% of patients with Williams syndrome and can range from trivial to severe. This stenosis may be isolated or may occur in multiple locations including the aortic arch, descending aorta, and arteries within the pulmonary, coronary, renal, mesenteric, and intracranial systems.

Other cardiac issues in patients with Williams syndrome include myxomatous degeneration of aortic or mitral valve leaflets, which occurs in 20% of patients. Hypertension occurs in 50% of patients. Animal models have suggested that the increase in blood pressure is due to a physiological adaptation to the abnormal blood vessels. Cardiovascular complications are the major cause of mortality in these patients. Also, precautions are mandatory for these patients prior to receiving general anesthesia, as reports of sudden cardiovascular collapse have been noted [49].

On average, children with Williams syndrome have mild to moderate intellectual disability. In addition, they have hyperacusis, severe impairments in visual-spatial and visual-motor skills, difficulties with socio-communication including declarative pointing, showing objects, and giving, as well as delays in acquisition of early motor skills and achieving language milestones [49, 58].

Strengths include facial recognition and discrimination, receptivity to music, auditory rote memory, selected aspects of language, and social and interpersonal skills. In fact, individuals have been described as having "cocktail party" personalities due to their highly social and empathetic nature. This includes being overfriendly, lacking a fear of strangers, having strong prosocial compulsion, having excessive talkativeness, and possessing expressive speech rich in vocabulary [58]. As a result, Williams syndrome and ASD are often felt to be complete opposites with respect to phenotype.

However, many studies exist that describe patients with Williams syndrome either having ASD or features of ASD. In addition, they are at risk for psychopathology including anxiety, obsessive-compulsive symptoms, distractibility, irritability, and ADHD. Social isolation is also common despite their typically outgoing personalities [49, 58].

A study of 20 individuals with Williams syndrome found a prevalence of 10% meeting criteria for ASD. The researchers noted that children not meeting full criteria for ASD still showed some ASD features. Those with Williams syndrome and ASD showed deficits in communication behaviors, showing, and initiating joint attention. However, compared to a cohort with ASD only, those with both conditions made social overtures and efforts to engage others, which was usually not seen in the ASD only group [38]. In addition, another study evaluating nine patients with both Williams and ASD noted that the group had severe impairments in verbal communication, with some individuals being nonverbal and others with language delay. Stereotypical behaviors were common, including toe walking and fascination with spinning objects. Other features seen in these subjects contrasted with those commonly attributed to Williams syndrome, including impairments in social interaction and severe intellectual disability [58].

Tuberous Sclerosis Complex

Tuberous sclerosis complex is a neurocutaneous syndrome caused by a genetic mutation inherited in an autosomal dominant manner or obtained as a spontaneous mutation. A mutation in *TSC1* on chromosome 9 or *TSC2* on chromosome 16 causes most cases, leading to abnormalities of the hamartin or tuberin proteins [30].

Tuberous sclerosis can lead to the presence of widespread abnormal growths of normal tissues called hamartomas. When these occur within the heart, they are termed cardiac rhabdomyomas. These are benign tumors made of cardiac myocytes that can be detected by echocardiography. In general, primary cardiac tumors occur in 0.2% of children, with cardiac rhabdomyomas being the most common type by far. Of those with rhabdomyomas, 70–90% have tuberous sclerosis. Conversely, 50% of patients with tuberous sclerosis will have rhabdomyomas.

These tumors commonly develop between 20 and 30 weeks' gestation, may increase in size as pregnancy progresses, and may result in arrhythmias, hydrops fetalis, or pericardial effusions. A small series of 44 cases described fetal loss occurring in approximately 11%. The tumors themselves are benign and more commonly located in the ventricle versus the atrium, but if located in a vital region, such as the outflow tract, they can result in hemodynamic compromise. The natural course is for rhabdomyomas to spontaneously resolve within the first 2 years of life.

Cardiac issues in patients with tuberous sclerosis complex include arrhythmias. Bradycardia may occur due to sinus node dysfunction and atrioventricular block. Tachycardia mechanisms include atrial tachycardia, accessory pathway-mediated tachycardia, and ventricular tachycardia. The mechanism underlying the arrhythmia may be linked to the presence of rhabdomyomas [26].

Among the psychiatric issues associated with tuberous sclerosis complex, ASD is the most common. Published prevalence estimates of ASD in individuals with tuberous sclerosis complex vary from 17% to 63%. In 1 study of 42 patients with tuberous sclerosis complex, 40.5% were found to have ASD. Those with and without ASD were tested with the SCQ. Both groups were found to have similar restricted, repetitive, and stereotyped behaviors and interest domain, whereas patients with ASD differed significantly with regard to deficits in reciprocal social interaction and language/communication domain.

Epilepsy has been considered a risk factor for those with tuberous sclerosis complex to develop ASD, and in this study, all of the patients with ASD had epilepsy. The mean age of seizure onset was significantly lower in patients with ASD (7.9 months) compared to those without ASD (16.9 months). In addition, psychiatric comorbidity is common with tuberous sclerosis complex, including anxiety and mood disorders, adjustment disorders, and ADHD [63].

Future Directions in the Genetics of CHD and ASD

There have been promising genetic links with regard to the causes of both CHD and ASD. Previous research had shown an unexpected overlap in genes harboring damaging de novo mutations in CHD and neurodevelopmental disorders. A recent study utilized whole exome analysis in 2871 individuals with CHD and their families. The genes from the CHD probands harboring damaging de novo mutations were compared to 4778 probands with ASD. Nineteen genes had de novo loss of function mutations in both cohorts, and 48 had damaging mutations in both, showing an overlap of mutated genes in individuals with CHD and others with ASD. Not every individual with the mutation had both conditions, so there are other factors that determine what disease manifestations occur with a particular gene mutation.

Of note, genes that are chromatin modifiers control events underlying the formation of neural connections, including neurogenesis and neural differentiation [17]. Eighty-seven percent of patients with CHD with loss of function de novo mutations in the chromatin modifier genes were also found to have neurodevelopmental disorders. Thus, potentially finding mutations in the overlapped chromatin modifier genes may identify CHD patients at risk for ASD and intellectual disability who may benefit from early diagnosis and treatment [31].

Clinical Evaluation

History

In treating patients with ASD, providers may need to rely heavily on history from the parents or caregivers, especially in working with nonverbal patients. Besides family members, having other treatment providers, such as staff from a residential treatment program, present for evaluations can be very helpful as they may have additional observations or questions to augment those from the family. Nonetheless, it is important to address the patient directly and give patients the opportunity to answer questions for themselves, noting that some patients with ASD may take longer than usual to respond to questions. In treating adult patients with ASD, it is important to clarify issues of guardianship and who has responsibility for medical decision-making, ideally prior to the appointment.

When evaluating patients with CHD, the clinician should obtain a thorough history to determine how well the patient is doing, focusing on questions involving the following symptoms:

Chest Pain Depending on the level of developmental disability, this may be the most difficult symptom to discuss as it typically involves descriptive factors such as location, quality, severity, and associated factors. Those with the patient may describe any physical changes associated with the pain including diaphoresis or change in color.

Chest pain is a very common presentation in pediatric cardiology, representing 5.2% of all inpatient and emergency room pediatric cardiology consultations [24] and 15% of outpatient visits. Fortunately, chances are unlikely that the symptom is associated with any significant heart disease, as an estimated 0–5% of pediatric patients with chest pain have a cardiac etiology [22]. Moreover, a review of 3700 patients in a pediatric cardiology clinic noted that 1% had a cardiac etiology [54]. Characteristics that should raise red flags include onset with exertion; association with palpitations, syncope, or fever; radiation of pain to the back, jaw, arm, or shoulder; and increased pain while supine. Other risk factors include a past medical or family history of cardiac disease [67].

Syncope Causes of syncope can vary from benign to life-threatening. The history can help determine the severity of an episode. Syncope that occurs while standing in a hot environment is much different than syncope that occurs while running down the basketball court. The evaluation in an individual with ASD can become very difficult without a clear history. In addition, the differential diagnosis includes seizures or altered mental status.

A careful history by witnesses may help guide initial steps of the workup, as does a review of past episodes. Vasovagal syncope is the most common type of benign etiology and involves an upright patient that is usually standing, walking, or changing positions. Prodromal symptoms are typical and include dizziness, blurry or darkened vision, muffled hearing or ringing in the ears, and a sensation of feeling hot with diaphoresis. Pallor is common as well. A history of poor oral intake, recent illness, or a hot environment is common.

Neurocardiogenic syncope is a less common form of benign syncope. This is often triggered by a "noxious stimulus" such as pain, nausea, or the sight of blood or a needle. This results in a cardioinhibitory (drop in heart rate), vasoinhibitory (drop in blood pressure), or mixed response, which results in syncope. Prodromal symptoms are less common in this situation, but often individuals with this type have had recurrent syncope since childhood of an unknown etiology. Once the trigger is determined, avoidance of the trigger is usually the best treatment.

Worrisome findings with syncope include lack of prodromal symptoms, injury while passing out (often those of a vasovagal etiology and prodromal symptoms are able to avoid injury, but not uniformly), and association with palpitations, exercise, or chest pain. "Seizure-like" activity at the onset of syncope often occurs due to transient decreased blood flow to the brain.

Palpitations Palpitations are risk-stratified based on the description and characteristics of the symptoms. Arrhythmias are more commonly associated with sudden onset and offset of symptoms, sustained symptoms, and random occurrences. While not always indicative, daily symptoms or episodes that gradually start and fade away are more likely to be sinus in origin. Often palpitations are confused for chest pain and vice versa, so those with ASD who cannot adequately describe the symptoms may end up being evaluated for the wrong symptom. Common noncardiac etiologies include anxiety and stress, which are more common in the ASD population. Red flags include an association with syncope or chest pain. Caregivers can look for neck pulsations, seeing the heart "beating through the chest" and feeling and counting the pulse if possible.

Cyanosis Cyanotic heart disease is increasingly detected during the neonatal period, particularly after establishing critical CHD screening protocols involving pulse oximetry usage in the newborn period. Critical CHD affects an estimated 2–3 per 1000 live births in the United States [8]. Those with cyanotic heart disease who do not receive corrective surgery may develop irreversible pulmonary hypertension known as Eisenmenger's syndrome. These patients are persistently cyanotic and can have physical findings such as clubbing of the nail beds. Regional discoloration of the extremities and perioral area with normal pulse oximetry is unlikely to be cardiac in nature and is due to changes in regional perfusion, commonly from environmental factors such as temperature.

Dyspnea and Activity Intolerance Shortness of breath may be due to a pulmonary process as well as a cardiac issue, so often evaluations by both specialties are indicated. Common etiologies including asthma and allergies should be considered, as well as a cardiac evaluation for any decrease in cardiac function, as seen in poor hemodynamic states with CHD as well as new onset cardiomyopathies in otherwise asymptomatic individuals. If feasible, exercise-related symptoms should be evaluated with stress testing to attempt to reproduce symptoms in a monitored setting.

After discussing the history of present illness, additional questions to ask include tolerance of medications and any changes to family history, social history, medications, and allergies. A detailed review of systems can help organize questions to make certain that any issues—whether cardiac or not—become known and handled appropriately.

The provider should screen for any issues with growth or development, as there is an increased risk of possible genetic issues in patients with CHD. A detailed family history is important due to the nature of multiple conditions being genetic in pediatric cardiology, including forms of cardiomyopathies and channelopathies. An important question to ask is the presence of any childhood deaths for any reason, sudden or unexpected deaths at any age, and unexplained accidents. In addition, it is important to determine whether any family members have had heart surgery or pacemaker or implantable cardiac defibrillator placement.

As always, a thorough social history is important, including who lives in the household and any school-related questions. Depending on the situation, questions concerning possible drug and substance abuse need to be asked, often without the patient's parents in the room to encourage truthfulness.

Physical Examination

In working with patients with ASD, the physical examination is often based on opportunity. Starting contact with the patient from a distance can make subsequent portions of the exam easier. For example, tapping a patient's feet first to "break the ice" can be a strategy used to gain acceptance rather than the first contact being a stethoscope on their chest.

The initial portion of the physical examination starts with the vital signs. A complete set of vital signs for cardiac evaluation includes height, weight, heart rate, respiratory rate, blood pressure, and oxygen saturation. Depending on the type of cardiac disease, patients often have a specific baseline that is considered their "normal" although the actual value is considered abnormal in general. A common example of this are oxygen saturations in the 80–90 percentile for patients with cyanotic conditions, such as hypoplastic left heart syndrome.

Anxiety is a common issue in those with ASD. Heart rate and blood pressure are easily influenced by stress. In cases where "white coat" issues are suspected, monitoring of blood pressure or heart rate at home or at school may be helpful in assessing the vital signs outside of the medical setting.

Patients with ASD prescribed certain psychopharmacologic agents are at risk for obesity and its resultant comorbidities, including hypertension and obstructive sleep apnea [1, 68]. Some antipsychotic medications may have a negative inotropic effect that reduces cardiac output and results in lowering of the blood pressure [19]. In addition, ADHD is a common comorbidity in ASD, and stimulant medications can result directly in an elevated blood pressure and heart rate. Alternatively, some non-stimulant ADHD treatments—such as guanfacine and clonidine—can result in decreased blood pressure or heart rate [57].

Auscultation of the heart sounds allows for a rapid assessment of the heart rate and rhythm and the presence of any extra heart sounds such as murmurs, clicks, or gallops. Features of concerning murmurs include loudness, timing in the cardiac cycle, harshness, and the presence of clicks, gallops, rubs, or thrills.

The finding of a vibratory systolic murmur without additional heart sounds and without a history of structural heart disease, failure to thrive, or cyanosis is likely a benign flow murmur. Physical maneuvers typically used to evaluate murmurs such as standing, squatting, and performing a Valsalva maneuver may be difficult for some patients with ASD to perform, so any unusual physical examination findings may need to be further evaluated with additional testing.

Palpation of pulses can detect irregular heart rhythm or abnormal rates. Usually the better tolerated areas by patients include the wrists and posterior tibial pulses in the lower extremities. Weaker distal pulses may be indicative of a condition limiting cardiac output, including severe aortic stenosis or coarctation of the aorta. Other physical findings include capillary refill times to assess for hydration status and perfusion as well as color and skin temperature.

The work of breathing is important to assess in younger children, as many cardiac issues create tachypnea and retractions may be seen between the ribs. The exam may need to be adapted based on the cooperation of the patient and the degree of their developmental delay, anxiety, and sensory issues that may be present with ASD.

Visual observation of jugular venous distension can suggest elevated venous pressure due to tricuspid disease, right atrial pathologies, large pericardial effusions, or complete heart block. Abdominal examinations are important to assess for hepatomegaly, which can suggest elevated venous pressures because of heart failure.

The patient's general appearance, size, and nutrition status can also be determined visually. Younger patients with CHD and heart failure can develop failure to thrive. Other related signs include pallor and diaphoresis due to increased circulating catecholamines.

Additional Testing

Cardiac testing is often employed to rule out commonly seen comorbidities. For patients with ASD, objective data from testing often needs to take the place of subjective reporting, and the timing of testing can be adjusted according to the needs of the patient. One example of this approach would be the evaluation of a teenager with tetralogy of Fallot and ASD with severe communication impairments. A known issue with patients with tetralogy of Fallot is arrhythmias or ectopic beats, which often foreshadow issues such as pulmonary valve insufficiency. Often, ambulatory 24-h Holter monitoring is performed serially to detect any rhythm issues. In a typical asymptomatic patient with no current hemodynamic issues, this is generally done every 3–5 years or as needed. However, in an individual with ASD, the monitoring may need to be performed more often given the patient's limited capacity to report symptoms such as palpitations.

Electrocardiogram One of the most common cardiac tests is the electrocardiogram (ECG). ECGs can evaluate conditions such as heart block, arrhythmias, and abnormal intervals, such as QT interval prolongation. In addition, certain arrhythmogenic conditions can be evaluated, such as the presence of a widened QRS representing preexcitation in Wolff-Parkinson-White syndrome.

Beyond rhythm conditions, ECGs can be useful in detecting a variety of other cardiac abnormalities. For example, due to changes in the formation of the conduction system with specific cardiac lesions, a left axis deviation can be seen in individuals with tricuspid atresia or atrioventricular septal defects. Deep Q waves, inverted T waves, or ST segment changes can all suggest perfusion issues. In addition, tall or prolonged P waves can indicate right or left atrial enlargement, respectively, and taller than normal QRS waves can indicate ventricular hypertrophy.

There are several ECG findings that are considered normal variants and typically do not require further intervention. These include sinus arrhythmia (an increase in heart rate with inspiration and a decrease with expiration), wandering atrial pacemaker (a change in P wave morphology without change in heart rate or P-QRS relationship commonly seen in pediatrics), and first-degree (PR interval above 200 ms) and second-degree (incremental increase in PR interval with a dropped P wave before resetting the cycle) AV Wenckebach. Depending on the comfort level of the practitioner, any deviation from normal sinus rhythm can be further evaluated by a cardiologist to determine the clinical significance.

Echocardiography This is the most common modality for the diagnosis of structural heart defects. Echocardiography uses ultrasound waves to create an image of the cardiac structure and function without the need for ionizing radiation. Echocardiography machines are portable and can be utilized in the inpatient and outpatient settings. Echocardiography is commonly used to further assess clinical findings such as murmurs or rhythm abnormalities.

Treatment

Interventions for the above cardiac conditions in those with ASD would be the same as in the regular population. Patients with clinically significant arrhythmias would undergo the same ablation procedure, and patients with CHD and ASD would have the same surgical repair.

However, the approach to care may need to be modified for patients with ASD. For example, after a cardiac catheterization, patients are asked to remain supine for 4–6 h after the procedure to avoid recurrent bleeding and hematomas from the femoral access sites. In some patients with ASD, this may not be feasible, so patients may need to be sedated during this time frame. In addition, sedation is often used when patients with cardiac histories are undergoing studies such as echocardiograms, computed tomography, or magnetic resonance imaging scans which require patients to be cooperative and relatively still.

In patients with ASD, the challenges of medication monitoring are very important. Considering that many psychotropic medications are commonly used to treat patients with ASD, knowledge of the cardiac side effects, particularly with respect to sudden death risk, of these medications becomes vital.

Patients with ASD often have ECGs performed for monitoring on psychotropic medications, especially those taking ADHD medications due to the recommendations from the American Heart Association [62]. Routine ECG screening for other psychotropic medications has been more controversial, with the primary concern being the prolongation of the QT interval.

A prolonged QT interval—whether congenital or acquired—represents delay in ventricular repolarization and thus increases the risk for the development of torsades de pointes (TdP), a dangerous ventricular arrhythmia that can lead to sudden death. In general, those with congenital long QT syndrome should avoid taking medications that prolong the QT interval, and normal individuals should refrain from taking multiple medications that prolong the QT interval simultaneously. Often, if the benefits outweigh the theoretical risks in starting a medication that can cause QT prolongation, a baseline ECG followed by a repeat ECG 1–2 weeks into therapy is recommended. There is a list of medications that prolong the QT interval on CredibleMeds' website (www.crediblemeds.org), which is updated regularly.

Several antipsychotics are known to affect the QT interval to varying degrees. A review article recommended ECG monitoring in the following scenarios:

- Evaluation of the patient suggests increased cardiac risk, including positive family history, symptoms, history of cardiac disease, other QT prolonging medications, or other medical conditions of concern.
- A patient's prescribed medications are listed as high risk for TdP.
- The patient has overdosed on antipsychotic medications [55].

Similar extrapolation of these recommendations to other classes of medications may be prudent, with referral to cardiology for evaluation on medication as needed. However, it is important to recognize that the information obtained by the ECG alone is not sufficient to determine the cardiac safety of a medication [25].

Researchers have found little evidence to indicate that psychotropic drug-associated QTc prolongation by itself is sufficient to predict TdP. Also, QTc prolongation was not found to be a dose-related phenomenon, as there was varying degrees of QTc interval prolongation in the studies reviewed. A review of 28 cases of TdP showed that 75% occurred at therapeutic drug doses and 21.4% occurred with a QTc of less than 500 ms, a threshold commonly used for concern [25]. The QTc interval depends upon the patient's gender, genetics, and health as well as other physiological variables [28].

Monitoring of the QTc includes a baseline ECG and follow-up ECGs while titrating the dose of the medication. The literature has recommended caution if the QTc is above the upper limit of normal or if there is a 10% increase in the QTc on a new medication [36].

Despite recommendations, there has been no evidence that ECG screening prior to starting ADHD medications has been cost-effective or appropriate to prevent sudden death in the pediatric population. The AHA reworded the recommendations to allow for *consideration* of obtaining an ECG prior to starting stimulant drug therapy but is clear to state that this is not mandatory [14].

Stimulant medications have also been shown to have possible cardiac side effects. In February 2006, the US Food and Drug Administration (FDA) convened its Drug Safety and Risk Management Advisory Committee to investigate a link between ADHD medications and cardiac problems in response to concern over sudden unexplained deaths in children taking stimulant medications. Controlled trials failed to show a correlation, but there was concern that the trials were not large enough or long enough to adequately discover a link. Accordingly, this committee voted to add a black box warning to ADHD medications. In March 2006, the FDA Pediatric Advisory Committee reviewed evidence and recommended warning labels instead of a black box warning [3]. Despite these findings, certain ADHD medications carry a black box warning, including the various forms of methylphenidate.

With that in mind, a multicenter study evaluated 1,200,438 individuals aged 2–24 years and demographically matched individuals who were taking ADHD medications with those who were not. Eighty-one individuals taking ADHD medications had a serious cardiovascular event (3.1 per 100,000 person-years), including 33 sudden cardiac deaths (1.3 per 100,000), 9 acute myocardial infarctions (0.3 per 100,000), and 39 strokes (1.5 per 100,000). Performing multiple analyses, ADHD medications were not associated with an increased risk of serious cardiovascular events in children and young adults [13].

Two conditions that have had scrutiny concerning ADHD medication use are Wolff-Parkinson-White (WPW) and long QT syndrome. The recent expert consensus statement allows for the use of ADHD medications in asymptomatic WPW patients with close observation for development of symptoms [48].

A review of patients with long QT syndrome was performed with 28 patients (8%) found also to have ADHD. None of the 15 patients who were treated with stimulants had long QT-triggered events in a combined 56 person-years of treatment. Paradoxically, there was a statistically lower long QT-triggered event rate in the stimulant-treated ADHD group compared to long QT-alone cohort. The authors stated that ADHD can be treated effectively and safely in mild- to moderate-risk long QT individuals [52].

However, another group reports that their experience with ADHD treatment in the long QT population has shown a threefold increase in non-fatal cardiac events when compared to long QT patients not receiving ADHD medications. For males, the increase is over sixfold. The causative relationship is further augmented by the fact that the two cohorts had similar cardiac event rates prior to the one group starting ADHD medications. The primary cardiac event noted was syncope [69].

Special Considerations in Adults with ASD

Although most of the ASD research focuses on children, most people living with ASD today are adults. The ASD adult literature focuses on morbidity and mortality over time and the relative risk of mortality conferred to individuals with ASD.

A 2011 study reviewed insurance data in 108 young adults with ASD and control matched this group for age, sex, and health insurance status. The purpose of the study was to evaluate chronic disease risk. Individuals with ASD were found to be more likely to have hyperlipidemia (31.5% versus 18.9%) than controls. There were no significant group differences concerning rates of hypertension, congestive heart failure, or coronary heart disease [60].

Research studies from 1992 to 2010 report increased risk of mortality in those with ASD compared to population controls as ranging from 0- to 5.6-fold. This risk was especially notable in females and those with severe intellectual disability.

A 2013 study following a cohort of 305 individuals with ASD for 20–29 years found a hazard rate ratio of 9.9. Twenty-nine individuals died during follow-up (9.5%), mostly due to respiratory, cardiac, and epileptic events. Five of the deaths were from cardiovascular causes and included cases of myocarditis, arrhythmia, congestive heart failure, and congenital heart disease [5].

Researchers in Denmark sought to compare the prevalence and types of circulatory system diseases in adults who were diagnosed with ASD as children. The study evaluated 118 adults with ASD and followed them for an average of 37.2 years to a mean age of 49.6 years. The group was matched to 336 sex- and age-matched population controls.

Eleven individuals from the ASD cohort were diagnosed with at least one or more diseases of the circulatory system (9.3%) compared to 54 in the control group (16.1%). This difference was not statistically significant, but looking more closely at the data, ischemic heart disease was diagnosed in 16 individuals from the control group and in no individuals in the ASD group.

The diagnosis of ischemic heart disease is usually a result of reporting associated symptoms including chest pain, discomfort, and distress. These are subjective symptoms that rely on proper identification and communication from the individuals affected. The authors thus speculate that those with ASD may not have the ability to recognize and communicate their needs due to various factors, including atypical sensory processing, intellectual disability, communication impairments, and resistance to new experiences [46].

In populations with special needs or significant medical conditions, parents commonly continue to accompany their adult children to medical visits and assume care in decision-making despite their child being over 18 years of age. Depending on the level of the patient's cognitive ability, providers should refrain from focusing on the parent initially and address the patient directly initially with the parent supplementing the conversation.

Conclusion

The prevalences of ASD and CHD are both increasing, resulting in a high likelihood that medical providers will care for patients with both conditions. In addition, there are many genetic syndromes that have both conditions as frequent comorbidities. Patients with CHD should undergo the proper developmental and

ASD screening to allow for timely interventions as indicated. The cardiac evaluation of an individual with ASD may need to be adapted depending on varying patient factors, such as cooperation.

ECG screening for those taking psychotropic medications is controversial and should be tailored to the individual patient depending on important factors such as symptomatology and family history.

Adults with ASD have been noted to have an increased risk of mortality compared to age- and sex-matched controls. Respiratory, cardiac, and neurologic causes are commonly noted. There is a relative paucity of research in adults with ASD compared to the pediatric literature. With the increasing incidence of ASD over time, additional research in adults with ASD will be important to help providers continue to provide quality care to this growing population.

Clinical Vignette # 1

A 14-year-old male with ASD with mild developmental delay presents to his primary care physician for follow-up of possible ADHD symptoms. His parents note that he is not performing well in school and that his grades have dropped. In addition, at home he often needs to be redirected to complete his chores and homework. The patient's parents and teachers have completed a Vanderbilt questionnaire, and the patient meets criteria for an ADHD diagnosis.

His primary care physician reviews the chart and notes that the patient has otherwise been healthy and he denies any symptoms in clinic today. However, the patient's parents note that one of the patient's cousins recently had heart surgery but for an unknown reason. The physician decides to order a screening ECG prior to initiating treatment. The ECG returns as abnormal for Wolff-Parkinson-White pattern, prompting a referral to cardiology.

The pediatric cardiologist evaluates the patient and notes that under the guidelines for asymptomatic patients with Wolff-Parkinson-White, treatment with stimulant medications for ADHD is acceptable if indicated. To be complete, a stress test is performed which shows clear loss of pre-excitation at heart rates above 150 bpm. The cardiologist sends a report to the primary physician clearing the patient for ADHD medications and arranges a follow-up visit for 1 month after the medication is started.

Clinical Vignette # 2

A pregnant female undergoes a routine fetal ultrasound and is informed that the fetus has what appears to be a large hole in the middle of the heart and other concerning findings, including echogenicity of the bowel. She is referred to a pediatric cardiologist who performs a fetal echocardiogram and confirms the diagnosis of a complete atrioventricular septal defect. The family is counseled on the increased risk of trisomy 21 with the fetal findings.

The family decides to defer additional testing, and the pregnancy proceeds to term gestation. The infant is delivered and confirmed to have both the heart defect on postnatal echocardiography and trisomy 21 by blood karyotype. After a brief stay in the neonatal intensive care unit for hyperbilirubinemia, the infant grows and thrives at home. He is regularly seen by pediatric cardiology, who recommends corrective surgery at 6 months of age. The family discusses comorbidities of trisomy 21 with their pediatrician, who recommends regular thyroid screening as well as referral for physical, occupational, and speech therapies. In addition, due to the risk of having a comorbid ASD diagnosis, the pediatrician recommends routine developmental screening at each well-child check and ASD-specific screening to be performed at 18 and 24 months with referral if indicated.

Clinical Pearls

- The prevalences of both congenital heart disease (CHD) and autism spectrum disorder (ASD) are increasing over time.
- Children with ASD have an increased frequency of congenital anomalies, including CHD.

- Children with CHD also have an increased risk of ASD compared to the general population.
- It is important for early screening for ASD to be carried out in children with CHD as appropriate and timely interventions can improve outcomes.
- There are many genetic syndromes which have both CHD and ASD as comorbidities.
- Recent advances in science have identified damaging de novo mutations that have overlap in causing both CHD and ASD.
- The cardiac evaluation of a child with ASD should be individually tailored based on what delays and sensory issues may be present.
- Symptoms to focus on include chest pain, palpitations, shortness of breath, dizziness, syncope, exercise intolerance, and pallor.
- Further diagnostic testing for a child with ASD also should be adjusted as needed, such as consideration of performing some studies under sedation.
- ECG screening for psychotropic medications is controversial and should be guided by risk factors such as symptoms and past medical and family histories.

References

1. Accordino RE, Kidd C, Politte LC, Henry CA, McDougle CJ. Psychopharmacological interventions in autism spectrum disorder. Expert Opin Pharmacother. 2016;17(7):937–52.
2. Antshel KM, Aneja A, Strunge L, Peebles J, Fremont WP, Stallone K, AbdulSabur N, Higgins AM, Shprintzen RJ, Kates WR. Autistic spectrum disorders in velo-cardio facial syndrome (22q11.2 deletion). J Autism Dev Disord. 2007;37(9):1776–86.
3. Barry CL, Martin A, Busch SH. ADHD medication use following FDA risk warnings. J Ment Health Policy Econ. 2012;15(3):119–25.
4. Bean Jaworski JL, Flynn T, Burnham N, Chittams JL, Sammarco T, Gerdes M, Bernbaum JC, Clancy RR, Solot CB, Zackai EH, McDonald-McGinn DM, Gaynor JW. Rates of autism and potential risk factors in children with congenital heart defects. Congenit Heart Dis. 2017;12(4):421–9.
5. Bilder D, Botts EL, Smith KR, Pimentel R, Farley M, Viskochil J, McMahon WM, Block H, Ritvo E, Ritvo RA, Coon H. Excess mortality and causes of death in autism spectrum disorders: a follow up of the 1980s Utah/UCLA autism epidemiologic study. J Autism Dev Disord. 2013;43(5):1196–204.
6. Bondy CA. Congenital cardiovascular disease in Turner syndrome. Congenit Heart Dis. 2008;3(1):2–15.
7. Botto LD, Correa A, Erickson JD. Racial and temporal variations in the prevalence of heart defects. Pediatrics. 2001;107(3):E32.
8. Bruno CJ, Havranek T. Screening for critical congenital heart disease in newborns. Adv Pediatr Infect Dis. 2015;62(1):211–26.
9. Burnett AC, Reutens DC, Wood AG. Social cognition in Turner's syndrome. J Clin Neurosci. 2010;17:283–6.
10. Carter JC, Capone GT, Gray RM, Cox CS, Kaufmann WE. Autistic-spectrum disorders in Down syndrome: further delineation and distinction from other behavioral abnormalities. Am J Med Genet B Neuropsychiatr Genet. 2007;144B(1):87–94.
11. Christensen D, Baio J, Braun K, Bilder D, Charles J, Constantino JN, Daniels J, et al. Prevalence and characteristics of autism spectrum disorder among children aged 8 years — autism and developmental disabilities monitoring network, 11 sites, United States, 2012. MMWR Surveill Summ. 2016a;65(3):1–23.
12. Christensen D, Bilder D, Zahorodny W, Pettygrove S, Durkin M, Fitzgerald RT, Rice C, Kurzius-Spencer M, Baio J, Yeargin-Allsopp M. Prevalence and characteristics of autism spectrum disorder among 4-year-old children in the autism and developmental disabilities monitoring network. J Dev Behav Pediatr. 2016b;37(1):1–8.
13. Cooper WO, Habel LA, Sox CM, Chan KA, Arbogast PG, Cheetham TC, Murray KT, Quinn VP, Stein CM, Callahan ST, Fireman BH, Fish FA, Kirshner HS, O'Duffy A, Connell FA, Ray WA. ADHD drugs and serious cardiovascular events in children and young adults. N Engl J Med. 2011;365(20):1896–904.
14. Cortese S, Holtmann M, Banaschewski T, Buitelaar J, Coghill D, Danckaerts M, Dittmann RW, Graham J, Taylor E, Sergeant J, European ADHD Guidelines Group. Practitioner review: current best practice in the management of adverse events during treatment with ADHD medications in children and adolescents. J Child Psychol Psychiatry. 2013;54(3):227–46.
15. Council on Children With Disabilities, Section on Developmental Behavioral Pediatrics, Bright Futures Steering Committee, Medical Home Initiatives for Children With Special Needs Project Advisory Committee. Identifying infants and young children with developmental disorders in the medical home: an algorithm for developmental surveillance and screening. Pediatrics. 2006;118(1):405–20.
16. Creswell CS, Skuse DH. Autism in association with Turner syndrome: genetic implications for male vulnerability to pervasive developmental disorders. Neurocase. 1999;5:511–8.

17. De Rubeis S, He X, Goldberg AP, Poultney CS, Samocha K, Cicek AE, Kou Y, Liu L, et al. Synaptic, transcriptional and chromatin genes disrupted in autism. Nature. 2014;515(7526):209–15.
18. DiGuiseppi C, Hepburn S, Davis JM, Fidler DJ, Hartway S, Lee NR, Miller L, Ruttenber M, Robinson C. Screening for autism spectrum disorders in children with Down syndrome: population prevalence and screening test characteristics. J Dev Behav Pediatr. 2010;31(3):181–91.
19. Fayek M, Kingsbury SJ, Zada J, Simpson GM. Cardiac effects of antipsychotic medications. Psychiatr Serv. 2001;52(5):607–9.
20. Fine SE, Weissman A, Gerdes M, Pinto-Martin J, Zackai EH, McDonald-McGinn DM, Emanuel BS. Autism spectrum disorders and symptoms in children with molecularly confirmed 22q11.2 deletion syndrome. J Autism Dev Disord. 2005 JAS;35(4):461–70.
21. Frid C, Drott P, Lundell B, Rasmussen F, Anneren G. Mortality in Down's syndrome in relation to congenital malformations. J Intellect Disabil Res. 1999;43:234–41.
22. Friedman KG, Alexander ME. Chest pain and syncope in children: a practical approach to the diagnosis of cardiac disease. J Pediatr. 2013;163(3):896–901. e1-3.
23. Fuller S, Nord AS, Gerdes M, Wernovsky G, Jarvik GP, Bernbaum J, Zackai E, Gaynor JW. Predictors of impaired neurodevelopmental outcomes at one year of age after infant cardiac surgery. Eur J Cardiothorac Surg. 2009;36:40–7.
24. Geggel RL. Conditions leading to pediatric cardiology consultation in a tertiary academic hospital. Pediatrics. 2004;114(4):e409–17.
25. Hasnain M, Vieweg WV. QTc interval prolongation and torsade de pointes associated with second-generation antipsychotics and antidepressants: a comprehensive review. CNS Drugs. 2014;28:887–920.
26. Hinton RB, Prakash A, Romp RL, Krueger DA, Knilans TK, International Tuberous Sclerosis Consensus Group. Cardiovascular manifestations of tuberous sclerosis complex and summary of the revised diagnostic criteria and surveillance and management recommendations from the International Tuberous Sclerosis Consensus Group. J Am Heart Assoc. 2014;3(6):e001493.
27. Hövels-Gürich H, Konrad K, Skorzenski D, Nacken C, Minkenberg R, Messmer BJ, Seghaye MC. Long-term neurodevelopmental outcome and exercise capacity after corrective surgery for tetralogy of Fallot or ventricular septal defect in infancy. Ann Thorac Surg. 2006;81(3):958–66.
28. Howland RH. Psychiatric medications and sudden cardiac death: putting the risk in perspective. J Psychosoc Nurs Ment Health Serv. 2015;53(2): 23–5.
29. Hsia T-Y, Gruber PJ. Factors influencing neurologic outcome after neonatal cardiopulmonary bypass: what we can and cannot control. Ann Thorac Surg. 2006;81(6):S2381–8.
30. Islam MP, Roach ES. Tuberous sclerosis complex. Handb Clin Neurol. 2015;132:97–109.
31. Jin SC, Homsy J, Zaidi S, Lu Q, Morton S, DePalma SR, Zeng X, Qi H, Chang W, Sierant MC, et al. Contribution of rare inherited and de novo variants in 2,871 congenital heart disease probands. Nat Genet. 2017;49(11):1593–601.
32. Kesler SR. Turner syndrome. Child Adolesc Psychiatr Clin N Am. 2007;16:709–22.
33. Khairy P, Ionescu-Ittu R, Mackie AS, Abrahamowicz M, Pilote L, Marelli AJ. Changing mortality in congenital heart disease. J Am Coll Cardiol. 2010;56:1149–57.
34. Khairy P, Van Hare GF, Balaji S, Berul CI, Cecchin F, Cohen MI, Daniels CJ, Deal BJ, et al. PACES/HRS Expert Consensus Statement on the Recognition and Management of Arrhythmias in Adult Congenital Heart Disease: developed in partnership between the Pediatric and Congenital Electrophysiology Society (PACES) and the Heart Rhythm Society (HRS). Endorsed by the governing bodies of PACES, HRS, the American College of Cardiology (ACC), the American Heart Association (AHA), the European Heart Rhythm Association (EHRA), the Canadian Heart Rhythm Society (CHRS), and the International Society for Adult Congenital Heart Disease (ISACHD). Heart Rhythm. 2014;11(10):e102–65.
35. Knickmeyer RC, Davenport M. Turner syndrome and sexual differentiation of the brain: implications for understanding male-biased neurodevelopmental disorders. J Neurodev Disord. 2011;3(4):293–306.
36. Labellarte MJ, Crosson JE, Riddle MA. The relevance of prolonged QTc measurement to pediatric psychopharmacology. J Am Acad Child Adolesc Psychiatry. 2003;42(6):642–50.
37. Lai MC, Lombardo MV, Autism B-CS. Lancet. 2014;383(9920):896–910.
38. Lincoln AJ, Searcy YM, Jones W, Lord C. Social interaction behaviors discriminate young children with autism and Williams syndrome. J Am Acad Child Adolesc Psychiatry. 2007;46(3):323–31.
39. Marelli A, Gilboa S, Devine O, et al. Estimated the Congenital Heart Disease Population in the United States in 2010 – What are the Numbers?. J Am Coll Cardiol. 2012;59:E787. https://doi.org/10.1016/S0735–1097(12)60788-8.
40. Marino BS, Lipkin PH, Newburger JW, Peacock G, Gerdes M, Gaynor JW, Mussatto KA, et al. Neurodevelopmental outcomes in children with congenital heart disease: evaluation and management: a scientific statement from the American Heart Association. Circulation. 2012;126(9):1143–72.
41. McDonald-McGinn DM, Sullivan KE. Chromosome 22q11.2 deletion syndrome (DiGeorge syndrome/velocardiofacial syndrome). Medicine. 2011;90(1): 1–18.

42. Miatton M, De Wolf D, Francois K, Thiery E, Vingerhoets G. Neuropsychological performance in school-aged children with surgically corrected congenital heart disease. J Pediatr. 2007;151(1):73–8. 78.e1
43. Miller SP, McQuillen PS, Vigneron DB, Glidden DV, Barkovich AJ, Ferriero DM, Hamrick SE, Azakie A, Karl TR. Preoperative brain injury in newborns with transposition of the great arteries. Ann Thorac Surg. 2004;77(5):1698–706.
44. Miodovnik A, Harstad E, Sideridis G, Huntington N. Timing of the diagnosis of attention-deficit/hyperactivity disorder and autism spectrum disorder. Pediatrics. 2015;136(4):e830–7.
45. Moss J, Richards C, Nelson L, Oliver C. Prevalence of autism spectrum disorder symptomatology and related behavioural characteristics in individuals with Down syndrome. Autism. 2013;17(4):390–404.
46. Mouridsen SE, Rich B, Isager T. Diseases of the circulatory system among adult people diagnosed with infantile autism as children: a longitudinal case control study. Res Dev Disabil. 2016;57: 193–200.
47. Niklasson L, Rasmussen P, Oskarsdóttir S, Gillberg C. Autism, ADHD, mental retardation and behavior problems in 100 individuals with 22q11 deletion syndrome. Res Dev Disabil. 2009;30(4):763–73.
48. Pediatric and Congenital Electrophysiology Society (PACES), Heart Rhythm Society (HRS), American College of Cardiology Foundation (ACCF), American Heart Association (AHA), American Academy of Pediatrics (AAP), Canadian Heart Rhythm Society (CHRS), et al. PACES/HRS expert consensus statement on the management of the asymptomatic young patient with a Wolff-Parkinson-White (WPW, ventricular preexcitation) electrocardiographic pattern: developed in partnership between the Pediatric and Congenital Electrophysiology Society (PACES) and the Heart Rhythm Society (HRS). Endorsed by the governing bodies of PACES, HRS, the American College of Cardiology Foundation (ACCF), the American Heart Association (AHA), the American Academy of Pediatrics (AAP), and the Canadian Heart Rhythm Society (CHRS). Heart Rhythm. 2012;9(6):1006–24.
49. Pober BR. Williams-Beuren syndrome. N Engl J Med. 2010;362(3):239–52.
50. Razzaghi H, Oster M, Reefhuis J. Long-term outcomes in children with congenital heart disease: National Health Interview Survey. J Pediatr. 2015;166(1):119–24.
51. Reilly C. Autism spectrum disorders in Down syndrome: a review. Res Autism Spectr Disord. 2009;3:829–39.
52. Rohatgi RK, Bos JM, Ackerman MJ. Stimulant therapy in children with attention-deficit/hyperactivity disorder and concomitant long QT syndrome: a safe combination? Heart Rhythm. 2015;12(8):1807–12.
53. Rutter M, Bailey A, Lord C, Berument SK. The social communication questionnaire. Los Angeles: Western Psychological Services; 2003.
54. Saleeb SF, Li WY, Warren SZ, Lock JE. Effectiveness of screening for life-threatening chest pain in children. Pediatrics. 2011;128(5):e1062–8.
55. Shah AA, Aftab A, Coverdale J. QTc prolongation with antipsychotics: is routine ECG monitoring recommended? J Psychiatr Pract. 2014;20(3):196–206.
56. Shuler CO, Black GB, Jerrell JM. Population-based treated prevalence of congenital heart disease in a pediatric cohort. Pediatr Cardiol. 2013;34:606–11.
57. Southammakosane C, Schmitz K. Pediatric psychopharmacology for treatment of ADHD, depression, and anxiety. Pediatrics. 2015;136(2):351–9.
58. Tordjman S, Anderson GM, Botbol M, Toutain A, Sarda P, Carlier M, Saugier-Veber P, et al. Autistic disorder in patients with Williams-Beuren syndrome: a reconsideration of the Williams-Beuren syndrome phenotype. PLoS One. 2012;7(3):e30778.
59. Tsao PC, Lee YS, Jeng MJ, Hsu JW, Huang KL, Tsai SJ, Chen MH, Soong WJ, Kou YR. Additive effect of congenital heart disease and early developmental disorders on attention-deficit/hyperactivity disorder and autism spectrum disorder: a nationwide population-based longitudinal study. Eur Child Adolesc Psychiatry. 2017;26(11):1351–9.
60. Tyler CV, Schramm SC, Karafa M, Tang AS, Jain AK. Chronic disease risks in young adults with autism spectrum disorder: forewarned is forearmed. Am J Intellect Dev Disabil. 2011;116(5):371–80.
61. van der Linde D, Konings EE, Slager MA, Witsenburg M, Helbing WA, Takkenberg JJ, Roos-Hesselink JW. Birth prevalence of congenital heart disease worldwide: a systematic review and meta-analysis. J Am Coll Cardiol. 2011;58:2241–7.
62. Vetter VL, Elia J, Erickson C, Berger S, Blum N, Uzark K, Webb CL, American Heart Association Council on Cardiovascular Disease in the Young Congenital Cardiac Defects Committee, American Heart Association Council on Cardiovascular Nursing. Cardiovascular monitoring of children and adolescents with heart disease receiving medications for attention deficit/hyperactivity disorder [corrected]: a scientific statement from the American Heart Association Council on Cardiovascular Disease in the Young Congenital Cardiac Defects Committee and the Council on Cardiovascular Nursing. Circulation. 2008;117(18):2407–23.
63. Vignoli A, La Briola F, Peron A, Turner K, Vannicola C, Saccani M, Magnaghi E, Scornavacca GF, Canevini MP. Autism spectrum disorder in tuberous sclerosis complex: searching for risk markers. Orphanet J Rare Dis. 2015;10:154.
64. Vis JC, Duffels MG, Winter MM, Weijerman ME, Cobbin JM, Huisman SA, Mulder BJ. Down syndrome: a cardiovascular perspective. J Intellect Disabil Res. 2009;53(5):419–25.

65. Wier ML, Yoshida CK, Odouli R, Grether JK, Croen LA. Congenital anomalies associated with autism spectrum disorders. Dev Med Child Neurol. 2006;48(6):500–7.
66. Wren C, Reinhardt Z, Khawaja K. Twenty-year trends in diagnosis of life-threatening neonatal cardiovascular malformations. Arch Dis Child Fetal Neonatal Ed. 2008;93(1):F33–5.
67. Yeh TK, Yeh J. Chest pain in pediatrics. Pediatr Ann. 2015;44(12):e274–8.
68. Yoon Y, Wink LK, Pedapati EV, Horn PS, Erickson CA. Weight gain effects of second-generation antipsychotic treatment in Autism Spectrum disorder. J Child Adolesc Psychopharmacol. 2016;26(9):822–7.
69. Zhang C, Kutyifa V, Moss AJ, McNitt S, Zareba W, Kaufman ES. Long-QT syndrome and therapy for attention deficit/hyperactivity disorder. J Cardiovasc Electrophysiol. 2015;26(10):1039–44.
70. Polyak A, Kubina RM, Girirajan S. Comorbidity of intellectual disability confounds ascertainment of autism: implications for genetic diagnosis. Am J Med Genet B Neuropsychiatr Genet. 2015;168(7):600–8.

Pulmonary and Sleep Disorders

11

T. Bernard Kinane and Jessica McCannon

Introduction

There is a limited published literature about the prevalence of respiratory disorders in children, adolescents, and adults with autism spectrum disorder (ASD), though the most common issues in clinical practice include sleep disturbances and asthma. There is also some common overlap with other disorders, including allergies and gastroesophageal reflux disease (GERD), whose manifestations impact sleep and may mimic asthma and cause nocturnal symptoms, difficulty sleeping, or cough. Treating sleep disturbances and respiratory disorders in patients with ASD is challenging for different reasons. In the case of sleep disturbances, treatment often requires behavioral, pharmacologic approaches and, on occasion, the use of noninvasive ventilation, i.e., continuous positive airway pressure ventilation (CPAP), which poses problems for individuals with tactile and auditory sensitivity. Medications required to treat common respiratory disorders such as asthma may cause behavior changes, and as many are inhaled, they may be more challenging to administer.

Sleep disturbances are prevalent in children and adolescents with ASD and have tremendous impact upon the child's behavior and family dynamics. Indeed, sleep disruption and ASD may be linked at a basic biological level. Sleep is regulated by a broad array of neuronal networks that use an assortment of neurotransmitters, including γ-aminobutyric acid (GABA) and melatonin. In ASD, a similar group of neurotransmitters play a role in its pathophysiology. GABA has a key role in the downregulation of neuronal networks [1, 2]. Thus disruption of this neurotransmitter system in patients with ASD is likely to be central to the pathophysiology of associated sleep disorders. Likewise, melatonin is an important regulator of sleep. Its synthesis is repressed by light and promotes sleep [3]. In ASD, there is a disruption of this hormone's natural circadian rhythm [4–6]. One study found that excretion of a metabolite of melatonin, 6-sulfoxymelatonin, thought to indicate lower levels of nocturnal plasma melatonin, is decreased in children with ASD [7]. However, genetic studies linking sleep pathophysiology and ASD have yielded conflicting results. The overall pattern is consistent with a central role for melatonin and GABA disruption in the sleep disorders commonly seen in this condition.

On the other hand, there are a few epidemiologic studies exploring the increased prevalence of asthma and ASD. Results of existing studies are conflicting; however, both conditions are likely to have a common inflammatory/immune basis [8]. For example, it was recently found that IL-17 is elevated in patients with both asthma and ASD [9].

T. B. Kinane (✉) · J. McCannon
Department of Pediatrics, Massachusetts General Hospital, Boston, MA, USA
e-mail: Kinane.Bernard@mgh.harvard.edu; jmccannon@mgh.harvard.edu

E. P. Hazen, C. J. McDougle (eds.), *The Massachusetts General Hospital Guide to Medical Care in Patients with Autism Spectrum Disorder*, Current Clinical Psychiatry,
https://doi.org/10.1007/978-3-319-94458-6_11

Common Conditions

Sleep Problems

Sleep problems are an important aspect of ASD and have prevalence rates of up to 80% of patients, with some studies indicating the highest rates occur in those with higher executive functioning [10]. A wide range of sleep disorders has been described in patients with ASD, with insomnia being the most frequent [11–13]. These disorders have important implications for the family and the patient's daytime function. A significant issue is that families with children with ASD who suffer from sleep disorders experience higher rates of stress, specifically maternal and marital stress, as a result of parental sleep disruption [14]. Disruption of sleep can also induce increased hyperactivity and lack of focus in the individual patient [15, 16]. The disruption of sleep and the resultant shorter sleep duration have been associated with increased severity of behavioral problems, which is consistent with effects of sleep disruption in a typical child [17]. Thus, the identification and management of sleep disorders are essential for the patient's and family's health and quality of life.

Insomnia has many forms, including prolonged sleep latency (sometimes related to bedtime resistance), decreased sleep efficiency (because of frequent arousals), and decreased sleep duration. All of these forms of insomnia are commonly observed in children with ASD [11, 18–20]. Parents often describe sleep-onset insomnia, which may be related to ASD patients perseverating over activities and a slow transition to a sleep routine [11, 18]. But the initiation of the normal sleep cycle may also be related to a similar background pathophysiology with altered GABA and melatonin metabolism. Reduced sleep duration has important implications for family routine, health, and quality of life, as patients may arouse from sleep in the very early morning.

Other sleep disorders have also been reported in patients with ASD. Parasomnias have been reported to have increased frequency in patients with ASD, but they are not a distinctive feature [18]. Rapid eye movement (REM) behavioral disorders, where individuals act out their dreams, may also occur [21]. A number of studies have shown decreased REM sleep in individuals with ASD [21]. This may in part be related to the usage of medications such as selective serotonin reuptake inhibitors (SSRIs) and serotonin-norepinephrine reuptake inhibitors (SNRIs) that are known to reduce REM sleep, and at times help the behavioral aspects of ASD and may also cause behavioral activation and thus sleep disturbance in some patients with ASD. Movement disorders such as restless leg syndrome (RLS) and periodic limb movement disorders (PLMD) are thought to occur with increased frequency in patients with ASD; however, no studies have directly assessed the prevalence [22]. Indeed, it may be difficult to establish the presence of RLS in ASD as patients may not be able to report symptoms and discomfort due to RLS. RLS and PLMD are usually associated with iron deficiency and low ferritin, and such a deficiency is likely to occur in ASD due to a restrictive diet [23]. Obstructive sleep apnea (OSA) is less common, though may be more likely in the presence of other risk factors, including obesity, large tonsils and adenoids, or comorbid developmental disorders like Down syndrome, in which there is a known risk of OSA. In a community sample, adolescents and adults with Down syndrome who also had ASD were more likely to have sleep problems [24].

Asthma

The links between asthma and ASD are currently unclear. Asthma may be underdiagnosed in children with ASD as the symptoms associated with asthma may be clouded by behavioral issues and communication difficulties. One case-control study including more than 5,000 cases demonstrated that while other immune-mediated conditions like allergies and autoimmune disease were diagnosed more often among children with ASD, asthma was diagnosed less often (13.7% vs. 15.9%; OR = 0.83, 95% CI 0.76–0.90) [25]. Another case-control study revealed that asthma was more common in control cases than in patients with ASD [26]. However, Kotey et al. (2014) found an unadjusted odds ratio of 1.35 for developing asthma among children with ASD [27]. The National Health Interview Survey assessed the prevalence of common medical conditions among children with developmental disabilities and reported that asthma exacerbations are more common among children with ASD compared to typical children [28]. It is presumed that this may be related to issues with adherence to therapy, though it is quite possibly related to unmet healthcare needs among patients with ASD and asthma. Additionally, asthma exacerbations pose problems by disrupting routines for children and adults with ASD (missed school, day programs), making adherence all the more important. Pharmacologic therapies, including both maintenance and controller medications and medications for acute exacerbations, have the potential to alter behavior in ASD patients, such as causing irritability and aggression.

Pneumonia

Swallowing disorders are frequently reported by patients, but systematic studies are lacking [29]. Such disorders could lead to increased risk of aspiration pneumonia, but no such increased risk has been shown in ASD. Immune dysfunction has been well described in ASD. While this seems related to the underlying pathophysiology of ASD, it does not appear to increase the risk of pulmonary infections [30].

Clinical Evaluation

History

Sleep Disorders Since sleep disorders are common in ASD, it is necessary to be vigilant for these disorders during clinical encounters. It is easy to overlook the role of sleep and its consequences in ASD. Hyperactivity may be a more common reflection of sleep deprivation than hypersomnia. A thorough sleep history should include sleep habits, sleep rituals, and daytime sleep-related symptoms. Understanding environmental contributors to poor sleep hygiene is important and requires asking parents to consider the impact of temperature, noise and light levels in the bedroom, and textures and other stimulation in the environment. Parents should be encouraged to keep a sleep diary to assess sleep latency, awakenings, and total sleep duration. This permits an assessment of the overall sleep patterns and can also be used to assess responses to therapy. A number of questionnaires are available and can provide useful insight. The Children's Sleep Habits Questionnaire and the Family Inventory of Sleep Habits are useful tools that assess overall sleep performance and help to identify areas of concern [31, 32]. A behavioral checklist can identify conditions such as depression and anxiety that can alter sleep. Most of the data can be obtained from the caregivers in cases where the patient is unable to communicate.

Asthma The clinical history for asthma requires assessment of symptoms (e.g., chest tightness, shortness of breath, cough, and wheezing), patterns of symptoms, and precipitating factors. While cough and wheezing are often apparent to caregivers of individuals with ASD, chest tightness and shortness of breath may not be reported. Nocturnal symptoms are also common in asthma, and while taking a sleep history, it is important to ascertain whether cough or shortness of breath is present during nocturnal awakenings. As with any patient with asthma, understanding the wide range of triggers is important, including weather and temperature (e.g., cold air, humidity), environmental triggers (e.g., dusts, molds, tobacco, pets, strong odors), and seasonal allergies. In a child or adult being considered for a diagnosis of asthma, a family history of asthma or atopy increases the likelihood that symptoms are related to asthma. Asking about ability to tolerate physical activities, including whether the child may struggle to keep up with same-age peers, is also important, as is understanding the impact of symptoms on school performance. It is also necessary to assess for other disorders that cause similar symptoms, such as GERD or chronic rhinitis.

Physical Examination

Sleep Disorders There are very few signs of sleep disorders on physical exam. Occasionally, patients may struggle to stay awake during a clinical interaction. Nocturnal bruxism may be apparent by worn dental enamel (see Chap. 7). Additionally, if patients are obese, or the oropharyngeal exam reveals large tonsils and a crowded posterior oropharynx, it is important to consider sleep disordered breathing or sleep apnea.

Asthma The pulmonary exam, like other components of the physical exam, can be difficult for some children and adults with ASD to tolerate. Auscultation, which permits detection of a prolonged expiratory phase or expiratory wheezes, typically described as high-pitched and musical in asthma, requires that the stethoscope be placed directly on the skin, which can be difficult for someone with tactile sensitivities. Some patients with ASD find it comforting to hold and help direct the stethoscope's movements and placement on the chest.

Studies

Sleep Disorders Iron studies, including ferritin, may be ordered to assess for iron deficiency, which is associated with RLS and PLMD. A sleep study/polysomnogram (PSG) is rarely indicated unless the clinical history is suggestive of obstructive sleep apnea (e.g., snoring, sleeping in unusual positions, daytime somnolence). PSG may be challenging to undertake in children and adults with ASD because of tactile and auditory sensitivities, but is not impossible. With ASD and other developmental disabilities, desensitization or visual aids are often helpful to prepare for the study. There are published protocols that have demonstrated efficacy in patients with ASD and other developmental disabilities, though patients with ASD may require longer time for desensitization [33].

Asthma The diagnosis of asthma should be suspected when appropriate symptoms (such as cough, chest tightness, shortness of breath, or wheeze) are precipitated by triggers such as exercise, allergens, cold air, or viral illnesses. Wheeze may be present on physical examination but should improve with bronchodilators. Pulmonary function tests are not required to diagnose asthma, and often the diagnosis is highly suggested and accepted when patients' symptoms improve with standard asthma therapies. Normal pulmonary function tests do not rule out asthma, as normal pulmonary function between exacerbations is the hallmark of asthma. However, the presence of airway obstruction (in the case of children 12 years and younger, with FEV1/FVC ratio <0.85; for children >12 years and adults, FEV1/FVC ratio <0.70) with bronchodilator reversal (improvement in FEV1 after the administration of albuterol) can confirm the diagnosis. In the appropriate clinical context, understanding the allergic triggers by skin testing or radioallergosorbent testing (RAST), can be helpful.

Treatment

Sleep Disorders Once medical and psychiatric conditions are addressed, with particular attention to major contributors like anxiety, tonsillitis, enlarged adenoids, seizures, and gastrointestinal conditions that may affect sleep, insomnia should be treated in a systematic way. Patients with ASD may have a number of behaviors that are not conducive to the establishment of a normal sleep pattern, including hypersensitivity to environmental stimuli, repetitive behaviors and thoughts, and difficulty following directions. Thus, improving sleep hygiene via sleep education and behavioral strategies is the core of the therapeutic approach. Key aspects of this approach include the utilization of activities that make it easier to fall asleep and stay asleep, such as a dark environment, eliminating caffeine ingestion, and providing a wind down period before bedtime [34]. The use of electronic devices such as televisions, computers, cell phones, and video-gaming devices that emit background light should be excluded from the bedroom and before bedtime. A small pilot study suggested a potential benefit from aerobic exercise training on improving sleep efficiency, decreasing sleep-onset latency, and decreasing wake time after sleep onset (as assessed by sleep-EEG) [35].

Insomnia is frequently resistant to therapy addressing sleep hygiene alone, and in some of these cases, it is necessary to resort to pharmacological intervention. Melatonin is the cornerstone of insomnia treatment in children with ASD. This treatment strategy has been shown to be effective at improving sleep initiation with minimal reports of adverse events [36, 37]. Melatonin is used as a sedative and is typically given in the 1–5 mg dose range 30 min prior to bedtime. As melatonin has a short half-life, it is less effective at treating nighttime awakenings, though a slow-release melatonin preparation offers some promise [38]. If melatonin is ineffective, additional pharmacologic treatment may be indicated, but few studies have been performed among children and adults with ASD.

A few psychotropic medications have been evaluated for the treatment of insomnia in individuals with ASD. Clonidine [39], mirtazapine [40], gabapentin [41], and risperidone [42] have been shown to improve sleep-onset latency in individuals with ASD, but no controlled studies have been completed. Risperidone, while effective, should be limited due to potential side effects, including weight gain, hyperprolactinemia, and tardive dyskinesia, except when it is indicated to treat a coexisting condition, like irritability. Benzodiazepines and over-the-counter medications like diphenhydramine can cause paradoxical excitation in some individuals with ASD and should be used with caution [28].

Movement disorders such as PLMD have been found to correlate with low serum ferritin. Iron deficiency is indeed more likely to develop in the ASD population due to mealtime rituals and restricted diets [43, 44]. Treatment with iron is beneficial, though it is important to keep in mind that iron can be constipating; comorbid gastrointestinal disorders are common among children and adults with ASD. If iron supplementation is unsuccessful, treatment with pramipexole (a non-ergot dopamine agonist) may be indicated; however this medication has not been studied in individuals with ASD, and its mechanism of action in RLS is unknown. Parasomnias should be treated in the usual way depending upon the sleep disruption. If medication is indicated, the common choices are benzodiazepines and tricyclic antidepressants (TCAs) such as amitriptyline, with benzodiazepines being particularly effective [34, 45]. TCAs can lower the seizure threshold and cause constipation. As mentioned earlier, benzodiazepines can cause paradoxical behavioral activation.

Obstructive sleep apnea can be addressed by surgical removal of enlarged tonsils or adenoids, the use of dental devices (which may require desensitization), or continuous positive airway pressure (CPAP). The use of CPAP can be problematic in patients with ASD because of tactile and auditory sensitivity. It is possible that the same desensitization protocols for dental devices and polysomnograms can help patients acclimate to ongoing treatment, though medical literature for desensitization approaches is lacking [33]. If surgery is undertaken, it is important to consider that some patients may have pain and swallowing difficulties postsurgery that may impact their ability to take medications that impact other important health issues (i.e., seizures). Further discussion of the treatment of OSA and enlarged tonsils and adenoids can be found in Chap. 9 on "Disorders of the Ear, Nose, and Throat."

Asthma Specific therapies for asthma depend on the severity of the symptoms, and there are well-established guidelines (see table). However, asthma medications may cause behavior changes among children and adults with ASD. Mild asthma is often treated with short-acting beta-agonists (albuterol) on an as needed basis. The challenge is that children with ASD may not be able to signal when they have symptoms and thus when they need an emergency medication. Using an inhaler with a spacer, a device to hold the medication released from the inhaler so that the child has the time to more effectively inhale the medication, can be challenging for any child, but even more so for a child with ASD. Beta-agonists can cause tremors, agitation, and aggression among children and adults with ASD.

More persistent asthma is treated with either inhaled corticosteroids alone or, when more severe, a combination of inhaled corticosteroids and a long-acting beta-agonist. Inhaled corticosteroids are traditionally not thought to be systemically absorbed in amounts that affect behavior, though anecdotally some typical adults report subtle changes in mood with their use. The same issues with short-acting beta-agonists occur with long-acting beta-agonists. Montelukast and other leukotriene inhibitors are used to treat allergic asthma but can cause nightmares, insomnia, and increased aggression, all of which can impact the behavior of patients with ASD. With acute exacerbations, systemic glucocorticoids (e.g., prednisone) are often required and may cause hyperactivity and irritability. Individuals with asthma often use nebulized therapy during an exacerbation, but nebulized medications including beta-agonists (e.g., albuterol) and anticholinergic medications (e.g., ipratropium) can cause behavioral issues.

Prevention of exacerbations of asthma is critically important in patients with ASD because of the impact of hospitalization and loss of routine with acute illness. Thus, maximizing the likelihood of adherence with maintenance medication is key. Ideally, the medications can be incorporated into a personalized routine for the patient. A case report describes how the medical team took advantage of one patient's interest in fire engines. A firefighter posed for a picture with a metered-dose inhaler (MDI). When it was time to use the MDI, the patient's care team showed him the picture, and the patient was permitted to put on a special firefighter hat, while he used his MDI with mask spacer, improving cooperation with the regimen [45].

Special Issues in Adults with ASD and Sleep Disorders or Asthma There are no major differences in the presentation or assessment of either sleep disorders or asthma in adults with ASD. With experienced parents and caregivers, there can be a much more nuanced understanding about communication style and techniques preferred by patients which can enhance education and awareness about diagnoses and their respective treatment plans.

Clinical Vignette # 1

A 4-year-old boy presented to the sleep clinic because he typically slept for just 3 h per night and some nights not at all. These findings were

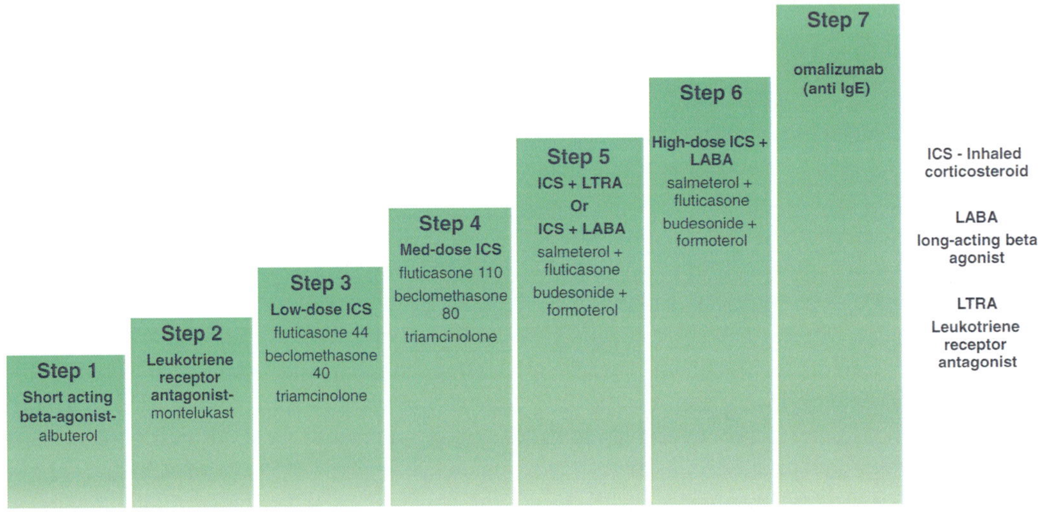

confirmed with a sleep diary filled out by his parents. Via a combination of clonidine (0.1 mg QHS) and melatonin (3 mg QHS), his sleep time was extended to 5–6 h. He functioned very well on this limited amount of sleep. The parents' major concern became the awakening time of 3 AM. After awakening, he would wander around the house and disrupt the rest of the family. His mother noticed that he could read the clock accurately and would perform certain daily activities at certain times. Via behavior modification and the use of a clock, he was taught that he could not leave his room until 6 AM, when the small hand of the clock pointed to 6 with a picture of the sun placed over it.

Clinical Vignette # 2

A 24-year-old male with ASD presented to a pulmonary clinic for evaluation of chronic cough of over a year. He was obese and unable to communicate and had a history of aggressive behavior, though this had improved with psychiatric treatment. He lived in a group home. Caregivers who knew him for years reported that he coughed predominantly at night, but that throughout the day he often cleared his throat more than coughing. They had never appreciated any audible wheezing, and he had never appeared to suffer from any respiratory distress, but they were quite concerned that he may have asthma. As part of his pulmonary visit, pulmonary function tests were attempted, but he could not reliably perform the required maneuvers, so testing was aborted before he became upset (since spirometry is not required to diagnose asthma). His lung exam was remarkable for good excursion and clear breath sounds without wheezes or prolonged expiratory phase. With obesity and nocturnal predominance of cough as well as daytime throat-clearing, suspicion was raised for gastroesophageal reflux disease (GERD) as a major contributor to his cough. Treatment with proton pump inhibitors and raising the head of bed (by putting the bed on risers) was recommended, with plans to try empiric treatment for asthma at the next visit if there was no improvement in his symptoms. At a follow-up visit 4 months later, the patient's cough had improved, and use of asthma medications was avoided, which may have negatively impacted his behavior.

Clinical Pearls

- Insomnia and other sleep disorders can present with a wide variety of symptoms, including behavioral difficulties. Careful history taking about sleep patterns, including the use of validated questionnaires or sleep diaries, can be helpful in diagnosis.
- Insomnia is the most common sleep disorder among individuals with ASD, and assessment and treatment of insomnia and other sleep disorders are critical given the cognitive and behavioral impact upon individuals and their families.
- Melatonin is the mainstay of pharmacologic treatment for insomnia for individuals with ASD given its benign side effect profile and based on numerous published controlled studies.
- Therapies for asthma, including both maintenance medications and emergency medications, may negatively impact the behaviors of individuals with ASD, and this should be closely monitored when managing asthma in this population.

References

1. Levitt P, Eagleson KL, Powell EM. Regulation of neocortical interneuron development and the implications for neurodevelopmental disorders. Trends Neurosci. 2004;27:400–6.
2. McCauley JL, Olson LM, Delahanty R, et al. A linkage disequilibrium map of the 1-Mb 15q12 GABA(A) receptor subunit cluster and association to autism. Am J Med Genet B Neuropsychiatr Genet. 2004;131B:51–9.
3. Gooley JJ. Treatment of circadian rhythm sleep disorders with light. Ann Acad Med Singap. 2008;37:669–76.
4. Melke J, Goubran Botros H, Chaste P, et al. Abnormal melatonin synthesis in autism spectrum disorders. Mol Psychiatry. 2008;13:90–8.

5. Rossignol DA, Frye RE. Melatonin in autism spectrum disorders: a systematic review and meta-analysis. Dev Med Child Neurol. 2011;53:783–92.
6. Rossignol DA, Frye RE. Melatonin in autism spectrum disorders. Curr Clin Pharmacol. 014;9:326–34.
7. Leu RM, Beyderman L, Botzolakis EJ, Surdyka K, Wang L, Malow BA. Relation of melatonin to sleep architecture in children with autism. J Autism Dev Disord. 2011;41:427–33.
8. Becker KG. Autism, asthma, inflammation, and the hygiene hypothesis. Med Hypotheses. 2007;69:731–40.
9. Akintunde ME, Rose M, Krakowiak P, et al. Increased production of IL-17 in children with autism spectrum disorders and co-morbid asthma. J Neuroimmunol. 2015;286:33–41.
10. Patzold LM, Richdale AL, Tonge BJ. An investigation into sleep characteristics of children with autism and Asperger's disorder. J Paediatr Child Health. 1998;34:528–33.
11. Krakowiak P, Goodlin-Jones B, Hertz-Picciotto I, Croen LA, Hansen RL. Sleep problems in children with autism spectrum disorders, developmental delays, and typical development: a population-based study. J Sleep Res. 2008;17:197–206.
12. Richdale AL, Schreck KA. Sleep problems in autism spectrum disorders: prevalence, nature, & possible biopsychosocial aetiologies. Sleep Med Rev. 2009;13:403–11.
13. Souders MC, Mason TB, Valladares O, et al. Sleep behaviors and sleep quality in children with autism spectrum disorders. Sleep. 2009;32:1566–78.
14. Honomichl RD, Goodlin-Jones BL, Burnham M, Gaylor E, Anders TF. Sleep patterns of children with pervasive developmental disorders. J Autism Dev Disord. 2002;32:553–61.
15. Chervin RD, Archbold KH. Hyperactivity and polysomnographic findings in children evaluated for sleep-disordered breathing. Sleep. 2001;24:313–20.
16. Chervin RD, Archbold KH, Dillon JE, et al. Inattention, hyperactivity, and symptoms of sleep-disordered breathing. Pediatrics. 2002;109:449–56.
17. Gabriels RL, Cuccaro ML, Hill DE, Ivers BJ, Goldson E. Repetitive behaviors in autism: relationships with associated clinical features. Res Dev Disabil. 2005;26:169–81.
18. Gail Williams P, Sears LL, Allard A. Sleep problems in children with autism. J Sleep Res. 2004;13:265–8.
19. Mazurek MO, Sohl K. Sleep and behavioral problems in children with autism spectrum disorder. J Autism Dev Disord. 2016;46:1906–15.
20. Richdale AL. Sleep problems in autism: prevalence, cause, and intervention. Dev Med Child Neurol. 1999;41:60–6.
21. Thirumalai SS, Shubin RA, Robinson R. Rapid eye movement sleep behavior disorder in children with autism. J Child Neurol. 2002;17:173–8.
22. Reynolds AM, Malow BA. Sleep and autism spectrum disorders. Pediatr Clin N Am. 2011;58:685–98.
23. Schreck KA, Williams K, Smith AF. A comparison of eating behaviors between children with and without autism. J Autism Dev Disord. 2004;34:433–8.
24. Hoffmire CA, Magyar CI, Connolly HV, Fernandez ID, van Wijngaarden E. High prevalence of sleep disorders and associated comorbidities in a community sample of children with Down syndrome. J Clin Sleep Med. 2014;10:411–9.
25. Zerbo O, Leong A, Barcellos L, Bernal P, Fireman B, Croen LA. Immune mediated conditions in autism spectrum disorders. Brain Behav Immun. 2015;46:232–6.
26. Lyall K, Van de Water J, Ashwood P, Hertz-Picciotto I. Asthma and allergies in children with autism spectrum disorders: results from the CHARGE study. Autism Res. 2015;8:567–74.
27. Kotey S, Ertel K, Whitcomb B. Co-occurrence of autism and asthma in a nationally-representative sample of children in the United States. J Autism Dev Disord. 2014;44:3083–8.
28. Schieve LA, Gonzalez V, Boulet SL, et al. Concurrent medical conditions and health care use and needs among children with learning and behavioral developmental disabilities, National Health Interview Survey, 2006–2010. Res Dev Disabil. 2012;33:467–76.
29. Heckathorn DE, Speyer R, Taylor J, Cordier R. Systematic review: non-instrumental swallowing and feeding assessments in pediatrics. Dysphagia. 2016;31:1–23.
30. Fatemi SH. The molecular basis of autism. New York: Springer; 2015.
31. Owens JA, Spirito A, McGuinn M. The Children's Sleep Habits Questionnaire (CSHQ): psychometric properties of a survey instrument for school-aged children. Sleep. 2000;23:1043–51.
32. Reed HE, McGrew SG, Artibee K, et al. Parent-based sleep education workshops in autism. J Child Neurol. 2009;24:936–45.
33. Primeau M, Gershon A, Talbot L, et al. Individuals with autism spectrum disorders have equal success rate but require longer periods of systematic desensitization than control patients to complete ambulatory polysomnography. J Clin Sleep Med. 2016;12:357–62.
34. Veatch OJ, Maxwell-Horn AC, Malow BA. Sleep in autism spectrum disorders. Curr Sleep Med Rep. 2015;1:131–40.
35. Brand S, Jossen S, Holsboer-Trachsler E, Puhse U, Gerber M. Impact of aerobic exercise on sleep and motor skills in children with autism spectrum disorders – a pilot study. Neuropsychiatr Dis Treat. 2015;11:1911–20.
36. Goldman SE, Adkins KW, Calcutt MW, et al. Melatonin in children with autism spectrum disorders: endogenous and pharmacokinetic profiles in relation to sleep. J Autism Dev Disord. 2014;44:2525–35.
37. Braam W, Smits MG, Didden R, Korzilius H, Van Geijlswijk IM, Curfs LM. Exogenous melatonin for sleep problems in individuals with intellectual disability: a meta-analysis. Dev Med Child Neurol. 2009;51:340–9.
38. Cortesi F, Giannotti F, Sebastiani T, Panunzi S, Valente D. Controlled-release melatonin, singly and

combined with cognitive behavioural therapy, for persistent insomnia in children with autism spectrum disorders: a randomized placebo-controlled trial. J Sleep Res. 2012;21:700–9.
39. Ming X, Gordon E, Kang N, Wagner GC. Use of clonidine in children with autism spectrum disorders. Brain Dev. 2008;30:454–60.
40. Posey DJ, Guenin KD, Kohn AE, Swiezy NB, McDougle CJ. A naturalistic open-label study of mirtazapine in autistic and other pervasive developmental disorders. J Child Adolesc Psychopharmacol. 2001;11:267–77.
41. Robinson AA, Malow BA. Gabapentin shows promise in treating refractory insomnia in children. J Child Neurol. 2013;28:1618–21.
42. Aman MG, Arnold LE, McDougle CJ, et al. Acute and long-term safety and tolerability of risperidone in children with autism. J Child Adolesc Psychopharmacol. 2005;15:869–84.
43. Allen RP. Restless legs syndrome/Willis Ekbom disease: evaluation and treatment. Int Rev Psychiatry. 2014;26:248–62.
44. Sharp WG, Berry RC, McCracken C, et al. Feeding problems and nutrient intake in children with autism spectrum disorders: a meta-analysis and comprehensive review of the literature. J Autism Dev Disord. 2013;43:2159–73.
45. Mason TB 2nd, Pack AI. Pediatric parasomnias. Sleep. 2007;30:141–51.

12 Gastroenterology

Nicole M. Benson and Sarah M. Kadzielski

Introduction

Gastrointestinal (GI) disorders in those with autism spectrum disorder (ASD) are common. This population undergoes hospitalization and treatment for GI conditions at significantly higher rates than their peers, making GI illnesses an important area to address with early detection and intervention [1]. In children in particular, the prevalence of GI symptoms may be at least 50%, although estimates have ranged from 9% to 70% [2, 3]. GI symptoms and illnesses do not always present with obvious signs and symptoms. Instead, those with ASD and GI conditions may present with new behavioral issues rather than specific GI symptoms, obscuring the underlying diagnosis [2, 3].

N. M. Benson (✉)
Child and Adolescent Psychiatry, Massachusetts General Hospital, Boston, MA, USA
e-mail: nbenson@mgh.harvard.edu

S. M. Kadzielski
Pediatric Gastroenterology and Nutrition, Massachusetts General Hospital, Boston, MA, USA

Lurie Center for Autism, Lexington, MA, USA
e-mail: smkadzielski@mgh.harvard.edu

Common Pediatric and Adult Gastrointestinal Conditions in ASD

Abdominal Pain or Discomfort

Chronic abdominal pain is defined as abdominal pain that persists or recurs frequently for a duration of at least 1 month [3]. Identifying the underlying cause requires a full medical work-up, including assessment of associated symptoms such as vomiting or diarrhea. The initial assessment of abdominal pain in the ASD population should be similar to the approach used with the non-ASD population because the pain may stem from a variety of etiologies. These can include GI disorders, such as gastroesophageal reflux disease (GERD), constipation, viral gastroenteritis, bacterial or parasitic infections, appendicitis, celiac disease, gallbladder disease, inflammatory bowel disease, cyclic vomiting syndrome, or malignancy (either intrinsic or extrinsic to the GI tract), as well as extraintestinal disorders, such as nephrolithiasis, musculoskeletal problems, streptococcal pharyngitis, viral illness, pneumonia, migraine headaches, or an intracranial process causing increased intracranial pressure.

Special consideration must be given to patients with ASD when assessing abdominal pain because these patients may demonstrate abdominal pain differently than the general population. Specifically, the pain may manifest in a variety of

E. P. Hazen, C. J. McDougle (eds.), *The Massachusetts General Hospital Guide to Medical Care in Patients with Autism Spectrum Disorder*, Current Clinical Psychiatry,
https://doi.org/10.1007/978-3-319-94458-6_12

ways particularly after meals or related to toileting and defecation. Some examples may include global changes in behavior, such as sleep disturbances or irritability; abnormal vocalizations or motor movements, such as unexplained crying or grimacing; self-injury, such as biting or head-banging; and repetitive movements, such as facial or vocal tics or rubbing the abdomen [2, 3].

Gastroesophageal Reflux Disease (GERD) and Reflux

Gastroesophageal reflux disease (GERD) is retrograde flow of gastric contents into the esophagus causing signs and symptoms that can include chest pain, abdominal pain, heartburn, nausea, vomiting or regurgitation, bad taste in the mouth, halitosis, and poor appetite or feeding refusal. As with abdominal pain in children with ASD, GERD in this population may present with nonspecific symptoms including irritability or aggressive behaviors, restriction of certain foods, or hitting or tapping on the chest. One study found that 43% of children with ASD and GERD exhibited irritability, much more often than the 13% rate of irritability found in those who did not have GERD [2]. Because aggressive or self-injurious behavior may be the primary clinical manifestation of GERD in patients with ASD, these symptoms may be misattributed to other causes, which can delay diagnosis and treatment [2].

Symptoms of GERD overlap with those of eosinophilic esophagitis (EoE). EoE is a chronic, immune-mediated disease characterized by inflammation and esophageal dysfunction. Symptoms of EoE may include pain with swallowing, the sensation of food getting stuck, nausea and vomiting, weight loss, abdominal pain, feeding refusal, and food aversions. Untreated EoE leads to sequelae of food impaction resulting from esophageal dysmotility, esophageal strictures, and fibrosis. EoE is more common in those with ASD than the general population (0.4% vs. 0.1%) and can present with food selectivity or feeding disorders [4]. Because of the atypical presentations of EoE in the ASD population, symptoms may be misdiagnosed as a food sensitivity, delaying treatment. EoE should be suspected in patients with symptoms of GERD that do not improve with antacid therapy. EoE should also be considered in patients with symptoms of GERD who also have a personal history of atopic disorders, such as asthma, reactive airway disease, allergic rhinitis, other environmental allergies, food allergies, or eczema.

The differential diagnosis of recurrent vomiting or regurgitation not only includes GERD and EoE but also rumination syndrome. Rumination syndrome is a functional disorder characterized by a persistent regurgitation of food into the mouth thought to be due to an increase in intragastric pressure which allows gastric contents to flow backward through the lower esophageal sphincter into the esophagus and up to the mouth [5].

Constipation

Constipation is diagnosed when patients have difficulty or delay in defecation with symptoms lasting at least 2 weeks [3]. The condition is more common in patients with ASD, although the true prevalence of constipation in this population has not been established. It has been estimated that 36% of individuals with ASD suffer moderate to severe constipation, significantly higher than the 3–10% found in the general population [6]. Long-term sequelae of chronic constipation include hemorrhoids, diverticulosis, and diverticulitis, making this an important condition to diagnose and treat.

The causes of constipation are multifactorial and should be fully investigated in any patient who presents with this common medical complaint. Up to 95% of childhood constipation has been estimated to be functional constipation with no clear physiologic or organic cause [1]. In children with ASD, special consideration must be given to behavioral issues relating to toileting and evacuation withholding behaviors. Those with ASD may also have sensory processing difficulties that alter GI motility and, in turn, change defecation physiology and pain with bowel movements [1, 3]. In this population, patients may suffer incomplete evacuation despite regular bowel movements without other symptoms, making this condition difficult to detect by caretakers in some cases. Patients with comorbid attention deficit hyperactivity disorder (ADHD) may also not pay close attention to internal body cues and put off using the bathroom until the last minute. Similarly, patients with attentional issues may not sit on the toilet for a long enough period to allow for complete evacuation.

Diarrhea

Diarrhea is diagnosed when patients have loose stools, and chronic diarrhea is diagnosed when loose stools persist for a period of at least 2 weeks [3]. In most cases, acute episodes are the result of self-limited infections and resolve within several days. With childhood chronic diarrhea, the causes in those with ASD are the same as in the general pediatric population and include functional disorders, infections, inflammatory bowel disease, structural abnormalities, and malabsorption syndromes [3]. Long-term sequelae of chronic diarrhea for those with ASD include poor weight gain and malnutrition; thus, diet and nutritional status should be assessed and monitored. At times, severe constipation with fecal impaction may present with overflow of loose stool, which can be perceived by patients and caregivers as diarrhea.

Food Sensitivities

Adverse reactions to food are a broad term to describe a negative response to ingesting a food item. Reactions can be further subdivided based on whether they are immune-mediated (food allergy, IgE-based reaction) or not (food intolerance or sensitivity). It is important to consider this when trying to understand an individual's food refusal or sensitivity [2].

The underlying cause of non-allergic adverse reactions is typically difficult to identify but may result from a prior bad experience or dislike of certain tastes or textures. Among individuals with ASD, one unpleasant experience may lead to generalized intolerance or sensitivity for certain foods or food groups, leading to self-selected broad dietary restrictions or food aversions [2]. Food intolerance or sensitivity may also be a sign of underlying GI disease, particularly GERD or EoE.

Lactose intolerance is common in the general population and not thought to be more common in patients with ASD [2]. An empiric trial of a lactose-free diet can be considered in patients with symptomatology that is consistent with lactose malabsorption or intolerance. Typically, within a few hours of ingestion of dairy products, patients with lactose malabsorption due to lactase deficiency develop intestinal gas, bloating, abdominal pain, diarrhea, or cramping. Not all patients with this condition have loose stools, so in patients with communication deficits who cannot convey bloating or cramping, discomfort may manifest in nonspecific pain behaviors.

Irritable bowel syndrome (IBS), as described by the Rome IV criteria, is a functional GI disorder that consists of recurrent abdominal pain associated with changes in stooling pattern. There are three subtypes of IBS: (i) IBS with predominant diarrhea (IBS-D), (ii) IBS with predominant constipation (IBS-C), and (iii) IBS with mixed bowel habits (IBS-M). IBS is felt to reflect a combination of factors including altered motility, visceral hypersensitivity, possible changes in the gut microbiome, and altered intestinal permeability. Patients with ASD can also have IBS, although it may be more difficult to identify.

Feeding Difficulties

Children with ASD have an estimated fivefold increased risk of developing a feeding issue compared to peers. Some experts have estimated that at least half of all children with ASD have feeding difficulties [1]. In this population, where there is a predisposition for having rigidity about behaviors and patterns, feeding issues that develop in childhood may persist into adulthood. Feeding difficulties in ASD range from self-restricted diets with little variety of foods (typically with a preference for starches and heavily processed foods and restricted intake of fruits, vegetables, and foods high in protein), elimination of an entire food group (or more than one), refusal of certain foods based on texture or color, or insistence on eating the same specific way each time. Abnormally low muscle tone can contribute to difficulties with chewing or swallowing and may lead to a preference for soft or smooth textured foods and away from meats. Other patients with sensory alterations might prefer crunchy foods such as raw vegetables or snack foods like crackers and chips. It is important to remember that, in addition to behavioral and sensory issues, feeding difficulties may reflect physical discomfort from a GI condition, such as GERD, EoE, esophageal dysmotility, or oropharyngeal dysphagia.

Feeding difficulties and restrictive feeding patterns may be associated with poor weight gain in children, weight loss in adults, or issues with development and growth. Evidence suggests that selective eating patterns put this population at risk for long-term nutritional complications [1].

On the other hand, obesity is common in people with ASD [7], just as it has reached epidemic proportions in the general US population. In the ASD population, obesity may result in part from self-restricted diets and preference for high-caloric foods. Use of edible rewards for behavior training can also contribute to excess weight gain. In addition, lack of physical activity due to patient preference, lack of a safe outdoor environment for patients, or affinity for electronic devices may contribute to this problem.

Both low appetite and overactive appetite may be side effects of psychiatric medications commonly used to treat comorbidities in patients with ASD. For example, appetite suppression and poor weight gain may be associated with stimulants given to treat ADHD. Other medications such as antipsychotics can increase appetite and cause significant weight gain.

Pica, Mouthing, and Foreign Body Ingestion

Pica, or ingestion of nonfood objects, is fairly common in patients with ASD. They may mouth or chew on objects such as toys, paper, clothing, plastic objects, dirt, or rocks and may also swallow the particles. These behaviors may be caused by sensory issues, confusion about what is food and what is not, nutritional deficiencies (e.g., iron, zinc), or abdominal pain or nausea related to GERD.

Individuals that can be impulsive or compulsive or who have a tendency to put nonfood objects in their mouths are at risk of foreign body ingestion. Many ingested objects will pass completely through the GI tract without requiring intervention, but there are a few objects that can be dangerous if ingested and need immediate medical care. These may include large, sharp, or pointed objects, button batteries, or multiple magnets. There are guidelines available for easy reference when evaluating a patient who has swallowed a foreign body [8]. Foreign body ingestions that may require urgent medical care include (1) sharp objects, which may perforate the bowel, (2) very large objects (>5 cm long), which may be too large to navigate the twists and turns of the intestinal tract, causing obstruction and/or perforation, (3) ingestion of multiple magnets, which may attract two loops of bowel together, causing pressure necrosis and perforation, (4) button batteries in the esophagus, which may cause mucosal burn, perforation, or fistula within very short periods of time, (5) superabsorbent polymers such as toy sponges, which may rapidly expand once in the body, and (6) lead objects, which may cause lead toxicity. Any ingestion causing airway symptoms or symptoms of esophageal obstruction such as an inability to handle oral secretions, should receive medical attention. Likewise, any patient with symptoms of bowel obstruction or perforation (fever, abdominal pain, vomiting) should also seek medical attention. In addition, ingestion of caustic substances may also cause mucosal damage; in this setting, we would recommend initial evaluation and close follow-up care to monitor for sequelae.

Genetic Disorders/Syndromes with ASD and GI Issues

There are several genetic disorders and syndromes that co-occur with ASD. It is important to note that some of these genetic disorders can predispose patients to GI conditions. In those with tuberous sclerosis complex (TSC), a genetic disorder characterized by the growth of hamartomas throughout multiple organ systems, co-occurring ASD has an estimated prevalence of 36% [9]. Patients with this syndrome are at risk for hamartomas of the GI tract. In those with neurofibromatosis type 1 (NF-1), characterized by café au lait spots and the growth of small tumors along the skin and nerves, co-occurring ASD has an estimated prevalence of 18% [9]. With this latter disorder, patients are at risk of developing GI tumors. Bannayan-Riley-Ruvalcaba syndrome (BRRS) is a rare genetic disorder that puts patients at risk for developing colonic and rectal polyps [10]. These patients also have an elevated risk for ASD.

Alterations in Microbiome

There has been growing interest in the gut-brain link to autism. Some families have initiated food elimination diets for ASD, such as a gluten-free casein-free (GFCF) diet, just as these diets have become more popular in the general population. Although there are many anecdotal reports of improvement in GI symptoms (e.g., abdominal pain, diarrhea, constipation, and bloating) and core features of ASD (e.g., stereotypies, communication, and response to therapies) with these dietary changes, no controlled studies to date have provided evidence to support this as a therapy for ASD [2, 11]. Children with ASD have been found to have disruptions in their microbiome, compared to non-ASD controls. These include decreased diversity of species, as well as a different balance of organisms (e.g., fewer *Bifidobacterium* species) [12]. The clinical significance of these alterations is unclear at present.

Clinical Evaluation

History

Any clinical evaluation must start with a thorough history of the presenting symptoms. This should include the age of symptom onset and the way in which each symptom first presented. The history should be obtained from as many of the patient's care providers as possible to ensure that the full array of symptoms is attained.

For those with ASD, it may be difficult to ascertain stooling patterns. A stool diary can be useful to keep track of bowel movement patterns and stool type/consistency. This is beneficial in a home setting, as well as for patients in residential programs where caregivers change constantly throughout the day. In addition, the stool diary can be paired with the Bristol Stool Scale to help patients and caretakers provide a more accurate and standardized description of stools. The goal is for patients to have one to two stools per day, with stool consistency of type three, four, or five on the scale.

In patients with impaired communication skills, the evaluation of symptoms can be particularly challenging and difficult. Some individuals are able to communicate symptoms of abdominal pain or discomfort fairly readily. Others may not be able to communicate such symptoms, necessitating a careful history to assess for behavioral changes including change in mood/irritability or changes in food preference/food sensitivity, particularly around mealtimes. Presence of these behavioral changes should prompt a work-up of underlying abdominal pain.

Physical Examination

The physical examination is an integral part of any work-up for a GI complaint. Prior to initiation of a physical exam of a patient with ASD, it is important to explain the planned exam and any procedure. Story boards or "If, Then" communication boards can be essential communication tools to describe upcoming exams to help them proceed smoothly (Fig. 12.1). Before beginning any exam, the procedure should be described to the patient and caretaker using simple words or pictures, then demonstrated, possibly on the caretaker, and then performed on the patient as it was just demonstrated and described. For more information on helping patients with ASD tolerate the physical exam, see Chap. 4 "Procedures."

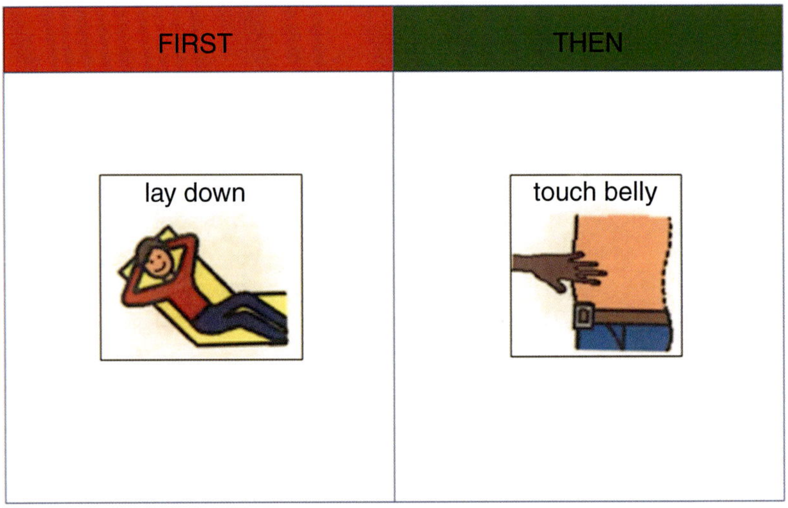

Fig. 12.1 Picture exchange communication board used in clinic to help with physical examination

Every attempt should be made to do a complete physical exam, including a rectal examination; however, this may not be feasible in all cases [2]. With a gentle approach and possibly some preparation by the caregiver prior to the visit, key aspects of physical examination may be accomplished. Involving the caregiver in the physical exam can be very helpful. Abdominal palpation is usually the most important part of the physical exam for GI problems, especially when evaluating for constipation. Caregivers should be asked if any part of the physical examination is particularly distressing to a given individual, in which case it should be left for last. Some patients will only allow a single aspect of physical examination before they stop cooperating, in which case abdominal palpation should be the first step of the exam. Some patients may refuse to lie on the examination table because they do not like the noise of the paper; in such cases, removing the paper may help. Some children may sit or lie across a caregiver's lap, which helps them feel more comfortable than being on the table. Other patients who refuse to get on the examination table may cooperate if they lie across several chairs placed next to each other to create a "bed." Some patients may respond well to a small prize or reward after each step of the examination or after all the steps have been completed.

Studies

Evaluation for GI problems should proceed similarly in patients with ASD as in those without. Depending on the presenting symptoms, this may involve bloodwork, lactose breath test, imaging studies (e.g., ultrasound, kidney, ureter, and bladder x-ray (KUB), computed tomography (CT), or magnetic resonance imaging (MRI)), diagnostic endoscopy or colonoscopy, pH/impedance monitoring, or anorectal manometry (ARM).

Special considerations must be given during the diagnostic approach depending on what tests the patient might tolerate. Sometimes, more challenging tests such as imaging can be accomplished with extra preparation ahead of the visit. However, if the patient cannot cooperate with a given diagnostic study, a provider might consider treating empirically for certain conditions, such as a trial of antacids for possible GERD or a lactose-free diet for possible lactose malabsorption.

For a patient with abdominal pain, diarrhea, weight loss, or poor weight gain, laboratory studies should include complete blood count with differential (CBC), erythrocyte sedimentation rate (ESR), C-reactive protein (CRP), complete metabolic panel, thyroid-stimulating hormone (TSH), celiac (TTG-IgA and total IgA), stool guaiac, stool calprotectin, and lactoferrin. This will evaluate for inflammatory bowel disease (IBD), celiac disease, metabolic disorders, or other inflammatory disorders.

For a patient with picky eating and food sensitivities, consider IgE tests for common food antigens, radioallergosorbent test ("RAST") for milk, soy, eggs, wheat, corn, beef, or other specific foods for which a caregiver reports intolerance.

Nutritional deficiencies due to poor intake should be evaluated with CBC, ferritin/iron studies, vitamin D level (25-OH-Vit D), vitamin B12 level, zinc, and folate. For patients with pica, a similar laboratory panel should be considered to rule out iron-deficiency anemia and zinc and lead abnormalities.

Treatment of Common Gastrointestinal Conditions in ASD

Medical therapy is similar for patients whether or not they have ASD. Additional behavioral considerations may need to be taken into account for patients with ASD. Changing behaviors or habits may require not only medications to address the underlying cause but also behavioral interventions to change the habits.

Abdominal Pain or Discomfort

The treatment of abdominal pain is driven primarily by the underlying cause. If the evaluation is unrevealing, the treatment is primarily symptomatic with emphasis on an understanding of the distress caused by the pain. It is important to recognize that, if pain persists over time, changes in signs or symptoms warrant reevaluation in most cases.

Gastroesophageal Reflux Disease (GERD) and Reflux

If a diagnosis of GERD is a consideration, one may treat empirically with acid suppression, typically a proton pump inhibitor. GERD is often a chronic condition, and because symptoms may be difficult to monitor in the ASD population, close follow-up and continued assessment is warranted to ensure that serious sequelae, such as Barrett's esophagus or esophageal strictures, do not develop over time. Wireless pH monitoring can be helpful in identifying whether or not certain behaviors are related to acid reflux events. The choice of specific medication may depend on the formulation the patient can tolerate, as well as what is covered by insurance or price of over-the-counter versions.

Constipation

When treating constipation in general, the goal is a pattern of one or two bowel movements per day, without pain or straining. Patients who have had hard or painful stool passage in the past may require several months (or longer) of a bowel regimen before their anxiety about defecation subsides.

For severely constipated patients, the initial treatment may require a full bowel cleanout, which can be difficult for patients with ASD to tolerate. Determination of the best cleanout regimen requires a conversation with the patient and caregiver to identify what would be most feasible for the individual. For example, some patients with taste sensitivities might refuse magnesium citrate but would be willing to drink a large volume of a preferred beverage with multiple doses of polyethylene glycol mixed into it. Other patients might do better with the smaller volume of magnesium citrate, despite the taste, as their caregivers can use rewards to help them finish the volume. The "ideal cleanout," which may be completed within a few hours for a patient without ASD, might require spacing of treatment over the course of 2 or 3 days for a patient with ASD.

Long-term treatment and prevention of constipation may require dietary changes and medications. When treating constipation in the ASD population, as with other conditions, finding a bowel regimen may take some trial and error in terms of dosage, formulation (suspension, liquid, capsules), and food preferences. Specific medication regimens for treatment of constipation in infants and children can be found in guidelines and involve osmotic stool softeners, stimulant laxatives, other medications to increase motility (such as magnesium), as well as newer agents that act on secretions of the gut (lubiprostone, linaclotide) [13].

Diarrhea

The treatment of diarrhea is highly dependent on the underlying cause. A full work-up should be completed to assess whether medical intervention is warranted. For example, patients with celiac disease should start a strict gluten-free diet. Patients who are diagnosed with IBD, either Crohn's disease or ulcerative colitis, should be treated accordingly by a qualified specialist. As with the treatment of constipation in the ASD population, experimentation with different formulations and tastes may be necessary when medications are indicated. Providers must be flexible and sensitive to the patient's tolerance for different drugs, and finding the correct regimen may take some time. Given how common constipation is in patients with ASD, fecal impaction with overflow of loose stool can be ruled out with a KUB to visualize stool in the colon. Treating loose stools might involve a trial of a lactose-free diet, even for a week as a starting point, to see if stool consistency improves. Nonspecific diarrhea of childhood, or "toddler's diarrhea", can be caused by fruit juice or excessive intake of fruit. Fiber supplements can sometimes be used as a bulking agent. Most infectious diarrhea is viral and will be self-resolved. Bacterial infections should be treated with the appropriate course of antibiotics.

Food Sensitivities and Feeding Difficulties

Evaluation in a multidisciplinary center can help to sort through the causes of food sensitivities or aversions and feeding difficulties in order to identify strategies to increase the variety of foods accepted by the patient. In addition to a gastroenterologist, the multidisciplinary team might involve a speech and language pathologist, occupational therapist, nutritionist, psychologist, and behavioral therapist.

Some reports have suggested that individuals with ASD may respond to dietary interventions with improvement in both GI symptoms and symptoms of ASD. At this time, available research and published studies do not support the use or effectiveness of gluten-free, casein-free (GFCF) diet in improving symptoms of ASD [2, 14].

Often treatment for food sensitivities and feeding difficulty requires dietary modification that is selected empirically and on an individual basis. For those with IBS, treatment is multimodal. Many patients with IBS without developmental delay, who are able to monitor and track their symptoms, identify specific foods that trigger their symptoms. It is recommended that any patients on special diets are supervised by a registered dietitian to ensure that the diet is nutritionally complete.

Pica and Mouthing

If nutritional deficiencies and GERD have been ruled out, management of pica is behavioral. Prevention includes prevention of opportunities by keeping the environment free of potential foreign objects, providing alternative sensory opportunities, educating the patient about what is food and nonfood, and distraction.

Foreign Body Ingestion

Guidelines about foreign body ingestion [8] are helpful to identify which patients can be monitored or observed at home for symptoms and those that need to come for urgent imaging and/or endoscopic or surgical removal. Poison Control should also be contacted for guidance on medical intervention for any ingestion, 1-800-222-1222 and www.PoisonHelp.org.

Genetic Disorders/Syndromes with ASD and GI Issues

Clinical evaluation and treatment of GI conditions in these patients require a combination of the same clinical evaluation and treatment of other patients with these genetic disorders and syndromes, as well as the specialized clinical evaluation and treatment needed for those with ASD and the same GI condition.

Alterations in Microbiome

Although dietary changes have not yet been shown to improve symptoms in ASD, new areas related to the microbiome are under investigation including dietary changes, probiotics, antibiotics, and fecal microbiota transplant (FMT). An association between ASD and alteration in the microbiome has been found, but a causal relationship has not been established. Research is ongoing to investigate the potential role of probiotics and FMT as future treatment considerations. Studies of the microbiome hold promise in terms of identifying a potential cause of some symptoms and/or a target for therapy [12].

Clinical Vignette # 1

An 8-year-old boy with ASD presents with changes in sleep patterns. He used to sleep through the night, but over the last few weeks, he has been waking up crying multiple times throughout the night. His parents have already put good sleep hygiene habits into place, such as consistent sleep/wake times, minimizing screen time before bed, and avoidance of caffeine. They had also tried melatonin, which helped him to fall asleep initially, but did not improve the multiple nocturnal awakenings. He had regular bowel movements without constipation. He was a very picky eater and milk was one of his preferred foods. He would sometimes ask for a glass of milk when he awoke in the middle of the night.

Due to consideration of possible GERD as a cause of the patient's nocturnal awakenings, the patient was started empirically on a proton pump inhibitor (PPI). A suspension was initially prescribed but the patient refused to take it. Multiple formulations of PPI were tried until his caregivers found success with a capsule that they could open and sprinkle into his food. His symptoms improved over the next few weeks, as did his sleep pattern. After a 3-month course of medication, he was weaned off the PPI but within a few weeks started to have gradual return of many of the previous symptoms.

He then underwent upper endoscopy which revealed esophagitis consistent with active GERD. He was restarted on a PPI for a longer course and after 6 months was very gradually weaned off the medication successfully.

His picky eating was addressed by feeding therapy by an occupational therapist to help him expand his diet.

Clinical Vignette # 2

A 4-year-old boy with ASD who is nonverbal develops increased aggressive behavior as well as self-injurious behavior. His caregivers do not note a pattern to the behaviors as they can occur even without demands being placed on him and during activities that he usually enjoys. He is evaluated thoroughly by his primary care physician who is unable to identify any obvious cause of pain, such as otitis media or strep throat. He is a picky eater and does not drink much water at baseline. His appetite has decreased. Lab work including celiac testing and inflammatory markers has been normal. A KUB shows significant stool burden throughout the entire colon including a large amount of formed stool in the rectum and sigmoid colon.

An outpatient "cleanout" regimen is discussed, with options including magnesium citrate or multiple stacked doses of polyethylene glycol. Parents choose the four ounces of magnesium citrate liquid (a rule of thumb is 1 oz per 1 year of life, up to maximum of 10 oz). He took a very small sip of the magnesium citrate but did not like the taste and refused to drink any more. His parents were unable to get him to take the full dose of medication. Instead, an alternative cleanout regimen was suggested, consisting of stacked doses of polyethylene glycol and senna as a stimulant laxative. The polyethylene glycol medication was mixed with lemonade, his preferred beverage. In order to get him to take multiple doses of the polyethylene glycol, his in-home behavioral therapist was able to use reinforcement to encourage him to continue drinking the rest. He was unable to swallow pills but willingly ate the senna given in "chocolate" square formulation. He repeated the same regimen the next day and eventually passed large amounts of liquid stool over the next 2 days.

After the cleanout, he continued on a daily dose of polyethylene glycol with titrations of the dose based on stool output. His aggressive and self-injurious behavior improved dramatically after the cleanout and continued to improve over the next few weeks.

Clinical Pearls

- Patients with ASD have the same GI conditions as the general population.
- Gastrointestinal conditions appear to be more prevalent in individuals with ASD as compared to the general population. Some of these may be mediated by increased sensory issues.
- Gastrointestinal problems in patients with ASD may present with behavioral changes alone, rather than classic symptoms for the condition, due to communication impairments. Nonspecific behavioral difficulties, such as self-injurious behavior, aggression, or sleep disruption, may herald underlying GI issues, particularly if there is a new onset of behavioral difficulties or if these behaviors have a relationship to meals or toileting patterns. Without a high index of suspicion, these behaviors might be incorrectly labeled as "autism behaviors" without identification of the true underlying GI cause.
- Clinicians may need to be willing to investigate certain symptoms more extensively in patients with communication difficulties. This may involve ordering more invasive testing than one would usually consider for a certain symptom or treating empirically for a given condition.
- Treatment for GI conditions should be the same for patients whether or not they have ASD.
- Evidence is inconclusive about the effectiveness of dietary interventions in patients with ASD. Although there may be a subgroup of patients with ASD for whom elimination diets may be useful, characterizing or predicting which patients will respond is not possible at this time. Any special diets should be done under the supervision of a nutritionist to ensure they are done safely.
- An association between ASD and alteration in microbiome has been found, but a causal relationship has not been established. Research is ongoing to investigate the potential role of probiotics and fecal microbiota transfer (FMT) as future treatment considerations.

Resources for Families and Providers of Those with Autism Spectrum Disorder and Gastrointestinal Issues

North American Society for Pediatric Gastroenterology, Hepatology, and Nutrition (NASPGHAN)
www.gikids.org
www.youtube.com
"The Poo in You – Constipation and Encopresis Educational Video"

American College of Gastroenterology (ACG)
http://patients.gi.org/

Autism Speaks Toolkits
https://www.autismspeaks.org/family-services/tool-kits
Guide for managing constipation in children
Guide to exploring feeding behavior in autism
Pica: a guide for parents
Pica: a guide for professionals
Parent's guide to toilet training in autism

References

1. McElhanon BO, McCracken C, Karpen S, Sharp WG. Gastrointestinal symptoms in autism spectrum disorder: a meta-analysis. Pediatrics. 2014;133(5):872–83.
2. Buie T, Campbell DB, Fuchs GJ 3rd, Furuta GT, Levy J, Vandewater J, et al. Evaluation, diagnosis, and treatment of gastrointestinal disorders in individuals with ASDs: a consensus report. Pediatrics. 2010;125(Suppl 1):S1–18.
3. Buie T, Fuchs GJ 3rd, Furuta GT, Kooros K, Levy J, Lewis JD, et al. Recommendations for evaluation and treatment of common gastrointestinal problems in children with ASDs. Pediatrics. 2010;125(Suppl 1):S19–29.
4. Heifert TA, Susi A, Hisle-Gorman E, Erdie-Lalena CR, Gorman G, Min SB, et al. Feeding disorders in children with autism spectrum disorders are associated with eosinophilic esophagitis. J Pediatr Gastroenterol Nutr. 2016;63(4):e69–73.
5. Kessing BF, Smout AJ, Bredenoord AJ. Current diagnosis and management of the rumination syndrome. J Clin Gastroenterol. 2014;48(6):478–83.
6. Afzal N, Murch S, Thirrupathy K, Berger L, Fagbemi A, Heuschkel R. Constipation with acquired megarectum in children with autism. Pediatrics. 2003;112(4):939–42.
7. de Vinck-Baroody O, Shui A, Macklin EA, Hyman SL, Leventhal JM, Weitzman C. Overweight and obesity in a sample of children with autism spectrum disorder. Acad Pediatr. 2015;15(4):396–404.
8. Kramer RE, Lerner DG, Lin T, Manfredi M, Shah M, Stephen TC, et al. Management of ingested foreign bodies in children: a clinical report of the NASPGHAN Endoscopy Committee. J Pediatr Gastroenterol Nutr. 2015;60(4):562–74.
9. Richards C, Jones C, Groves L, Moss J, Oliver C. Prevalence of autism spectrum disorder phenomenology in genetic disorders: a systematic review and meta-analysis. Lancet Psychiatr. 2015;2(10):909–16.
10. Lowichik A, White FV, Timmons CF, Weinberg AG, Gunasekaran TS, Nathan K, et al. Bannayan-Riley-Ruvalcaba syndrome: spectrum of intestinal pathology including juvenile polyps. Pediatr Dev Pathol. 2000;3(2):155–61.
11. Srinivasan P. A review of dietary interventions in autism. Ann Clin Psychiatry. 2009;21(4):237–47.
12. Kang DW, Adams JB, Gregory AC, Borody T, Chittick L, Fasano A, et al. Microbiota Transfer Therapy alters gut ecosystem and improves gastrointestinal and autism symptoms: an open-label study. Microbiome. 2017;5(1):10.
13. Constipation Guideline Committee of the North American Society for Pediatric Gastroenterology H, Nutrition. Evaluation and treatment of constipation in infants and children: recommendations of the North American Society for Pediatric Gastroenterology, Hepatology and Nutrition. J Pediatr Gastroenterol Nutr. 2006;43(3):e1–13.
14. Sathe N, Andrews JC, McPheeters ML, Warren ZE. Nutritional and Dietary Interventions for Autism Spectrum Disorder: A Systematic Review. Pediatrics. 2017;139(6):e20170346.

Nephrology

13

Amita Sharma and Jonathan Paolino

Introduction

The approach to the diagnosis and treatment of renal disorders in children and adults with autism spectrum disorder (ASD) is not unlike that of the general population. There are, however, some topics that need to be highlighted because patients with ASD may be at increased risk of these disorders. These include tuberous sclerosis complex, lithium toxicity, juvenile nephronophthisis, enuresis, and urinary tract infections. Because of the important role of the kidney both in the metabolism of commonly used medications and in the overall health of an individual, an understanding of these conditions is essential for both primary care and subspecialty healthcare providers caring for patients with ASD.

Common Conditions

Clinical Vignette # 1

A 7-year-old boy with ASD is referred for evaluation of kidney cysts seen on a recent abdominal ultrasound that was performed to evaluate abdominal pain. The parents report that the child has had delays in his language development. On physical exam, facial angiofibromas and hypopigmented macules on the torso and arms were observed. On neurological examination, gait, reflexes as well as muscle bulk, tone, and power were normal. The remainder of the physical examination was normal.

Complete blood count and tests for renal and liver function were normal, as were levels of plasma electrolytes, glucose, calcium, magnesium, total protein, albumin, and the urinary protein to creatinine ratio and urinalysis.

A kidney ultrasound showed irregularly shaped kidneys measuring 9 cm bilaterally, with several simple cysts in each kidney.

Diagnosis: Tuberous Sclerosis Complex Tuberous sclerosis complex (TSC) is an autosomal dominant genetic syndrome characterized by benign tumor (hamartoma) formation in multiple organs. The term tuberous describes the potato-like appearance of brain lesions observed by the French neurologist

A. Sharma · J. Paolino (✉)
Department of Pediatrics, Massachusetts General Hospital, Boston, MA, USA
e-mail: asharma5@mgh.harvard.edu; jpaolino1@mgh.harvard.edu

E. P. Hazen, C. J. McDougle (eds.), *The Massachusetts General Hospital Guide to Medical Care in Patients with Autism Spectrum Disorder*, Current Clinical Psychiatry,
https://doi.org/10.1007/978-3-319-94458-6_13

Bourneville in the late 1880s. The diagnosis of TSC can be challenging because clinical manifestations are varied, few are specific to the disorder, and some only become evident in childhood. TSC affects approximately 1 in 6,000 individuals, involving all racial and ethnic groups. The disorder is caused by mutations in the genes *TSC1* (located on chromosome 9q34) [1] and *TSC2* (located on chromosome 16p13.3) encoding for the proteins hamartin and tuberin, respectively. These proteins bind and form the hamartin-tuberin complex that antagonizes an insulin-signaling pathway, which plays a role in regulation of cell size, cell number, and organ size.

When a new mutation occurs in a family, TSC resulting from the *TSC2* gene is four times more common than that arising from *TSC1* or approximately 80% of TSC cases. By contrast, the prevalence of *TSC1* and *TSC2* mutations is equal in familial cases. Two-thirds of affected individuals have a de novo pathogenic variant. Most de novo mutations are a consequence of a spontaneous mutation in the egg or sperm before fertilization, thus initiating a potential autosomal dominant inheritance pattern. However, in some cases, the somatic mosaic or a gonad mosaic may reside in the parental germline. When a germline mutation is present, more than one sibling can be affected, consistent with autosomal dominant inheritance; consequently, subsequent generations have a 50% chance of inheriting the disease. TSC disease exhibits high variability of severity between families and within families with the same mutation.

The diagnosis of TSC may be facilitated by the clinical criteria which are well defined and recently have been updated [2] and may be corroborated by genetic studies. TSC is a heterogeneous disease of variable severity affecting almost all organ systems. The main organs involved are the brain, skin, lungs, and kidneys, with a wide diversity of symptoms and severity across patients.

Central nervous system involvement is most common. TSC causes disorganization of the brain's laminar structure, hypomyelination, epilepsy, and social behavior deficits in addition to tumorigenesis. Cortical tubers in the temporal lobe may be related to the increased likelihood of an ASD diagnosis in patients with TSC. While 2–9% of individuals with ASD are diagnosed with TSC, as many as 50% of individuals with TSC present with features of ASD [3].

Renal disease is the second leading cause of early death in individuals with TSC. Almost universally, children with TSC are born with normal kidneys, with the exception of those with the TSC2/PKD1 contiguous gene syndrome. With age, however, proliferative renal disease develops, resulting in renal cysts and angiomyolipomas (AMLs). Both of these can cause chronic kidney disease (CKD) and progress to ESRD (end-stage renal disease). It is estimated that approximately 1,000,000 individuals worldwide have CKD attributable to TSC, with *TSC2* mutations generally producing a more severe renal phenotype [4]. An estimated 80% of children with TSC have an identifiable renal lesion by a mean age of 10.5 years. Less common renal manifestations of TSC include oncocytomas, malignant AMLs, renal cell carcinoma (RCC), interstitial renal disease, and focal segmental glomerulosclerosis (FSGS).

The incidence of AMLs and renal cysts increases with age, with an incidence of 38–55% at preschool age ($\leq$ 6 years), increasing to 75–80% in the school-age group and reaching 86–100% in adults [6]. TSC-associated AMLs are typically multiple and bilateral unlike sporadic AMLs. The majority of patients with TSC are asymptomatic with regard to renal manifestations, but serious complications do occur. In a series of 149 patients, 69% had AMLs, of which 9% bled [5]. The potential for developing hemorrhage is directly related to the AML size and vascularity. As AMLs grow, there may be a destructive mass effect within the renal parenchyma, hemorrhage, or outward growth that becomes exophytic with extension into renal fat, thus causing hematuria, intra-tumoral or retroperitoneal bleeding, and mass effect that can cause abdominal pain [6].

For asymptomatic AMLs measuring > 4 cm in diameter or > 3 cm and growing rapidly, treatment with a mammalian target of rapamycin (mTOR) inhibitor has been successful in the short term [7]. Current treatment options for AMLs are focused on conserving kidney function and limiting potentially fatal hemorrhage by embolization [8]. The risk of hemorrhage is 25–50%. Corticosteroid therapy decreases post-embolization syndrome. Nephrectomy is to be avoided because of the high incidence of complications and increased risk of chronic renal insufficiency.

Epithelial cysts are generally asymptomatic and are more often associated with hypertension and renal failure than are AMLs. In addition, an estimated 2–3% of patients with TSC carry a contiguous germline deletion that affects both the *TSC2* gene and adjacent PKD1 gene on chromosome 16p13, resulting in a polycystic kidney phenotype that is detectable in infancy or early childhood and that generally leads to renal insufficiency in the late teens to early 20s.

Glomerulocystic kidney disease is a rare presentation that is usually diagnosed in the neonatal period [9]. Typically, it is characterized by glomerular cysts involving about 5% of nephrons without tubular dilation. Glomeruli show large abnormal parietal epithelial cells piled up against Bowman's capsule with abnormal podocytes attached to the glomerular tuft. Because the cysts are small, the kidneys are typically normal or slightly increased in size. There may be loss of corticomedullary differentiation on imaging.

Oncocytomas are benign epithelial tumors that are fat poor and composed of polygonal cells with abundant, finely granular, eosinophilic cytoplasm with closely packed mitochondria. The intercalated cell of the cortical collecting duct is thought to be the cell of origin. Oncocytomas are usually noticed on evaluation of renal complications such as flank pain and hematuria or during surveillance with ultrasonography. Oncocytomas are usually multiple and bilateral and are a more common cause of RCC in patients with TSC compared with sporadic oncocytomas in the general population. Nephron-sparing surgery is the treatment of choice because diagnosis cannot be definitively made with noninvasive testing [10].

The overall incidence of RCC in patients with TSC is similar to that in the general population, with a lifetime risk of 2–3%. However, the cancer is diagnosed at a younger age in patients with TSC. RCC may be difficult to distinguish radiographically from fat poor AMLs and may require tissue diagnosis. There are case reports of RCC in children and even in one infant with TSC [11].

Renal replacement choice is guided by TSC-related behavioral difficulties. When aggressive outbursts and significant hyperactivity preclude the possibility of undergoing dialysis, preemptive renal transplant may be the modality of choice [12].

A variety of other renal lesions have been inadequately described in patients with TS. These include parapelvic or perirenal lymphatic cysts in patients with extra pulmonary lymphangioleiomyomatosis AMLs [13], renal artery stenosis, and aortic coarctation [14]. Incidental finding of a horseshoe kidney has also been described in patients with TSC [15].

Clinical Vignette # 2

A 17-year-old boy with ASD was seen in the Emergency Department for a suicide attempt by overdose of psychiatric medications. The patient was transferred from an inpatient psychiatry facility because of significant drowsiness. His medications were citalopram, lithium, and aripiprazole. He has been on lithium for the last 10 years.

On examination, the patient was obtunded with dysarthric speech. There were no neurocutaneous stigmata. The reflexes were brisk; muscle bulk and tone were normal. The rest of the physical examination was normal.

The patient's serum creatinine was 2.5 mg/dL with a serum uric acid of 10 mg/dL. Complete blood count and tests for liver function were normal, as were levels of plasma electrolytes, glucose, calcium, magnesium, total protein, and albumin; the urinary protein to creatinine ratio and urinalysis were normal as well. Urine-specific gravity was < 1005. Serum lithium level was 3 mEq/L.

The electrocardiogram (ECG) showed sinus bradycardia and T wave flattening with a normal QTc interval. Renal ultrasound showed bilateral echogenic kidneys. The patient underwent renal dialysis, with a reduction in the lithium level to 0.3 mEq/L.

Diagnosis: Acute Lithium Toxicity with Acute Kidney Injury Mood stabilizer and antidepressant medication use is common and often long term in individuals with ASD. It correlates with age, number of physical illnesses, and number of comorbid psychiatric diagnoses.

Lithium salts are commonly used mood stabilizers. Normally, lithium is not present in significant amounts in body fluids (< 0.2 mEq/L). However, lithium salts have been used therapeutically for almost 150 years. Lithium affects inositol monophosphate and glycogen synthase kinase-3 pathways, affecting energy metabolism, neuroprotection, and neuroplasticity, though the precise mechanism of mood stabilization is not well understood.

Unfortunately, lithium also has a narrow therapeutic index, with therapeutic levels between 0.6 and 1.5 mEq/L. The optimal steady-state concentration of lithium for maintenance treatment of bipolar disorder is generally considered to be 0.6–1.2 mEq/L, with slightly elevated steady-state concentrations (0.8–1.5 mEq/L) indicated for the acute management of manic episodes. Because toxicity can occur at levels > 1.5 mEq/L, lithium levels must be carefully monitored and lithium dosage adjusted as necessary.

Lithium is excreted almost entirely by the kidneys. Lithium is freely filtered by the glomerulus since it is not bound to serum proteins. In the proximal tubule, lithium is handled similarly to sodium. Approximately 80% of the lithium that is filtered by the glomerulus is reabsorbed, mostly in the proximal convoluted tubule. The remainder is excreted in the urine. Lithium has an elimination half-life of 12–27 h after a single dose, but its elimination half-life can increase to as long as 58 h in patients taking lithium chronically. Thus, one must measure lithium levels several times after a toxic ingestion, because its rate of elimination is variable and cannot be predicted in any given patient. Volume depletion or renal impairment from any cause increases lithium reabsorption.

There are three types of lithium poisoning: acute, acute on chronic, and chronic. Acute on chronic poisoning occurs in patients being treated with lithium who take an overdose, like the patient in Case 2. The symptoms and signs of toxicity differ based upon the total body burden of lithium and the rate of onset of toxicity. Chronic lithium intoxication starts insidiously with silent affliction of the kidneys followed by "prodromal" symptoms, and when moderate severity has been reached, an accelerating renal vicious circle with decreasing kidney function is imminent. After this point the chronic intoxication resembles acute intoxication. However, the clinical presentation of lithium toxicity is only loosely correlated with serum drug concentrations, and there is great variability in severity associated with a given concentration in acute on chronic vs. chronic where serum levels correlate more closely with clinical signs as drug distribution has reached a steady state. The severity of chronic lithium intoxication correlates directly with the serum lithium concentration and may be categorized as mild (1.5–2.0 mEq/L), moderate (2.0–2.5 mEq/L), or severe (> 2.5 mEq/L). Of note, lithium must be measured in a lithium-free tube; blood tubes anticoagulated with lithiated heparin can cause falsely positive lithium levels [16]. Toxic symptoms may be present even when concentrations are well within the recommended therapeutic range. Symptoms associated with mild poisoning include lethargy, drowsiness, coarse hand tremor, muscle weakness, nausea, vomiting, and diarrhea. Moderate toxicity is associated with confusion, dysarthria, nystagmus, ataxia, myoclonic twitches, and ECG changes (flat or inverted T waves). Severe toxicity, which can be life-threatening, is associated with grossly impaired consciousness, increased deep tendon reflexes, seizures, syncope, renal insufficiency, coma, and death.

Treatment of acute lithium intoxication includes general care and hydration. The quantity and quality of fluid are guided by the patient's fluid status, concomitant nephrogenic diabetes insipidus (NDI), and renal status [17]. Also, other organ involvement including thyroid function and potential hypercalcemia needs to be addressed.

Extracorporeal removal by prolonged hemodialysis is the treatment of choice for severe lithium toxicity, as lithium is readily dialyzable due to its low molecular weight, negligible protein binding, and small volume of distribution [18]. Lithium clearance with hemodialysis ranges from 70 to 170 mL/min, compared to normal renal clearance of 10–40 mL/min (due to extensive reabsorption of lithium in the proximal tubules) and only 15 mL/min with peritoneal dialysis [19]. Nine hours of hemodialysis removes approximately 60% of the total lithium stores. However, in most cases, unless serum lithium concentrations are extremely high, one session of hemodialysis over 4–6 h is usually sufficient. It is important to make sure that lithium levels remain below 1 mEq/L (1 mmol/L) for 6–8 h after treatment [20].

NDI, with an estimated prevalence of 20–70%, is the most common chronic side effect of lithium on the kidneys [21]. Acute onset of nocturia is an important clue to the presence of NDI. A water restriction test should be performed to establish the correct diagnosis and to exclude central diabetes insipidus or primary polydipsia which may be coexistent. Lithium causes dysregulation of the aquaporin system in principal cells of the collecting duct [22]. Initially the defect is reversible, but on chronic use it becomes irreversible [23]. If maximum urine osmolality is below 200 mosmol/kg, the tubular damage is often permanent, even if lithium is discontinued. When lithium-induced NDI is diagnosed, the medication should be discontinued if possible. If lithium therapy is absolutely necessary, amiloride should be instituted alone [24] or in combination with hydrochlorothiazide [25]. Serum lithium concentrations must be carefully monitored since diuretic-induced volume depletion may increase proximal sodium and lithium reabsorption. The ensuing fall in lithium excretion may then require a reduction in drug dose. It is also postulated that NDI can further enhance the pathological effects of lithium on proximal tubules, contributing to proximal tubule atrophy and interstitial fibrosis.

Long-term lithium therapy can cause chronic tubulointerstitial nephritis (TIN), which may lead to chronic kidney disease [26] that occasionally progresses to ESRD [27]. Chronic lithium-induced TIN is characterized by the presence of tubular atrophy and interstitial fibrosis. In the initial stages, distal and collecting tubules form microcysts which can be detected with magnetic resonance imaging [28]. Major risk factors for nephrotoxicity appear to be the duration and cumulative dose of lithium exposure. Mean loss of glomerular filtration rate (GFR) is about 2.3 mL/min/year with an average latent period between the onset of lithium therapy and ESRD of 20 years [29]. It has been suggested that 15–20% of patients develop a slowly progressive decline in GFR, which usually does not fall below 40–60 mL/min. Progressive renal failure with a serum creatinine concentration above 2 mg/dL due solely to lithium is uncommon. The course of the renal disease after discontinuation of lithium is unpredictable as progression may occur due to other comorbidities or ongoing secondary factors, such as systemic and intraglomerular hypertension, possibly resulting in secondary glomerulosclerosis.

Proteinuria is an uncommon manifestation of lithium toxicity and is usually less than a gram/day. However, lithium is also known to cause minimal change disease [30] and focal segmental sclerosis (FSGS) [31] as well as incomplete distal renal tubular acidosis (RTA).

Lithium-associated ESRD is an uncommon but not rare complication. The safe and effective use of lithium requires regular monitoring of kidney function. Current strategies for minimizing the renal effects of lithium include (i) assiduously avoiding episodes of renal toxicity, (ii) monitoring serum lithium concentrations in order to achieve optimal efficacy at the lowest possible concentration, (iii) adding amiloride and/or hydrochlorothiazide, (iv) monitoring urine osmolality and serum creatinine levels on a yearly basis and getting further medical evaluation when the serum creatinine level consistently rises, and (v) possibly administering lithium once a day.

Clinical Vignette # 3

An 8-year-old boy with a history of language delay and social impairment was referred for nocturnal enuresis. His birth history was unremarkable. Review of systems was positive for failure to thrive, polyuria, polydipsia, and night blindness.

The physical exam was unremarkable, with the exception of some hand-flapping gestures when the patient appeared to be nervous.

Laboratory evaluation revealed a serum creatinine of 2.5 mg/dL with marked anemia. Urine dipstick showed no blood or protein with a specific gravity of 1005. Tests of liver function were normal as were levels of plasma electrolytes, glucose, calcium, magnesium, total protein, albumin, and the urinary protein to creatinine ratio and a urinalysis.

A kidney ultrasound showed symmetrical kidneys with increased echogenicity and loss of corticomedullary differentiation. The kidney sizes were at the lower limit of normal. The bladder and the collecting system were unremarkable.

The differential diagnosis considered included juvenile nephronophthisis (NPHP) as well as congenital anomalies of kidney and urinary tract (CAKUT).

Renal biopsy showed tubular basement membrane disruption, tubulointerstitial infiltrates, and corticomedullary cysts.

Genetic studies showed that the patient had a homozygous NPHP1 mutation.

Diagnosis: Juvenile Nephronophthisis (NPHP) CAKUT cover a wide range of structural malformations that result from defects in the morphogenesis of the kidney and/or urinary tract. These anomalies account for about 40–50% of children with chronic kidney disease worldwide. Currently, more than 20 monogenic CAKUT-causing genes have been identified [32]. Currently, *HNF1B* and *PAX2* are considered to be the most frequent CAKUT-causing genes [33]. Deletion of *HNF1B on chromosome 17 (which encodes HNF1B transcription factor) is associated with both ASD and schizophrenia* [34]. Further, in another study the neurodevelopmental phenotype of 38 patients with *HNF1B* associated renal disease due to intragenic mutations (18/38) vs. 17q12 deletion in (20/38) was studied. It was found that 17q12 deletions, not *HNF1B* intragenic mutations, are involved in the neurodevelopmental phenotype of these patients [35].

In addition to the targeted mutations of these individual genes, a recent report evaluated copy number variation (CNV) as a possible cause of renal hypodysplasia (RHD). The CNVs examined were 100 kb and occurred at a frequency of 1% in the whole population. The authors determined that although the overall frequency of CNVs was similar in the RHD group compared with controls, the number of rare CNVs was increased, as was the size of the CNVs observed in affected individuals. Many of the genetic regions affected by the CNVs harbor genes that plausibly contribute to these phenotypes. These findings imply that CNVs may contribute to the pathogenesis of up to 16% of individuals with kidney malformations characterized by RHD and neurodevelopmental phenotype. Individuals with kidney malformations and ASD may have a molecular diagnosis attributable to a rare CNV [36]. Kidney malformations may be a sentinel manifestation of pathogenic genomic imbalances. The authors advocate a search for pathogenic CNVs in this population of patients with RHD for the diagnosis of their specific genomic disorders and for the evaluation of potential developmental delay.

NPHP represents an autosomal recessive kidney disease and is one of the common genetic disorders causing ESRD in children and adolescents. NHPH is a genetically heterogeneous disorder with 20 identified genes. Though mostly an isolated kidney disease, in about 15% of patients additional extrarenal organs may be affected, including the eyes, central nervous system, bones, and liver, leading to variant syndromes. Advances in molecular genetics over the last two decades have given rise to multiple etiologies of NPHP disorders. Autosomal recessive hereditary renal cystic ciliopathies account for approximately 5% of CKD in the pediatric population. The phenotypic variants reflect mutations in distinct genes encoding for a variety of protein products that invariably have a ciliary or basal body localization.

The nature of mutations (e.g., truncating mutations vs. missense mutations), modifier effects, and oligo-genetic inheritance have also been proposed as an explanation for the clinical variability within ciliopathies and within families suffering from these disorders [37]. In 1997, the first genetic cause of nephronophthisis was identified through the detection of a deletion that covered the *NPHP1* gene [38]. Later, it became apparent that *NPHP1* is not only mutated in isolated nephronophthisis but that a significant number of patients with *NPHP1* mutations also display neurological symptoms, including ASD [39, 40].

Another group of cystic diseases is autosomal dominant interstitial kidney disease (ADIKD). ADIKD can be the result of several different identified genetic mutations, such as *MUC1*, *REN*, *HNF1B* (hepatocyte nuclear factor-1b), and *UMOD* (uromodulin), as well as unidentified hereditary disorders. Clinical features vary, but common features include progressive renal insufficiency, bland urine sediment, and small kidneys with varying frequency of corticomedullary cysts and the absence of hypertension. Other distinguishing features including hyperuricemia and gout may be present in individuals with *UMOD* and *REN* mutations [41].

Though normally patients with ADIKD are not hypertensive, hypertension may occur later in the disease course secondary to loss of kidney function. Also, there is an increased prevalence of obesity and related medical comorbidities in children with ADIKD and ASD. In addition to traditional obesogenic risk factors common to typically developing children, children with ASD have additional risk factors including psychopharmacological treatment, disorders of sleep, atypical eating patterns, and decreased physical activity. Obesity and its associated sequelae can pose a significant threat to the self-care, quality of life, and health of individuals with ASD [42].

Management requires taking care of CKD and related comorbidities of anemia, hypertension, and hyperphosphatemia. As with TSC complex, preemptive renal transplant is often preferred to dialysis.

Clinical Vignette # 4

An 8-year-old girl with ASD is referred for diurnal enuresis. Her birth history was unremarkable. Review of systems was positive for constipation, epilepsy, and stereotypic behavior. The physical examination was normal.

Urine dipstick showed no glucose, blood, or protein with a random specific gravity of 1030.

Diagnosis: Enuresis Urinary incontinence is a common problem in the pediatric population and is well described in the medical literature. According to the definitions clarified by the International Children's Continence Society, urinary incontinence is defined as intermittent urine leakage in a child 5 years of age or older [43]. It is described as *enuresis* when occurring during sleep and *daytime incontinence* when occurring during the day.

While urinary incontinence is common in children, it appears to be both more prevalent and more persistent in children with ASD. Epidemiological studies suggest that the prevalence of urinary incontinence in the general pediatric population is approximately 20% at age 5 years with a spontaneous cure rate of approximately 15% annually [44–46]. In a study of children with ASD aged 10–14 years, 11% were found to have symptoms of enuresis [47]. Similarly, another study of 40 children over the age of 5 years with ASD found that 30% exhibited symptoms of enuresis and 25% showed symptoms of daytime incontinence [48]. Despite the evidence that enuresis is a common and persistent issue in the ASD population, the research on therapeutic approach remains relatively modest.

Before treatment is started, it is important to understand the motivations of the patient and whether urinary incontinence represents a significant problem in the patient's life. Motivation for change will be contingent on this perception of impact on the patient's day-to-day activities and is a critical determinant in the success or failure of treatment strategies. Before beginning a treatment regimen, patients should be screened for other common comorbidities which may predispose them to symptoms of incontinence, including diabetes, urinary tract infection (UTI), obstructive sleep apnea, and constipation. It is important to distinguish whether symptoms have been present since childhood or whether they are new in origin, as this may reveal the cause of episodes of incontinence. A diary of fluid intake should be maintained and can be helpful in revealing an underlying etiology, such as polydipsia. A voiding history may reveal a pattern of voiding successes and episodes of incontinence which may help to guide a treatment strategy. Examination should focus on determining the presence of organic causes of incontinence which may require a more specific treatment regimen. A urine dipstick should be collected on all patients prior to initiation of treatment to look for evidence of UTI, proteinuria, or glycosuria. If the history and urine dipstick are normal, additional labs or imaging is unlikely to be revealing and is therefore unnecessary. Treatment should only be initiated once other more concerning etiologies of incontinence are ruled out.

The principles of treatment of enuresis for children with ASD are similar to treatment for those without. As with all children with urinary incontinence, it is important to educate patients and parents on the normal function of the bladder and the causes of urinary incontinence. Both should understand that incontinence is a common problem among children and is not the fault of the patient. Families should be advised to keep a symptom diary throughout treatment to help follow progress, while therapy is ongoing. Regularly scheduled toilet sitting should be implemented to provide the opportunity for children to practice voiding, and positive feedback should be provided for the desired behavior. When appropriate, children may be provided a motivating reward for continent voids [49]. Conversely, punitive feedback should be avoided for episodes of incontinence. Rather, the child should be redirected and allowed to have the opportunity to void. For children with significant difficulty tolerating scheduled toilet sitting, it is reasonable to provide a toy or other non-stimulating activity to overcome resistance to the activity [49]. A concerted effort should be made to continue with this training regimen despite setbacks, which may occur and should be coordinated with care takers both at home and in school [50]. The management of enuresis is discussed in more detail in Chapter 14: Genitourinary Disorders.

Clinical Vignette # 5

A 6-year-old female was seen by her pediatrician for fever. Urinalysis is positive for leucocyte esterase and nitrites with positive WBC screen. Urine culture is positive for pan-sensitive *E. coli.*

Diagnosis: Febrile UTI UTIs are common in children, occurring in approximately 7% of febrile infants under age 2 years and 7.8% of febrile or symptomatic children aged 2–19 years old [51]. While there is little data available looking at rates of genitourinary infections in children with ASD as they age, a study of infections focused on the first 2 years of life revealed an increased rate of genitourinary tract infections in children with ASD as compared to age-matched controls (OR 2.2) [52]. The origin of this increased incidence of UTI is unknown however may be related to other comorbidities in the population, such as constipation. It is well known that children with ASD are at increased risk for chronic constipation [53]. There is a strong association between UTIs and chronic constipation with one study showing rates of UTI as high as 11% in children with chronic constipation [54]. This same study showed resolution in all patients without urinary tract abnormality following 12 months of treatment for constipation. It is proposed that chronic constipation causes detrusor instability and incomplete bladder emptying, predisposing these patients to UTIs [55, 56]. For this reason children with UTI should be screened for constipation, and the constipation should be treated if present.

It is important to make the diagnosis of UTI early in its course to avoid complications of urosepsis, renal scarring, and acute kidney injury [57]. It may be more difficult, however, to make this diagnosis in children with ASD, particularly when they are unable to verbalize symptoms. UTI should remain on the differential for nonverbal children who exhibit worsening agitation or behavior dysregulation and should be investigated in all children who develop symptoms of urinary incontinence.

The approach to treatment of children with ASD is similar to that of the general pediatric population. Children should begin an antibiotic regimen tailored to specific organisms identified in the urine culture or treated with an empiric course appropriate for age. Following appropriate treatment, efforts should be aimed at preventing future episodes by addressing underlying comorbidities that may predispose to recurrent UTIs.

Clinical Pearls

- Children with renal cysts and/or AMLs should be screened for ASD to allow for timely neurocognitive intervention.
- Nephron-sparing surgery may be necessary in the treatment of renal complications of TSC. In patients with ASD and ESRD, preemptive renal transplant is often the modality of choice rather than dialysis.
- Lithium levels need to be followed closely in patients with ASD with mood disorders.
- Nocturnal polyuria is often the first sign of lithium toxicity in a previously continent individual.
- Amiloride may be used with lithium to decrease toxicity.
- Lithium should be discontinued if NDI or proteinuria develops.
- Echogenic kidneys in ASD children require workup for autosomal recessive and dominant interstitial diseases.
- Renal hypodysplasia (RHD) and ASD may occur due to HGF1 beta mutations.
- Enuresis is common and can be challenging to treat in ASD children.
- Associated constipation and voiding dysfunction make patients with ASD more prone to developing a UTI.

References

1. van Slegtenhorst M, de Hoogt R, Hermans C, Nellist M, Janssen B, Verhoef S, et al. Identification of the tuberous sclerosis gene TSC1 on chromosome 9q34. Science (New York, NY). 1997;277(5327):805–8.
2. Krueger DA, Northrup H. Tuberous sclerosis complex surveillance and management: recommendations of the 2012 International Tuberous Sclerosis Complex Consensus Conference. Pediatr Neurol. 2013;49(4):255–65.
3. Franz DN, Bissler JJ, McCormack FX. Tuberous sclerosis complex: neurological, renal and pulmonary manifestations. Neuropediatrics. 2010;41(5):199–208.
4. Dabora SL, Jozwiak S, Franz DN, Roberts PS, Nieto A, Chung J, et al. Mutational analysis in a cohort of 224 tuberous sclerosis patients indicates increased severity of TSC2, compared with TSC1, disease in multiple organs. Am J Human Genet. 2001;68(1):64–80.
5. O'Callaghan FJ, Noakes MJ, Martyn CN, Osborne JP. An epidemiological study of renal pathology in tuberous sclerosis complex. BJU Int. 2004;94(6):853–7.
6. Crino PB, Nathanson KL, Henske EP. The tuberous sclerosis complex. N Engl J Med. 2006;355:1345.
7. Bissler JJ, Kingswood JC, Radzikowska E, Zonnenberg BA, Frost M, Belousova E, et al. Everolimus for angiomyolipoma associated with tuberous sclerosis complex or sporadic lymphangioleiomyomatosis (EXIST-2): a multicentre, randomised, double-blind, placebo-controlled trial. Lancet. 2013;381(9869):817–24.
8. Pirson Y. Tuberous sclerosis complex-associated kidney angiomyolipoma: from contemplation to action. Nephrol Dial Transplant. 2013;28(7):1680–5.
9. Murakami A, Gomi K, Tanaka M, Ohyama M, Itani Y, Ishikawa H, et al. Unilateral glomerulocystic kidney disease associated with tuberous sclerosis complex in a neonate. Pathol Int. 2012;62(3):209–15.
10. Srinivas V, Herr HW, Hajdu EO. Partial nephrectomy for a renal oncocytoma associated with tuberous sclerosis. J Urol. 1985;133(2):263–5.
11. Washecka R, Hanna M. Malignant renal tumors in tuberous sclerosis. Urology. 1991;37(4):340–3.
12. Paul E, Thiele EA, Shailam R, Rosales AM, Sadow PM. Case records of the Massachusetts General Hospital. Case 26-2011. A 7-year-old boy with a complex cyst in the kidney. N Engl J Med. 2011;365(8):743–51.
13. Matsui K, Tatsuguchi A, Valencia J, Yu Z, Bechtle J, Beasley MB, et al. Extrapulmonary lymphangioleiomyomatosis (LAM): clinicopathologic features in 22 cases. Hum Pathol. 2000;31(10):1242–8.

14. Flynn PM, Robinson MB, Stapleton FB, Roy S 3rd, Koh G, Tonkin IL. Coarctation of the aorta and renal artery stenosis in tuberous sclerosis. Pediatr Radiol. 1984;14(5):337–9.
15. Niemi AK, Northrup H, Hudgins L, Bernstein JA. Horseshoe kidney and a rare TSC2 variant in two unrelated individuals with tuberous sclerosis complex. Am J Med Genet A. 2011;155a(10):2534–7.
16. Wills BK, Mycyk MB, Mazor S, Zell-Kanter M, Brace L, Erickson T. Factitious lithium toxicity secondary to lithium heparin-containing blood tubes. J Med Toxicol. 2006;2(2):61–3.
17. Fenves AZ, Emmett M, White MG. Lithium intoxication associated with acute renal failure. South Med J. 1984;77(11):1472–4.
18. Clendeninn NJ, Pond SM, Kaysen G, Barraza JJ, Farrell T, Becker CE. Potential pitfalls in the evaluation of the usefulness of hemodialysis for the removal of lithium. J Toxicol Clin Toxicol. 1982;19(4):341–52.
19. Okusa MD, Crystal LJ. Clinical manifestations and management of acute lithium intoxication. Am J Med. 1994;97(4):383–9.
20. Lavonas EJ, Buchanan J. Hemodialysis for lithium poisoning. Cochrane Database Syst Rev. 2015;(9):Cd007951.
21. Boton R, Gaviria M, Batlle DC. Prevalence, pathogenesis, and treatment of renal dysfunction associated with chronic lithium therapy. Am J Kidney Dis. 1987;10(5):329–45.
22. Trepiccione F, Christensen BM. Lithium-induced nephrogenic diabetes insipidus: new clinical and experimental findings. J Nephrol. 2010;23(Suppl 16):S43–8.
23. Christensen BM, Kim YH, Kwon TH, Nielsen S. Lithium treatment induces a marked proliferation of primarily principal cells in rat kidney inner medullary collecting duct. Am J Physiol Renal Physiol. 2006;291(1):F39–48.
24. Batlle DC, von Riotte AB, Gaviria M, Grupp M. Amelioration of polyuria by amiloride in patients receiving long-term lithium therapy. N Engl J Med. 1985;312(7):408–14.
25. Sinke AP, Kortenoeven ML, de Groot T, Baumgarten R, Devuyst O, Wetzels JF, et al. Hydrochlorothiazide attenuates lithium-induced nephrogenic diabetes insipidus independently of the sodium-chloride cotransporter. Am J Physiol Renal Physiol. 2014;306(5):F525–33.
26. Markowitz GS, Radhakrishnan J, Kambham N, Valeri AM, Hines WH, D'Agati VD. Lithium nephrotoxicity: a progressive combined glomerular and tubulointerstitial nephropathy. J Am Soc Nephrol: JASN. 2000;11(8):1439–48.
27. Aiff H, Attman PO, Aurell M, Bendz H, Schon S, Svedlund J. End-stage renal disease associated with prophylactic lithium treatment. Eur Neuropsychopharmacol: J Eur Coll Neuropsychopharmacol. 2014;24(4):540–4.
28. Farres MT, Ronco P, Saadoun D, Remy P, Vincent F, Khalil A, et al. Chronic lithium nephropathy: MR imaging for diagnosis. Radiology. 2003;229(2):570–4.
29. Presne C, Fakhouri F, Noel LH, Stengel B, Even C, Kreis H, et al. Lithium-induced nephropathy: rate of progression and prognostic factors. Kidney Int. 2003;64(2):585–92.
30. Wood IK, Parmelee DX, Foreman JW. Lithium-induced nephrotic syndrome. Am J Psychiatry. 1989;146(1):84–7.
31. Santella RN, Rimmer JM, MacPherson BR. Focal segmental glomerulosclerosis in patients receiving lithium carbonate. Am J Med. 1988;84(5):951–4.
32. Vivante A, Kohl S, Hwang DY, Dworschak GC, Hildebrandt F. Single-gene causes of congenital anomalies of the kidney and urinary tract (CAKUT) in humans. Pediatr Nephrol (Berlin Germany). 2014;29(4):695–704.
33. Thomas R, Sanna-Cherchi S, Warady BA, Furth SL, Kaskel FJ, Gharavi AG. HNF1B and PAX2 mutations are a common cause of renal hypodysplasia in the CKiD cohort. Pediatr Nephrol (Berlin Germany). 2011;26(6):897–903.
34. Moreno-De-Luca D, Mulle JG, Kaminsky EB, Sanders SJ, Myers SM, Adam MP, et al. Deletion 17q12 is a recurrent copy number variant that confers high risk of autism and schizophrenia. Am J Hum Genet. 2010;87(5):618–30.
35. Clissold RL, Shaw-Smith C, Turnpenny P, Bunce B, Bockenhauer D, Kerecuk L, et al. Chromosome 17q12 microdeletions but not intragenic HNF1B mutations link developmental kidney disease and psychiatric disorder. Kidney Int. 2016;90(1):203–11.
36. Sanna-Cherchi S, Kiryluk K, Burgess KE, Bodria M, Sampson MG, Hadley D, et al. Copy-number disorders are a common cause of congenital kidney malformations. Am J Hum Genet. 2012;91(6):987–97.
37. Arts HH, Knoers NVAM. Current insights into renal ciliopathies: what can genetics teach us? Pediatr Nephrol. 2013;28(6):863–74.
38. Hildebrandt F, Otto E, Rensing C, Nothwang HG, Vollmer M, Adolphs J, et al. A novel gene encoding an SH3 domain protein is mutated in nephronophthisis type 1. Nat Genet. 1997;17(2):149–53.
39. Yasuda Y, Hashimoto R, Fukai R, Okamoto N, Hiraki Y, Yamamori H, et al. Duplication of the NPHP1 gene in patients with autism spectrum disorder and normal intellectual ability: a case series. Ann General Psychiatry. 2014;13:22.
40. Roberts JL, Hovanes K, Dasouki M, Manzardo AM, Butler MG. Chromosomal microarray analysis of consecutive individuals with autism spectrum disorders or learning disability presenting for genetic services. Gene. 2014;535(1):70–8.
41. Eckardt KU, Alper SL, Antignac C, Bleyer AJ, Chauveau D, Dahan K, et al. Autosomal dominant tubulointerstitial kidney disease: diagnosis, classification, and management – a KDIGO consensus report. Kidney Int. 2015;88(4):676–83.

42. Curtin C, Jojic M, Bandini LG. Obesity in children with autism spectrum disorder. Harv Rev Psychiatry. 2014;22(2):93–103.
43. Neveus T, Eggert P, Evans J, Macedo A, Rittig S, Tekgul S, et al. Evaluation of and treatment for monosymptomatic enuresis: a standardization document from the International Children's Continence Society. J Urol. 2010;183(2):441–7.
44. Forsythe WI, Redmond A. Enuresis and spontaneous cure rate. Study of 1129 enuretis. Arch Dis Child. 1974;49(4):259–63.
45. Hunskaar S, Arnold EP, Burgio K, Diokno AC, Herzog AR, Mallett VT. Epidemiology and natural history of urinary incontinence. Int Urogynecol J Pelvic Floor Dysfunct. 2000;11(5):301–19.
46. von Gontard A. Urinary incontinence in children with special needs. Nat Rev Urol. 2013;10(11):667–74.
47. Simonoff E, Pickles A, Charman T, Chandler S, Loucas T, Baird G. Psychiatric disorders in children with autism spectrum disorders: prevalence, comorbidity, and associated factors in a population-derived sample. J Am Acad Child Adolesc Psychiatry. 2008;47(8):921–9.
48. von Gontard A, Pirrung M, Niemczyk J, Equit M. Incontinence in children with autism spectrum disorder. J Pediatr Urol. 2015;11(5):264.e1-7.
49. Kroeger K, Sorensen R. A parent training model for toilet training children with autism. J Intellect Disabil Res: JIDR. 2010;54(6):556–67.
50. Zaffanello M, Giacomello L, Brugnara M, Fanos V. Therapeutic options in childhood nocturnal enuresis. Minerva Urol Nefrol = Ital J Urol Nephrol. 2007;59(2):199–205.
51. Shaikh N, Morone NE, Bost JE, Farrell MH. Prevalence of urinary tract infection in childhood: a meta-analysis. Pediatr Infect Dis J. 2008;27(4):302–8.
52. Rosen NJ, Yoshida CK, Croen LA. Infection in the first 2 years of life and autism spectrum disorders. Pediatrics. 2007;119(1):e61–9.
53. Pang KH, Croaker GD. Constipation in children with autism and autistic spectrum disorder. Pediatr Surg Int. 2011;27(4):353–8.
54. Loening-Baucke V. Urinary incontinence and urinary tract infection and their resolution with treatment of chronic constipation of childhood. Pediatrics. 1997;100(2 Pt 1):228–32.
55. Hellerstein S, Linebarger JS. Voiding dysfunction in pediatric patients. Clin Pediatr. 2003;42(1):43–9.
56. Jones E, Dimmock PW, Spencer SA. A randomised controlled trial to compare methods of milk expression after preterm delivery. Arch Dis Child Fetal Neonatal Ed. 2001;85(2):F91–5.
57. Jahnukainen T, Chen M, Celsi G. Mechanisms of renal damage owing to infection. Pediatr Nephrol (Berlin Germany). 2005;20(8):1043–53.

Urology

14

Shelly King, Melissa Young, Hillary Risk, and Taylor Wang

Introduction

In this chapter, the urologic clinical evaluation, associated conditions, and treatment for individuals with autism spectrum disorder (ASD) will be discussed. Urologic conditions can affect both children and adults with ASD. The limitations of a patient's ability to communicate and behavioral symptoms associated with ASD can present challenges to the management of a patient with ASD. There has been little research done on urologic issues in children and adults with ASD. This chapter will provide a basic understanding of how to conduct a urologic-focused exam, common testing, and treatment of urologic-related problems. Individuals with ASD may have associated genetic disorders or syndromes that may also affect the urologic system; the most common are discussed in this chapter.

Clinical Evaluation

In general, the clinical evaluation of urological conditions in patients with ASD is the same as that for all the pediatric population and adult population, although there are some special recommendations and indications for children and adults with ASD.

General

Basic initial observations of the patient are important, including attention to the appearance, activity level, and behavior of the patient as well as interactions with parents or caregivers [4]. The patient with ASD may have limited eye contact or may not offer a greeting to the provider.

Strong evidence shows that abuse in men and women with developmental disabilities is more likely to occur than in the general population. Abuse or violence can come from intimate partners, caregivers, or peers. When evaluating a patient with ASD in the urologic setting, the clinician should regularly screen for abuse and violence [12].

History

History of Present Illness

The history should be gathered in the usual fashion, including the onset, type of symptoms, location, duration, triggers, voiding history

S. King · M. Young (✉) · H. Risk · T. Wang
Pediatric Urology, Riley Hospital for Children, Indiana University School of Medicine, Indianapolis, IN, USA
e-mail: myoung1@iuhealth.org

E. P. Hazen, C. J. McDougle (eds.), *The Massachusetts General Hospital Guide to Medical Care in Patients with Autism Spectrum Disorder*, Current Clinical Psychiatry,
https://doi.org/10.1007/978-3-319-94458-6_14

and habits, and details about urinary incontinence (daytime, nighttime, or both), urinary retention, and/or urinary tract infection (UTI). If UTI is suspected, ask about associated febrile history, specifically temperatures > 101.5 °F. If the patient has had fever associated with UTI, if possible obtain all past urine culture reports [4].

Obtaining a thorough history will be important as it will help the clinician decide what testing, if any, needs to be performed. If the patient is past the developmental age for toilet training and is not toilet trained, determining whether the problem is behavioral or physiologic will help guide interventions and the treatment plan. Enuresis and daytime voiding symptoms can have an impact not only a child's social experiences but his academic and psychological development as well. These urologic issues only confound and may further affect the developmental delays that may be present in a patient with ASD [6] (Tables 14.1).

Depending upon the patient's chronological age and the degree of language and intellectual impairments, the patient may have limited capacity to report his own history. In this case, the history should be gathered from parents or caregivers. When taking a history, keep in mind that the patient may have a difficult time processing information quickly. Stress and anxiety may occur if the patient feels as if they cannot answer the question. Being concrete and specific or giving answer options may help the patient to provide an answer [12]. Using images and having the patient point to the area of pain or concern may also be helpful.

Table 14.1 Age of attaining urinary continence [3, 4]

26% are continent by 24 months.
85% continent by 30 months.
98% continent by 36 months.
Children have until age 5 years to attain night continence
Urinary control occurs when there is:
Increase in bladder capacity
Brain development that allows bladder and sphincter to work in concert
Volitional control of the external sphincter

Past Medical History

A thorough past medical history should include birth history, past surgeries, family history, social history, living environment, sexual abuse history, psychiatric history, past and present treatment approaches, and past diagnosis of genetic syndrome(s) [4].

Medications

Review all medications and their intended use and any potential side effects. Many psychiatric medications commonly used to treat patients with ASD are quite sedating and can promote deep sleep, which can lead to nocturnal enuresis [4].

Review of Systems

Important factors to consider in the review of systems are as follows:

- Weight: Recent weight change (certain psychiatric medications can influence appetite and weight).
- HEENT: Low set or abnormally shaped ears can be associated with renal involvement/abnormalities.
- Neurological: Hydrocephalus, abnormal limb movement, seizure history, headaches, developmental delay, repetitive movements, and spastic or flaccid muscles.
- Endocrine: Failure to thrive, thyroid and/or pituitary abnormalities.
- Cardiovascular: Murmurs, cardiac structural abnormalities, such as atrial or ventricular septal defects (midline anomalies can be a predisposition for renal abnormalities).
- Hematology: Bleeding disorders (personal or family history).
- Respiratory: Asthma, reactive airway disease.
- Gastrointestinal: Bowel habits, history of constipation (which can be a significant source of lower urinary tract symptoms).
- Psychiatric: Additional psychiatric diagnoses such as attention-deficit/hyperactivity disorder, anxiety disorders, or mood disorders [4].

Physical Examination

Particular strategies may need to be used for successful examinations or tests for a patient with ASD. More discussion of helpful approaches to examination and testing is provided in Chap. 4: Procedures.

- Explain what you are going to do before you do it; warn before you touch.
- Show the patient what you are going to do on a doll or dummy.
- Tell the patient how long the exam or test will take.
- Limit the amount of time the patient must be undressed.
- Give the patient adequate time to process what you are saying.
- Use numbing jelly or cream for invasive testing such as catheter placement.
- Use resources such as involvement of a child life specialist who can work with the patient on accommodating stressful sensory stimuli [12].

Consider the chronological age, developmental stage, sex, and family dynamics of the patient before performing the exam. For example, it is important to ask adolescents their preferences regarding having parents or caregivers in the room during the exam [4].

A urologic-focused physical exam includes the abdomen, back/spine, lower extremities, neuromuscular evaluation, and genitalia. Observe the patient's gait, and ask the caregiver about a history of toe walking, unsteady gait, coordination issues, and frequent falling. Assess the abdomen for retained stool and palpate the kidneys and bladder. Turn the patient on his side, and assess the lumbosacral region for dimples, hair patches, hemangiomas, sacral agenesis, or subcutaneous lipomas. After undressing the patient, inspect underwear for dampness or fecal soiling [4]. Assess the external genitalia last, looking at the anatomy, noting any rashes, and observing any leakage of urine with cough or valsalva [2] (Tables 14.2, and 14.3).

Table 14.2 Tanner stages: male development [3, 4]

Stage	Pubic hair	Testes and penis
Stage I Prepubertal	There is no androgen-sensitive coarse, pigmented pubic hair	Testes, scrotum, penis size and proportion same as early childhood. Testes smaller than 4 mL or less than 2.5 cm
Stage II Age 11.5 years (9.9–14.5 years)	Development of minimal pigmented curled or straight hair at the base of the penis	Begin to have enlargement of scrotum and testes with change in the texture of the scrotal skin. Testes 4 mL or 2.5–3.2 cm
Stage III Age 12.4 years (10.1–16.5 years)	Hair spread over the junction of the pubis, darker, coarser, and curlier	Penis grows in length with some increase in circumference. Testes 12 mL or 3.6 cm Gynecomastia (13.2 years) Voice fluctuates (13.5 years) Increase in muscle mass
Stage IV Age 13.2 years (11.2–15.8 years)	Increase in hair distribution, with none on the medial thigh	Penis size increase, further development of the glans, scrotum, skin darkens. Testes 4.1–4.5 cm Voice changes Acne Axillary hair
Stage V Age 15.3 years to adult	Hair increase in quantity and size, and spread to the medial surface of the inner thigh, adult in appearance; described as inverse triangle	Penis, testes, and scrotum are adult in size and shape. Facial hair Male build Gynecomastia resolves

Table 14.3 Tanner stages: female development [4]

Stage	Genitalia	Breast
Stage I Prepubertal	Soft (villus) hair develops, no coarse pigmented hair	Papilla is elevated above the level of the chest wall
Stage II Age 10.9 years (8.9–12.9 years)	Sparse coarse pigmented hair along the labia	Breast buds palpable and areolae enlarge. Adrenarche 6 to 8 years
Stage III Age 11.9 years (9.9–13.9 years)	Hair becomes darker, coarser, and curlier and begins to spread along the mons pubis	Breasts and areolae continue to grow without separation of contour
Stage IV Age 12.9 years (10.5–15.3 years)	Hair increases in surface area without spread to the medial thighs	Areolae and papillae rise above the level of the breasts and form secondary mounds
Stage V Age 15.3 years to adult	Hair appears as inverse triangle with spread to the medial surface of the thighs Adult hair quantity and type	Adult female breasts; Areola recesses to the contour of the breast

Table 14.4 Urine output per day according to age [2]

Age	Output (cc)
1–3 years	500–600
3–5 years	600–700
5–8 years	650–1000
8–14 years	800–1400

Labs

- Urinalysis (UA): Screening urine dipstick to evaluate urine for infection.
- Urine culture: Urine collected in sterile cup as clean catch midstream, catheter, or bag sample is sent to the microbiology lab for identification of bacteria in the urine and sensitivities to antibiotics. A urine culture is considered positive if > 100,000 bacteria are present on a clean catch urine.
- Urine calcium/creatinine ratio: Used when evaluating hematuria and dysuria.

Radiology

- Renal bladder ultrasound: Basic ultrasound to evaluate the kidneys and bladder anatomically. This should also include a pre- and post-void bladder volume to assess ability to adequately empty.
- Post-void residual (PVR) ultrasound: Used to assess the ability to empty the bladder. After voiding to completion, an acceptable PVR is < 30 mL of urine present in the bladder. Incomplete bladder emptying can put the patient at greater risk for UTI and bladder dysfunction.
- MAG 3 with Lasix: A nuclear medicine test that is completed to evaluate renal function, renal size, renal shape, renal location, and the ability to drain the kidneys. This can reveal blockages that do not allow the kidney to drain properly. Blockages in the kidney can be minor, moderate, or severe and sometimes require surgery to correct.
- Voiding cystourethrogram: This is a type of X-ray that is done with fluoroscopy to evaluate the shape of the bladder, filling process of the bladder, and emptying process of the bladder. This test also evaluates the structure of the urethra and ureters and whether any vesicoureteral reflux is present when the bladder is filling or emptying.

Other

- Voiding diary: This is a very basic log of urinary output (Table 14.4). This provides the provider with frequency of bathroom visits as well as any episodes of urinary incontinence and urinary frequency.
- Uroflowmetry: This is a test that measures the amount of urine voided at a time and the speed of urination. It also provides details of the urine stream and indicates whether pelvic floor muscles are recruited when voiding.
- Urodynamics: This is a very specialized test that evaluates how the bladder functions when filling and emptying with urine. This test also provides pressures within the bladder as it is filling and emptying. This test is used to assist

with the evaluation of several common complaints like urinary incontinence, retention, and frequency as well as UTIs.

Common Conditions

Autism Spectrum Disorder, Associated Comorbidities, and Urological Significance

The literature does not describe specific urological comorbidities directly related to a diagnosis of ASD. However, many individuals with ASD have an identified underlying genetic disorder. Many of these genetic disorders also have associated urological comorbidities that need to be taken into consideration when providing urological care and examination. We will discuss the most common of these disorders in detail below.

Tuberous Sclerosis Complex (TSC)

Tuberous sclerosis is an autosomal dominant genetic disorder that affects multiple organ systems, primarily with the development of benign neoplasms of the brain, skin, and kidneys. The incidence of TSC is 1 in 5,800 and the disorder is inherited in 30% of cases [19]. The prevalence of ASD in TSC has been estimated from 16% to 65%, and conversely, the prevalence of TSC in ASD is 1–4% (possibly up to 8–14% in the subgroup of individuals with ASD and a seizure disorder) [20]. Angiomyolipomas can occur in up to 80% of TSC patients, usually with multiple tumors occurring in both kidneys. These tumors are usually asymptomatic, but when they are symptomatic, patients usually present with renal failure or hypertension, as the angiomyolipoma may alter normal kidney function or may lead to hemorrhage due to aneurysm formation [19]. Angiomyolipomas greater than 4 cm are often treated with embolization. Renal cysts are also common in these patients and usually affect both kidneys but are less likely to present with hemorrhage. It is recommended that renal ultrasound be performed at diagnosis and then repeated every 1–3 years, depending on findings, and that an MRI or CT scan is performed if there is concern for malignancy [19]. Further discussion of TSC with regard to renal manifestations in ASD patients can be found in Chap. 13: Nephrology.

Fragile X Syndrome

Fragile X syndrome (FXS) is a genetic condition that results in a range of developmental and cognitive delays. Males with this condition are more severely affected than females [5]. The prevalence of ASD among patients with FXS is between 25% and 33%; conversely, the prevalence of FXS in ASD is estimated at 2% [20]. Patients with FXS often have significant delays with toilet training, which may occur one to several years later than normal. In treating patients with FXS, special attention should be paid to issues with anxiety, sensory processing, and poor sequential learning skills [5]. Patients with FXS frequently have genitourinary abnormalities, including enlarged testes after puberty in men and primary ovarian insufficiency in women [20], which may be best managed by a referral to an endocrinologist for evaluation and treatment.

Down Syndrome

Down syndrome, or Trisomy 21, is the most common chromosomal cause of intellectual disability and occurs in 1/1,000 live births. The prevalence of Down syndrome in children with ASD is estimated to be as high as 16.7%, and the rate of ASD among patients with Down syndrome ranges between 1–10% [20]. Outside of a delay in toilet training, patients with Down syndrome can have a range of urological comorbidities. Common kidney abnormalities include renal hypoplasia (20%), glomerular microcysts (over 20%), simple renal cysts (6%), and obstructive uropathy (7%) with decreased creatinine clearance [10]. Ureteral abnormalities can include an obstructed megaureter, ureteral atresia, and vesicoureteral reflux [10]. An increased incidence of posterior urethral valves and hypospadias has been found, along with dysfunctional voiding and urinary retention [10]. Among males with Down syndrome, there is an increased incidence of cryptorchidism, which occurs in at least 25% of patients, and hypogonadism, resulting in an increased risk for testicular cancer and infertility [10]. For this reason, males with Down syndrome should be closely monitored by testicular examination at each well-child visit by their primary care provider, and if the testicles are not descended by age 1 year, surgical intervention should be considered [1]. There are currently no recommended urological screening guidelines, but a screening renal ultrasound is a widely accepted practice, and other radiological studies, such as a voiding cystourethrogram, urodynamic testing, and renal scan, may be required based on patient presentation and concerns.

Neurofibromatosis Type 1

Neurofibromatosis type 1 (NF1) is an autosomal dominant condition occurring in 1/3,000 live births caused by decreased production of the protein neurofibromin, which is a tumor suppressor [14]. This condition is characterized by cafe-au-lait spots, neurofibromas, optic pathway tumors, Lisch nodules, and dysplastic skeletal findings [20]. Individuals with ASD have been shown to have a 100–190-fold increased risk of neurofibromatosis when compared to the general population [20]. The incidence of urological manifestations in NF1 patients has been estimated at around 8%, usually in the form of retroperitoneal tumor development in or surrounding the urinary tract [14], so a renal bladder/abdominal ultrasound is recommended as part of these patients' annual examination.

Prader-Willi Syndrome

Signs and symptoms of Prader-Willi syndrome can vary among individuals, but they often include low muscle tone, intellectual disability, and developmental delay [20]. Patients with this syndrome often struggle with a constant craving for food and have significant weight gain. Hypogonadism in these patients results in males having underdeveloped genitals, incomplete or delayed puberty, and infertility [9]. Males may have a small penis and scrotum and small or undescended testicles. In females, the clitoris and labia may be small, and menstruation may not start until women are in their 30s [9]. These findings warrant a referral for evaluation by pediatric endocrinology for additional testing and management.

CHARGE Syndrome

CHARGE (Coloboma, Heart defect, Atresia of the choanae, Retarded growth and development, Genitourinary anomalies, and Ear anomalies or deafness) syndrome occurs in 1/8,500 live births, and the prevalence of ASD in CHARGE syndrome has been estimated to be as high as 27.5–40% [20]. Urinary tract abnormalities can occur in up to 40% of these patients and include findings of solitary kidney, ectopic kidney, renal hypoplasia, vesicoureteral reflux, and increased risk for UTI [18]. A baseline renal bladder ultrasound at birth to evaluate anatomy is recommended, and additional functional studies may be indicated.

Genital abnormalities are common in patients with CHARGE syndrome. Up to 85% of males will have an underdeveloped (micro)penis, and 60% will have undescended testes; 25% of females will have small labia and a small or missing uterus; and 90% of all patients will have a lack of puberty without hormone intervention [7]. These findings warrant a referral for evaluation by pediatric endocrinology for additional testing and management.

Urinary Incontinence and Autism Spectrum Disorder

It's widely accepted that patients with neuropsychiatric and intellectual disabilities, including those diagnosed with ASD, are more affected by urinary incontinence than typically developing children [17]. Urinary incontinence is defined as any involuntary or uncontrollable leakage of urine [11] and can occur in a variety of situations. Incontinence that occurs while sleeping is referred to as enuresis or nocturnal enuresis [11]. Studies have shown that around 10% of children in the United States between age 3 and 12 years have daytime incontinence [13]. Nocturnal enuresis is also very common, with 6% of 7-year-old girls and 9% of 7-year-old boys as well as 3% of 10-year-old girls and 7% of 10-year-old boys affected [13].

Only a few studies have focused on urinary incontinence in pediatric patients with

ASD. These studies have shown increased rates of nocturnal enuresis, daytime urinary incontinence, and fecal incontinence as well as behavioral and emotional disorders [17]. Forty percent of children with ASD have at least one type of incontinence: 30–41% have nocturnal enuresis, 25–41% have daytime urinary incontinence, and 12.5–31% have fecal incontinence [8, 17] . Twenty to thirty percent of children with nocturnal enuresis have at least one psychiatric disorder, twice the rate of children without nocturnal enuresis [16].

Delayed urinary continence occurs in 20.5% of children with ASD, and lower urinary tract symptom scores (based on completed International Consultation on Incontinence Questionnaire-Pediatric LUTSs) were significantly higher: 6.6 versus 3.9 in a control group [17]. These lower urinary tract symptoms included increased rates of urinary urgency (30%), postponement of voiding (15.4%), and straining to void (5.1%) [17]. Despite an increased prevalence of incontinence and enuresis, children with ASD have also shown increased therapy resistance and often have disrupted sleep [16].

Genitourinary Conditions in Adults with ASD

While it can be said that the current literature regarding ASD and urological symptoms and findings in children is sparse, it is unfortunate that even less can be found concerning adults with ASD. Studies examining physical health-related issues in adults with ASD in general are limited, and what is available has not specifically addressed urological issues or concerns. This disparity provides an opportunity for future examination and study.

Treatment

Urinary Incontinence

As noted above, toileting issues have been noted in people with ASD regardless of their cognitive ability. Many show a substantial degree of control of toileting, even exhibiting withholding behaviors. The authors have had experience with patients who would only urinate into the toilet and required incontinence pads, pull-ups, or diapers to stool. In some situations the inability to become continent can be related to anxiety to the toileting experience rather than a failure to learn toileting behaviors.

Day accidents can create constant anxiety and the fear of public embarrassment. Nocturnal enuresis can prevent children from attending sleepovers and camps, leading to increased social isolation. Incontinence can also have a negative impact on an individual's healthy psychological development, for example, by interfering with a child's sense of mastery and independence. Support and education necessary to achieve continence in children with ASD are essential to physical and emotional health.

Successful toilet training can be achieved by using small systematic steps. Table 14.5 identifies signs that a child is ready for toilet training.

Structured teaching is an important strategy for patients with ASD. This approach allows the learner to follow steps as independently as possible. Table 14.6 shows a structured breakdown of toilet training steps. The steps could be posted in a place accessible to the patient with pictures to assist with visual learning.

How the child will generalize a new activity should be considered and planned for from the outset of teaching. The phrase "train and hope" was identified in Stokes and Baer's classic review of treatment generalization strategies [15]. "Train and hope" refers to teaching individuals a desired skill within a treatment session and hoping that the individual will generalize the use of that skill without implementation of a predetermined plan or strategy to facilitate generalization.

Nocturnal Enuresis

Nocturnal enuresis (bedwetting) is a common problem in children both with and without ASD. Treatment should be considered whenever the problem is causing significant distress or interfering with activities, such as sleepovers or

Table 14.5 Toilet training readiness

1. Holds urine close to 2 h without accident, may be dry at night
2. Bowel movements seem predictable, child may hide to stool or urinate
3. Child can pull pants up and down independently
4. Understands what/where the bathroom is
5. Takes off soiled or wet clothing quickly/independently
6. Can identify wet versus dry
7. Can follow simple one step instruction
8. Can communicate desire to use the toilet using words, signs, or pictures.

Parents/family must be ready to invest time, patience and energy into process

Table 14.6 Toilet training steps

Breakdown of teachable toilet training steps represented with pictures
Enter bathroom
Pull pants/underwear down (parent may assist initially if necessary)
Sit on toilet (if fearful start with clothes on)
Tear off toilet paper
Wipe off with toilet paper
Pull up pants/underwear
Flush toilet
Wash hands
Generalize steps in other locations/situations
Verbal praise reward for success with each step, larger predetermined reward for completion of the sequence (sometimes referred to as the super reward).

If excessive concern arises with a particular step in the sequence such as tearing off toilet paper or flushing, redirect reward pattern to deter repetition of the same step

camps, self-esteem, or healthy psychological intervention. Particularly for children over the age of 7 years, intervention is preferable to the "wait it out" approach.

Treatment of nocturnal enuresis typically starts with a simple behavioral plan that includes five steps:

1. Encouraging the child to drink more fluid during the day and less at night, which is referred to as "fluid shifting." Suggested volumes for young children are 6–8 oz every 60–90 min throughout the day until 4–5 h before bedtime, after which intake should be limited to only 12 oz. It should be noted that children involved in sports need to drink to stay hydrated. Children should go to games and practices well hydrated and not wait until they are finished playing to consume a large volume of fluid just before bed.
2. Encourage adequate fiber intake such that the child has at least one soft bowel movement daily.
3. Avoid carbonated beverage, caffeine, and citric acid, as these drinks can irritate the bladder or increase urine production. Also avoid milk or milk-based products in the evening.
4. Void on a regular schedule during the day to promote good bladder health.
5. Double void (urinate) at bedtime to ensure that the child is going to bed with an empty bladder. This typically involves attempting to void once at the start of the bedtime routine and again immediately prior to going to bed.

When the above steps alone are not sufficient, the use of an enuresis alarm can be helpful. The enuresis alarm is a device used to help a child learn to wake up in response to the urge to urinate. The device alarms with a loud noise and/or vibration when it senses the first few drops of urine. There are many different alarms on the market, including some that can play a recorded message from a parent. The latter may be better tolerated for some children with ASD, who may be very sensitive to loud alarm sounds.

The child wakes to the sound and is encouraged to go to the bathroom to finish urinating. Over time, the child associates the sensation of a full bladder with the alarm going off and waking up to void. This can take up to 3–4 months of regular use to be successful, so it is important for the clinician to encourage patience and support families to stick with the process.

In some cases, it can be helpful to have the child sleep on the floor in the parent's bedroom for the first couple of weeks of treatment, so the parent can make sure the child learns to respond promptly when the device goes off. If a child refuses to get up to the alarm and bedwetting does not improve despite a few months of consistent use, the child is likely not ready to work with the enuresis alarm at that time.

When nocturnal enuresis is causing significant distress and is not responding to behavioral approaches alone, treatment with medications should be considered. Medications are much more likely to be successful when used in conjunction with a behavioral plan.

Desmopressin is the most commonly prescribed medication for nocturnal enuresis. Once given primarily via a nasal spray, it is now available in 0.1 mg and 0.2 mg oral tablets, with a typical pediatric dose range of 0.1–0.6 mg, given as a single dose at bedtime. Our recommended approach is to start at a midrange dose of 0.4 mg (two of the 0.2 mg tablets). If this dose is effective, an attempt can be made to decrease the dose to 0.2 mg. If 0.4 mg is not effective, the dose can then be increased to 0.6 mg. Side effects must be reviewed with the family, most significantly the risk of hyponatremia water intoxication syndrome if excess fluid is consumed after taking the medication. The patient must stop drinking fluids 2 h before taking the medication and continue to take minimal fluids for 8 h after.

Anticholinergic medications, such as oxybutynin and tolterodine, reduce abnormal bladder contractions that can be associated with an overactive bladder and can be helpful in treating urinary frequency, leakage of urine, and daytime incontinence. They can be used in combination with desmopressin to treat nocturnal enuresis. There are many on the market, and the longer-acting versions are most useful as most children sleep longer than 8 h. Side effects are similar to other anticholinergic medications and include dry mouth and constipation.

Imipramine, a tricyclic antidepressant with anticholinergic activity, has also been shown to be effective in the treatment of nocturnal enuresis. In addition to its anticholinergic effects, it is thought to shorten the time of the sleep stage where nocturnal enuresis happens. A dose of 25–50 mg, or 2.5 mg/kg/d, is typically given approximately 1 h before bedtime. Care must be taken to avoid using imipramine in combination with other medications that decrease tricyclic metabolism or medications that prolong the QT interval.

Clinical Vignette # 1

Child with ASD

Jay, an 8-year-old male with persistent urinary incontinence, presented to the urology clinic. His parents reported that he was voiding 12–15 times a day. They believed that he sensed the need to void and would become very anxious. The frequency of urination and his overall level of anxiety both seemed to have escalated over the last year.

The physical exam revealed urinary meatal stenosis and palpable stool in the abdomen. His parents reported that he would have a bowel movement about once every 3 days. Jay often hid to defecate and his stools were large and hard. His parents also reported an upward deflection to a very strong but thin urinary stream. He had never had a urinary tract infection and urinalysis performed in the office was normal. A screening renal/bladder ultrasound was normal except for large post-void residual urine.

A meatotomy was done to correct meatal stenosis. This is often done in the office with EMLA cream, a topical anesthetic. However, in children with ASD, it is typically done under a general anesthetic. This provides a safer environment and avoids frightening the patient by forcefully holding him down for the procedure.

Constipation can contribute to urinary frequency. For this patient, a cleanout regimen with polyethylene glycol 68 g in 32 oz of a sports drink was given for 2 days. The patient was continued on 17 g of polyethylene glycol daily to prevent constipation. A strict timed voiding schedule was started at once every hour, and the parents gradually tried to increase the scheduled interval of voiding to every 2–3 h.

The frequency and urgency of the patient's urination improved with bowel management but did not completely resolve, so he was started on an anticholinergic medication, tolterodine (preferred dose is 0.1 mg/kg/d). He continued the stool softener and timed voiding regimen.

His urinary frequency improved with treatment, and he was able to work on his voiding schedule and toilet training steps without anxiety.

Jay continued to have accidents and didn't seem to identify the urge to urinate with the necessary next step, going to the bathroom. The parents were instructed to use a voice-activated enuresis alarm which has a small sensor that fits in underwear and a small speaker that attaches to the patient's shirt. The voice on the alarm can be recorded to say whatever phrase the family uses to direct the patient to use the bathroom. The first few drops of urine activate the device, reminding the child he is starting to void and needs to go to the bathroom. Over approximately 3 months, Jay learned to associate the urge to urinate with his parent's voice directing him to the bathroom. The parents were able to eliminate the alarm after 3 months. They continue to monitor Jay closely to ensure mastery of this skill.

Clinical Vignette # 2

Adult with ASD

Evan is a 22-year-old young man with Down syndrome and ASD with minimal verbal skills who presented to an outpatient urology clinic with his parents, who reported issues with enuresis and encopresis.

Records obtained from an outside facility show that Evan was initially evaluated at the age of 10 years with concerns regarding lack of toilet training. At that time, he struggled with both enuresis and encopresis. He never took himself to the bathroom and had to be directed to do so. Even with direction and timed sitting, he remained incontinent. He had no history of urinary tract infection, kidney stones, or issues with starting or maintaining his stream. A screening renal/bladder ultrasound was done and was normal other than a moderate post-void residual volume of urine. The physical exam was deferred at the initial visit due to the patient's anxiety. His enuresis and encopresis were thought to be behaviorally related, as opposed to a physiologic problem, so a recommendation was made to work with their behavior therapist and return to clinic as needed.

Unfortunately, the family had relocated multiple times over the last 10 years and reported inconsistent follow-up. They hoped to reestablish urologic care and address his continued issues of enuresis and encopresis. They reported that they have worked diligently for years with behavior therapists on behavior modification, timed voiding, and relaxation with no success. At the time of the appointment, Evan was able to sit and attempt to void every 2 h, but he was constantly wet in between. He did have bowel movements in the toilet every 2–3 days, with intermittent fecal smearing. He's had no urinary tract infections, and a recent repeat renal/bladder ultrasound showed a slightly thickened bladder wall, grade 1 hydronephrosis on the left, and a large post-void residual. After discussing his specific anxiety and sensory issues, a physical examination was done. On exam, it was noted that he had a right undescended testicle, a small sacral dimple and a bifid gluteal crease. Evan's mother reported that these findings had never been brought to her attention but that very few providers had performed full examinations over the years due to his anxiety and lack of cooperation.

Due to the fact that Evan had never been fully continent of bladder and only somewhat continent of bowel, had changes on renal/bladder ultrasound, and had an abnormal spine exam, there was concern for neurogenic bladder and bowel related to a tethered spinal cord. An MRI of the lumbosacral spine and video urodynamic testing was ordered. The MRI showed a fatty filum, likely causing a tethered spinal cord. Urodynamic testing showed a small capacity, high-pressure bladder, which was trabeculated in appearance, and a patent urethra. Evan was started on anticholinergic medication, his family was taught intermittent catheterization in case of urinary retention, and a referral for evaluation by a neurosurgeon was made. Evan underwent a tethered cord release and had a right orchiopexy done at the same time by a urology surgeon. Three months postoperatively, Evan was doing well and was having only two small urinary accidents daily and no bowel issues with continued behavior modification and anticholinergic therapy. Repeated urodynamic testing showed decreased bladder pressures and increased capacity. His progress will continue to be monitored with repeat renal/bladder ultrasounds at least yearly and urodynamic testing as needed for changes in symptoms, and the dose of his anticholinergic medication will be weaned down as his progress allows. Yearly testicular exams will also occur.

Clinical Pearls

- The recommended clinical urological evaluation in patients with ASD does not differ from that of typically developing patients, but patient-specific strategies to decrease anxiety and improve cooperation should always be utilized.
- While an ASD diagnosis alone is not correlated with specific urological issues, individuals with some genetic syndromes related to ASD can have increased risk for urologic comorbidities and should be fully evaluated.
- When working with a patient on urinary continence training, behavioral training is the primary focus. Structured teaching, guided by a patient's level of development, has proven to be a successful approach for many patients with ASD.
- Treatment of constipation is imperative to achieving urinary continence.
- Currently there is a lack of data and resources regarding the urologic care of adults with ASD, and there is a great need for more knowledge in this area.

References

1. American Academy of Pediatrics. Undescended testicles. Retrieved November 2017, from caring for your baby and young child: birth to age 5. 2015. https://www.healthychildren.org/English/health-issues/conditions/genitourinary-tract/Pages/Undescended-Testicles.aspx.
2. Baskin LS, Kogan BA, editors. Handbook of pediatric urology. Philadelphia: Lippincott Williams & Wilkins; 2005.
3. Chemaitilly W, Escobar O, Witchel SF. Endocrinology. In: Zitelli BJ, McIntire SC, Nowalk AJ, editors. Zitelli and Davis' atlas of pediatric physical diagnosis. 6th ed. Philadelphia: Elsevier Saunders; 2012. p. 369–400.
4. Diaz-Saldano D. Assessment of children. In: Core curriculum for urologic nursing, 2017. 1st ed. Pitman: Anthony J. Janetti Inc/Society of Urologic Nurses and Associates; 2017. p. 37–47.
5. Fragile X Clinical & Research Consortium. Consensus of the fragile X clinical & research consortium on clinical practices. Retrieved October 2017, from National Fragile X Foundation: 2012. https://fragilex.org/2017/treatment-and-intervention/consensus-fragile-x-clinical-research-consortium-clinical-practices/.
6. Gor RA, Fuhrer J, Schober JM. A retrospective observational study of enuresis, daytime voiding symptoms, and response to medical therapy in children with attention deficit hyperactivity disorder and autism spectrum disorder. J Pediatr Urol. 2010;2012(8):314–7. https://doi.org/10.1016/j.jpurol.2010.10.009.
7. Kirk J. Genital abnormalities. Retrieved October 2017, from The Charge Syndrome Foundation: https://www.chargesyndrome.org/genital-abnormalities. 2017.
8. Kroeger KA, Sorensen-Burnworth R. Toilet training individuals with autism and other developmental disabilities: A critical review. Res Autism Spectr Disord. 2009;3:607–18.
9. Mayo Clinic. Prader-Willi syndrome. Retrieved October 2017, from MayoClinic.org: http://www.mayoclinic.org/diseases-conditions/prader-willi-syndrome. 2017.
10. Mercer ES, Broecker B, Smith E, Kirsch AJ, Scherz HC, Massad CA. Urological manifestations of Down syndrome. J Urol. 2004;171:1250–3.
11. Neveus T, von Gontard A, Hoebeke P, Hjalmas K, Bauer S, Bower W, Jorgensen TM, Rittig S, Walle JV, Yeung CK, Djurhuus JC. The standardization of terminology of lower urinary tract function in children and adolescents. Report from the standardization committee of the International Children's Continence Society (ICCS). J Urol. 2006;176(1):314–24.
12. Nicolaidis C, Kripke CC, Raymaker D. Primary care for adults on the autism spectrum. Med Clin North Am. 2014;98(5) https://doi.org/10.1016/j.mcna.2014.06.011.
13. Schaeffer AJ, Diamond DA. Pediatric urinary incontinence: classification, evaluation, & management. Afr J Urol. 2013;20:1–13.
14. Schroder A, Stein R, Thuroff J, Gutjahr P. Neurofibromatosis type 1 and its urological manifestation. Eur Urol. 2006;5(2):302.
15. Stokes TF, Baer DM. On implicit technology of generalization. J Appl Behav Anal. 1977;10:349–67.
16. Van Herzeele C, Vande Walle J. Incontinence and psychological problems in children: a common central nervous pathway? Pediatr Nephrol. 2016;31(5):689–92.
17. von Gontard A, Pirrung M, Niemczyk J, Equit M. Incontinence in children with autism spectrum disorder. J Pediatr Urol. 2015;11(5):264–7.
18. Williams MS. Kidney abnormalities. Retrieved October 2017, from The Charge Syndrome Foundation: https://www.chargesyndrome.org/kidney-abnormalities. 2017.
19. Yohay K, Keros ST. Tuberous sclerosis. Retrieved October 2017, from Clinical Advisor: http://www.clinicaladvisor.com/pediatrics/tuberous-sclerosis. 2013.
20. Zafeiriou DI, Ververi A, Vargiami E. Childhood autism and associated comorbidities. Brain and Development. 2006;29(5):257–72.

15 Gynecology

Kathryn S. Brigham and Anne Althausen Plante

Introduction

Gynecology care is essential for promoting and maintaining health in all women. It must be provided to all women in a confidential and comprehensive way. We must strive to affirm each woman's dignity by avoiding emotional and physical harm during our interactions and examinations. Due to multiple obstacles, it is more challenging to deliver consistent and high-quality gynecology care to women with intellectual and emotional disabilities. The emotional and cognitive limitations of each woman's unique impairment directly impact how and where routine counseling and examinations can best be delivered.

Communication is central to providing appropriate care. Barriers can exist in communicating with the patient, obtaining consent for the examination and testing, and providing appropriate patient autonomy in decision making when treating patients with autism spectrum disorder (ASD). In order to maximize communication with a patient with ASD, we must elicit information about her preferred method of communication (e.g., verbal vs. pictorial). We must endeavor to communicate with the patient and her care providers directly. We must use simple, basic, and straightforward language that the patient is familiar with, such as the words they use to refer to different body parts.

Each patient will have a different degree of cognitive capability that will determine how much she can participate in her care. It is our responsibility to determine whether the goals of the patient and her caregivers are the same and, when appropriate, provide the patient the opportunity to discuss concerns confidentially. In this chapter, we will provide an overview of gynecologic care for both pediatric and adult patients with ASD.

Well Visit

A complete pelvic exam includes the following elements: (1) thorough inspection of the external genitalia, urethral meatus, vaginal introitus, and perianal region, (2) speculum examination of the vagina and cervix, and (3) bimanual examination of the cervix, uterus, and adnexa. While asymptomatic pediatric and adolescent patients will likely not need a full pelvic exam, external genital examination should be conducted in order to

K. S. Brigham
Department of Pediatrics, Division of Adolescent and Young Adult Medicine, Massachusetts General Hospital, Boston, MA, USA

A. A. Plante (✉)
Department of Obstetrics and Gynecology, Massachusetts General Hospital, Boston, MA, USA
e-mail: amalthausen@mgh.harvard.edu

E. P. Hazen, C. J. McDougle (eds.), *The Massachusetts General Hospital Guide to Medical Care in Patients with Autism Spectrum Disorder*, Current Clinical Psychiatry,
https://doi.org/10.1007/978-3-319-94458-6_15

evaluate the patient for normal anatomy, issues of personal hygiene, and any abnormalities of the vulva, introitus, and perineum that might require further investigation [3]. Conducting this type of exam is an important opportunity to review with the patient with ASD and her caregivers the "rules" of appropriate touching and how to perform basic toileting and menstrual hygiene.

Vulvar Care

Vulvar skin can be quite sensitive. It can react to products that are well-tolerated in other parts of the body. Once the vulva is irritated, a cycle of itching and scratching can develop that leads to more irritation, itching, and scratching. The table below provides some helpful information about basic vulvar care and prevention of skin irritation and breakdown (Table 1).

Internal Pelvic Exam

The American College of Obstetricians and Gynecologists (ACOG) recommends that annual pelvic exams be performed on patients 21 years and older [2]. Internal pelvic examinations are not necessary before initiating oral contraceptives in an otherwise asymptomatic patient. Screening for sexually transmitted diseases can also be completed using urine samples or vaginal swabs and deferring an internal pelvic exam [45].

Although providers may identify pelvic pathology in asymptomatic patients under the age of 21 years, there is no evidence that supports routine internal examination of a healthy asymptomatic patient. Pelvic exams are indicated as part of a thorough evaluation of any patient in this age group who has symptoms of menstrual disorders, vaginal discharge, or pelvic pain [3, 51].

All patients age 21 years or older should receive a yearly internal and external pelvic exam [2]. In asymptomatic patients, the decision whether or not to perform an internal pelvic examination should be a shared decision with the patient and her caregivers. Patients with menstrual disorders, abnormal uterine bleeding, persistent vaginal discharge, or pelvic pain should undergo an internal exam.

Cervical cancer screening guidelines published by ACOG and the American Society for Colposcopy and Cervical Pathology (ASCCP) in 2012/2013 recommend beginning PAP smear screening at the age of 21 years, irrespective of sexual activity of the patient [8, 31, 35]. These recommendations are based on the most current

Table 1 General vulvar care

Do	Do not
Wear cotton underwear or no underwear when possible	Wash the vulva. If you feel like the area needs to be washed, do not scrub
Wash with lukewarm water	Use feminine wipes, powders, creams, or other over-the-counter products
Use Vaseline, olive oil, or coconut oil on the vulvar skin daily to keep it hydrated	Douche
Avoid scented laundry detergents or fabric softeners for clothes that touch the vulvar skin	Use tea tree oil, witch hazel, gold bond powder, Epsom salts, or other "cleansing" products because they irritate the skin
Apply ice or cool compress to soothe the area if irritated	Use over-the-counter yeast treatments without talking to the provider because they can be irritating to the vulva and may not treat the underlying condition
Sleep with gloves or socks on your hands if you scratch in your sleep	
Use tampons for menses if possible. Constant contact with a pad causes more irritation	
If you use pads, avoid pads with high latex content such as Always	
Use lubricant to make intercourse more comfortable	

Mitchell, C MD and Pascal, A DNP General Vulvar Care
Department of Obstetrics and Gynecology, Massachusetts General Hospital, Boston, MA
Harvard Medical School, Boston, MA. General Vulvar Care. 12/2015

understanding of the human papilloma virus infection in the adolescent and the pathophysiology of invasive cervical cancer.

In the ASD population, the ability of the patient to consent to and comply with an office examination can vary widely. Every effort should be made to avoid physical and emotional trauma during office examinations. Although often a challenge for patients' caregivers, multiple visits to the office may allow the patient to gradually become familiar with her provider, the exam table, and the experience of a stranger looking at and touching her pelvic area. Patients with ASD will benefit from appointments with extra time and adequate support staff who are comfortable treating them. Appointments scheduled when the office is relatively calm and quiet may also increase the comfort of these patients and their care providers. Successful completion of an exam may require providing the patient with a mild oral sedative, or it may require that examinations are performed under anesthesia in an operating room setting. Proper instruments such as extra narrow or pediatric speculums should be available in the office to enable the most comfortable exam possible. Topical anesthetic applied prior to the exam may also provide some comfort.

A basic pelvic exam, PAP smear, cervical cultures, and endometrial biopsies can be performed in conjunction with other procedures that require moderate sedation, such as dental cleanings or colonoscopy, and this is also often most convenient for the physicians or nurse practitioners providing the patient care. Limiting repeated exposure to the risks of general anesthesia is also an important consideration.

Breast examination is an important component of the well woman exam. The occurrence of breast cancer prior to the age of 20 years is rare and uncommon before the age of 30 years [35]. Between the ages of 20 and 39 years, screening breast exam is recommended by the American Cancer Society, ACOG, and the National Comprehensive Cancer Network every 1–3 years [5, 42, 45]. All three organizations recommend yearly clinical breast exams for patients ages 40 years and older. Yearly mammogram screening over the age of 40 years is also recommended. Family history of breast and ovarian cancers may influence the frequency of mammogram screening and age at which they should start.

Adolescent Care

The ASD adolescent population and their caregivers may benefit significantly from an initial "reproductive healthy visit" with an obstetrician/gynecologist for in-depth discussion of basic genital hygiene, menstrual hygiene and management, contraception, and fertility (ACOG 2012, [31, 47]).

Sexual Activity and Education

Forty-seven percent of neurotypical females aged 15–19 years have engaged in intercourse (vaginal, oral, and anal), which increases with age from 31% of females ages 15–17 years to 67% of females ages 18–19 years [10]. There is, however, limited sexuality data available in adolescents with intellectual and developmental disabilities, including those with ASD [3, 6]. Data regarding risk factors for high-risk behaviors among adolescents with mobility impairments and learning and emotional disabilities are presented in Table 2.

Table 2 Prevalence of risk factors for high-risk behavior among 15–19-year-olds with disabilities

Factors	Controls (n = 167)	Mobility impairment[a] (n = 15,689)	Learning disability (n = 1301)
Welfare status	9.5%	20%*	17.1%*
Repeated a grade	18.2%	34%*	49.6*
Appears old for age	12.1%	13.8%*	11.5%*
Sexually experienced	36.9%	45.7%*	38.5%*
Non-heterosexual	5.3%	11.3%**	6.7%***

Data from Blum et al. [6]

[a]Mobility impairment includes but is not limited to paraplegia, quadriplegia, and spasticity

*$p < 0.001$

**$P < 0.01$

***$p < 0.05$

Adolescents with disabilities will have concerns about their sexuality which are similar to those of their peers without disabilities. The objective of sexual education should not be to eliminate sexual interest but to encourage each patient to understand and take responsibility for her sexual feelings and desires. The provider should explore and discuss normal anatomy, sexuality, contraception, and sexually transmitted diseases. Healthy and safe sexual behaviors should be discussed with the patient with the involvement of her caregivers depending on her degree of intellectual and developmental disabilities. Assessing an individual's ability to consent to voluntary sexual activity is central to her safety and well-being.Persons with disabilities experience rates of sexual assault ranging from 25% to 83%, and most (up to 93%) of those abused know the perpetrators [43, 48]. Assessing patients for signs and symptoms of sexual abuse or changes in behavior that may be indicators of sexual abuse is vital to the health and well-being of women with ASD who may not be able to communicate the details of their experiences [3]. Physical indicators may include bruising, infection, acute or chronic bleeding, irritation of the genitals, rectum, mouth or breasts, new difficulty sitting or walking, or unexplained stomachaches or headaches. Any significant behavior change without other explanation may also be a sign of abuse.

Human papillomavirus vaccination is recommended for the ASD population because of the high risk of sexual assault in any adolescent with disabilities [18]. The target age for vaccination is 11–12 years old, but it can be given as early as age 9 years. There are three types of vaccination available (bivalent, quadrivalent, and nine-valent), which are all given in a two-dose series (0 and 6 months) if started before age 15 and three dose-series if started at age 15 or older (0, 1-2, and 6 months). The safety profiles for each of the formulations are very similar (CDC, Vaccine Safety [7]).

Menstruation Challenges and Management

Menstruation, defined as ovulation followed by withdrawal bleeding, is not physiologically necessary [26]. The concept that monthly bleeding is healthy has been perpetuated by the use of oral contraceptives that were initially designed to mimic the average length of a normal menstrual cycle [21, 22]. The reduction in the volume and frequency of uterine bleeding and the reduction in normal cyclic hormonal fluctuations can prevent and treat multiple medical conditions including heavy bleeding (menorrhagia), painful cramping (dysmenorrhea), and pelvic pain related to endometriosis, irregular menses, anemia, menstrual-related headaches, and mood changes (PMS) and reduce the risk of ovarian and endometrial cancer.

Menarche generally occurs between ages 12 and 13 years in well-nourished populations in developed countries [9]. Menarche typically occurs within 2–3 years after thelarche (breast budding) at Tanner stage IV breast development. By age 15 years, 98% of girls will have experienced menarche. Age of menarche in patients with ASD may vary from the general population. A single study showed delay of menarche by 8 months compared with age-matched controls [24].

All adolescents have intermittent anovulatory cycles for the first 2–5 years after menarche. Their cycle intervals are generally 21–45 days. Bleeding generally lasts 2–7 days and requires 3–6 tampons or pads a day. Patients that fall outside of this general development pattern may require additional evaluation [32]. Conditions that may require further evaluation are outlined in Table 3.

Hygiene

For patients with ASD and their caregivers, menstrual hygiene can be a significant challenge. The ability of patients to change and dispose of their

Table 3 Menstrual conditions that may require evaluation

	Age (years)	Sign/symptom
Amenorrhea	13	Onset of thelarche 3 years prior
		No signs of pubertal development
	14	Signs of hirsutism
		History or exam suggestive of excessive exercise or an eating disorder
		Concerns of genital outflow tract obstruction or anomaly
	15	Primary amenorrhea regardless of additional history
Specific complaints	Any	Were regular but then became markedly irregular
		Occur more frequently than every 21 days
		Occur less frequently than every 45 days
		Occur 90 days apart even once
		Last more than 7 days
		Require frequent pad or tampon changes (soaking more than one every 1–2 h)

Table from American College of Obstetricians and Gynecologists [32]

own pad or tampon may vary. For some patients, the bleeding may be very distressing because blood may be associated with injury or pain, and the concept of "normal blood" may be difficult for them to understand [38]. The presence of a pad may cause agitation leading to removal of the pad and not replacing it or improperly disposing of it. The opportunity for caregivers to give adequate support for toileting at home or school may also be limited. Menstrual hygiene can be discussed proactively, and plans for management can be developed with the patient and her care providers prior to the predicted menarche. Most patients who can use the toilet without assistance can learn how to use menstrual products correctly. The privacy of the patient should be respected and supported as much as possible.

Behavior Changes

It is common for women in the reproductive age group to experience premenstrual mood syndrome (PMS). Changes in mood may be related to increased central nervous system sensitivity to alternations in steroid hormone levels during ovulation and just prior to menstruation [3]. The diagnosis of PMS should be made by observing and recording behavior changes on a menstrual calendar for 2–3 months to establish the cyclic recurrence of the symptoms [36]. Continuing to document symptoms following the initiation of treatment can help determine its effectiveness and guide adjustments in the treatment.

In the ASD population, mood changes associated with cyclic hormone changes can be particularly challenging to manage. In one study, 18% of women with developmental delay were found to have cyclic behavior changes which may include self-abusive behavior, temper tantrums, crying spells, and "autistic" behavior [37]. Patients may also experience increased frequency of seizures, migraine headaches, irritable bowel syndrome, or worsening fatigue. There is no epidemiologic data comparing menstrual mood changes in adolescents with disabilities with other teenagers. It is not uncommon for caregivers to pursue gynecologic intervention when these multiple symptoms persist.

It is common to use hormonal suppression of ovulation to treat PMS. Although this practice is not well supported in the literature, it is accepted as a reasonable approach in adolescents with mood, behavior, or medical problems [3]. Hormonal suppression with oral contraceptive pills can be used cyclically to manage behavior changes prior to the menstrual withdrawal week or continuously if the patient has symptoms that persist during the withdrawal week. There are multiple options available which allow the provider to tailor the treatment to each specific patient (see Table 4). One must consider the risks and benefits of each choice in the context of each patient's medical and social needs.

Table 4 Options for menstrual manipulation in adolescents with disabilities

Treatment	Specific Benefits	Disability Concerns
NSAIDs	Decreases flow and pain	GI issues
Combined oral contraceptives	Can use extended or continuous regimen	If immobile: possible risk of VTE Daily reminders Interfere with certain EI-AED
Contraceptive patch	Weekly application Can use extended or continuous regimen	If immobile: possible risk of VTE Patient can remove from skin Interfere with certain EI-AED
Contraceptive ring	Monthly Can use extended or continuous regimen	If immobile: possible risk of VTE Placement by others (privacy) Interfere with certain EI-AED
Oral progestin	Decreased flow	BTB Daily reminders Interfere with certain EI-AED
Depot medroxyprogesterone acetate	Every 3 months	Weight gain in obese adolescents
Progesterone implant	Every 3 years Decreased dysmenorrhea	BTB Insertion may be challenging
LNG-IUD	Every 3-5 years	Challenging insertion, may need anesthesia Initial BTB
Surgical methods: hysterectomy	Complete amenorrhea	Legal and ethical implications Major surgery

Modified from Quint [39]
Abbreviations: *BTB* breakthrough bleeding, *EI-AED* enzyme-inducing antiepileptic drugs, *GI* gastrointestinal, *LNG-IUD* levonorgestrel intrauterine device, *NSAIDs* nonsteroidal antiinflammatory drugs, *VTE* venous thromboembolism

Treatment for pain during menses may mediate changes in behavior due to discomfort. Nonsteroidal anti-inflammatory drugs (NSAIDs) are the first line of treatment in both neurotypical women and women with ASD. NSAIDs were found to be effective in 65% of 45 adult women with intellectual and developmental disabilities with cyclic behavior changes [37].

Menstrual Suppression

Cyclic menstrual bleeding can be very challenging to manage in the ASD population. Decreased menstrual flow may markedly improve the symptoms and ease with which the patient with ASD can navigate her menses.

Due to comorbid medical conditions, medications, and hygiene issues, adolescents and adults with ASD are at higher risk for abnormal menstrual bleeding [50]. Irregular menstrual bleeding should be thoroughly evaluated, including ruling out pregnancy, prior to initiating any hormonal treatment. Following a complete evaluation, it is important to determine if predictable heavier and longer bleeding is easier to manage than sporadic, irregular light bleeding [3].

Nonhormonal Methods

Oral tranexamic acid (brand name: Lysteda) reduces menstrual blood loss by decreasing fibrinolysis with the reduction in bleeding ranging from 26% to 60% [29]. It is taken for a maximum of 5 days during menses. The use of anti-prostaglandin medications, such as ibuprofen or Ponstel, may decrease ovulatory bleeding while avoiding the risks, drug interactions, and side effects of the hormone-containing treatment options [15]. The risk of thrombotic events with tranexamic acid is controversial. Its use is generally contraindicated in patients with a history of thromboembolic disease and in those using estrogen- and progestin-containing oral contraceptive pills (OCPs) [38].

Estrogen- and Progesterone-Containing Methods

Estrogen-containing contraceptives appear to have adverse effects on coagulation factors, placing users at increased risk of venous thromboembolism [23]. Each patient's level of physical activity must be assessed in order to avoid giving sedentary patients treatment options that increase their risk of deep vein thrombosis (DVT) [41]. Comprehensive lists of contraindications for the various forms of contraception medications can be found in the US Medical Eligibility Criteria for Contraceptive Use, 2010 Centers for Disease Control and Prevention (CDC) [49].

ASD patients may be taking medications that can alter the efficacy of oral contraceptive pills, such as anticonvulsants. The OCPs can also affect the metabolism of other medications (e.g., antibiotics) necessitating close monitoring and potential dose adjustments of the other medications.

Combination Oral Contraceptives

Estrogen- and progestin-containing OCPs can be used cyclically to decrease menstrual blood loss in patients with ovulatory and anovulatory cycles. Continuous OCPs may also be used to decrease the total days of menstrual bleeding. It is common to have an increased incidence of irregular bleeding with continuous use of OCPs, and anticipatory counseling is very important to reassure the patient and her caregivers that it is not uncommon or pathologic [3].

It can be difficult for some patients with ASD to swallow pills. There are chewable formulations, and many of the pills can be crushed and mixed in apple sauce to be swallowed more easily [31].

Contraceptive Patch

Contraceptive patches contain ethinyl estradiol (EE) and norelgestromin (progesterone component). The patch is placed once a week for 3 weeks and then removed for a week to allow for menses. It can also be used continuously to suppress menstruation completely. There is a higher estrogen exposure with the use of the patch compared with OCPs or the vaginal ring. The presence of the patch itself may be an irritant to some patients which could result in an unscheduled removal. The patch may also be less effective in women with high body weight (>90 Kg/200lbs) [31].

Contraceptive Ring

The contraceptive ring is inserted into the vagina and most often left in place for 3 weeks followed by an interval-free week. It can also be used continuously. The limitation of the ring is in its vaginal insertion and removal, which may be very difficult for some patients with ASD, especially those with physical limitations. While it can be inserted by a partner, caregiver, or provider, this may present a significant safety issue and compliance challenge. For patients who are comfortable placing and removing the ring themselves, the ring is an excellent option because it only requires changing every 4 weeks and obviates the need to take an oral daily medication.

Progesterone-Only Methods

Oral Progesterone

Progesterone-only oral pills (POPs) can reduce blood loss and regulate menstrual cycles. The progestin (norethindrone) dose is substantially lower than the dose in any combination oral contraceptive. It is dispensed in packs of 28 active pills, which are taken continuously (i.e., no pill-free or nonhormonal pill week). Progestin-only contraceptive pills work by thickening the cervical mucus, suppressing ovulation, and thinning the endometrium. Ovulation is not consistently suppressed with norethindrone POPs [33]. Due to the lower dose of progesterone and the absence of estrogen, POPs may have a higher incidence of breakthrough bleeding when taken continuously, but they are safely used in patients who are at higher risk of DVT [4]. Because of the short duration of action and the short half-life of POPs, it is essential that the pill be taken at the same time each day to maximize contraceptive efficacy. This can prove to be a challenge for those patients with ASD who are unable to manage their own medications.

Other options for oral progesterone pills to produce amenorrhea include medroxyprogesterone acetate (10–20 mg two times per day), megestrol acetate (20–60 mg two times per day), and norethindrone acetate (5 mg once or twice per day). Prolonged use of these medications can cause acne, mood changes, weight gain, headaches, and lipid abnormalities.

Intramuscular Progesterone

Depot medroxyprogesterone acetate (DMPA), given intramuscularly or subcutaneously, has a high rate of amenorrhea after 90 days, 50–60% at 1 year, and approximately 70% at 2 years of use [37, 38]. It is administered in the doctors' office every 3 months, which improves compliance with the medication but requires a trip to the provider's office.

Irregular bleeding is common up to 90 days. During the 1st months of use, episodes of unpredictable bleeding and spotting lasting 7 days or longer are common. The frequency and duration of such unscheduled bleeding decrease with increasing duration of use [20]. One can consider giving combination OCPs for 1–2 months following the first dose of DMPA in an effort to eliminate breakthrough bleeding for patients for whom menstrual hygiene is an issue.

Most studies of weight gain associated with DMPA concluded there was a mean gain of <2 kg lasting up to 12 months. The weight gain in the DMPA group in the studies was generally similar to the comparison group using another form of contraception [27]. Because of the associated decrease in bone density, DPMA should be used for short-term suppression in those women for whom it is the best option [13, 16].

Progesterone Implant

The etonogestrel implant (Nexplanon) is a single-rod progestin contraceptive placed subdermally in the inner upper arm for long-acting (3 years) reversible cycle suppression and contraception. Irregular bleeding is a common side effect, which may or may not decrease with continued use. During the first 2 years of use of the single-rod etonogestrel implant, 22% of women developed amenorrhea, 34% had fewer than three bleeding/spotting episodes in 90 days, and the remainder had frequent or prolonged episodes of uterine bleeding [11, 12]. Etonogestrel implant does not induce significant bone loss, despite creation of a relatively hypoestrogenic state, so it may be safely used for prolonged menstrual suppression. Placement must be performed in a doctor's office with local anesthesia. If the patient is unable to cooperate, sedation may be required.

Progesterone Intrauterine Device

The levonorgestrel-releasing intrauterine devices (IUDs) are approved by the FDA for the treatment of heavy uterine bleeding. Although irregular bleeding is common in the first 3–6 months, it has an amenorrhea rate of up to 50% at 1 year [46]. There has been one meta-analysis of levonorgestrel-releasing intrauterine devices (Liletta®, Mirena®, and Skyla®) in the general population that reported 70–80% reduction of blood loss [28].

While effective for 3–5 years (Skyla® 3 years; Liletta®, Mirena®, and Kyleena® for 5 years), the IUD most often requires placement under anesthesia in the ASD population because the procedure requires prolonged speculum placement and produces painful uterine cramping. The presence of a narrow vagina, small uterus, or significant contractures also increases the difficulty of placement. The IUDs need to be removed/exchanged every 3–5 years, which could also require an examination under anesthesia.

IUD expulsion rates range from 5% to 22% (11.2% reported in teenagers with disabilities) [1, 22] (ACOG 2012). All patients with IUDs are instructed to monitor symptoms, such as increased cramping and irregular bleeding, both of which can be signs of IUD malposition. Any patient who returns to her normal menstruation pattern following IUD placement should be evaluated for a malpositioned and/or expulsed IUD with a pelvic exam and/or a pelvic ultrasound to confirm proper placement. Caregivers of patients with ASD who are unable to communicate changes in their symptoms should be encouraged to be vigilant in their observations and recording of symptoms.

Gonadotropin-Releasing Hormone Analogues

While most commonly used to manage pelvic pain associated with endometriosis, gonadotropin-releasing hormone (GnRH) analogues, such as DepoLupron, can be used for menstrual suppression [34]. The use of GnRH analogues is limited because of the menopausal symptoms and bone thinning side effects. Norethindrone acetate is often given in conjunction to mitigate the hot flashes, irregular bleeding, and bone thinning side effects. If all other forms of medical menstrual management have been ineffective or are contraindicated, it should be considered as a short-term "last resort" prior to surgical intervention.

Hormone Use with Antiepileptic Drugs

Catamenial epilepsy is a condition in which women experience changes in seizure patterns related to their menstrual cycles. Because adolescents with intellectual disabilities have a high rate of seizure disorders, it is important to understand the effect of estrogen and progesterone on seizures. Up to 30% of these patients will manifest their seizure disorder after the onset of puberty [38]. The change in seizure activity may be related to changes in estrogen (proconvulsant effect) and progesterone (anticonvulsant effect).

Because suppression of menses may be of significant benefit in managing increased seizure activity during the menstrual cycle, clinicians should pay attention to potential interactions between antiepileptic medications and hormone medications [17, 30]. Antiepileptic medications that affect hepatic cytochrome p450 can decrease the levels of some hormonal-based medications including combination OCPs, depot medroxyprogesterone acetate, and progestin implants. The most common resulting symptoms are breakthrough bleeding and decreased contraceptive effect [25, 40]. Interactions between OCPs and antiepileptic medications are summarized in Table 5.

The oral contraceptive medications may also alter the metabolism of the anticonvulsant medications (e.g., estrogen increases the rate of metabolism of lamotrigine), which can influence their efficacy.

Table 5 Effects of anticonvulsant medications on estrogen-containing oral contraceptive pills

Anticonvulsants that decrease OCP efficacy	Barbiturates (e.g., phenobarbital and primidone)
	Carbamazepine and oxcarbazepine
	Felbamate
	Phenytoin
	Topiramate
	Vigabatrin
Anticonvulsants that do not decrease OCP efficacy	Ethosuximide
	Tiagabine
	Gabapentin
	Valproic acid[a]
	Zonisamide
	Levetiracetam

Data from Harden and Leppik [17], Jentick et al. [19], Krauss et al. [25], and Mattson et al. [30]

[a]Use of valproic acid has been linked to serious neurologic conditions and major fetal malformations. Use of valproic acid in women at risk of pregnancy should be greatly cautioned [19]

Surgical Methods

Endometrial Ablation

Selective destruction of the endometrial lining via ablation procedures can be used to treat heavy menses. Rates of amenorrhea 1 year following ablation range from 13% to 75% [14]. Failure rates are higher for women under 45 years of age. The destruction of the endometrium significantly decreases the patient's fertility, but it is not a method of birth control. The technology for this procedure was designed for women who have completed their childbearing, and it is not supported by ACOG for use in adolescents [31].

Hysterectomy

Hysterectomy for management of menstrual bleeding is rarely indicated. While removing the uterus will eliminate menstrual bleeding and the risk of pregnancy, it will not protect the ASD patient from sexual abuse or sexually transmitted diseases. Hysterectomy will not treat behavioral changes related to hormone fluctuations. It is always irreversible and has the highest potential for morbidity and mortality of all the methods of menstrual suppression. Caregivers who request hysterectomy should be thoroughly counseled that hysterectomy is only indicated in extreme situations such as a cancer diagnosis.

Contraception

The choice of contraceptive methods for any patient should be directed by the effectiveness, convenience, reversibility, and cost (see Table 4). The need for protection from sexually transmitted diseases should also be considered. The degree of intellectual impairment in each patient greatly affects the contraceptive method choice.

Most of the methods of menstrual suppression discussed above serve as excellent forms of contraception. The exceptions are the progesterone-only methods medroxyprogesterone acetate (Provera), megestrol acetate (Megace), norethindrone acetate (Aygestin), and the GnRH analogue DepoLupron. While these medications effectively suppress menstruation, they are not approved as methods of contraception.

Condoms are not the most effective method of contraception but should be discussed and offered as an excellent strategy to prevent sexually transmitted infections. In addition to teaching patents with ASD how to use condoms properly, they should also be taught how to encourage and expect their sexual partners to use condoms [3].

Patients with ASD and their caregivers should be aware of the availability of emergency contraception in the form of levonorgestrel (Plan B). Available over the counter, it can effectively prevent an unwanted pregnancy with very few side effects. It can be considered for occasional use even in those patients for whom hormonal contraception is contraindicated [3].

Sterilization

Surgical sterilization is usually performed electively for family planning and not for medical indications. Consent for sterilization should be based on the ability of the patient to voluntarily request to end their reproduction capacity. The presence of a mental disability does not, however, in itself justify either sterilization *or* its denial [44]. Federal, state, and local laws and regulations vary widely and must be taken into consideration if the patient is not her own legal guardian. A sterilization procedure can be considered after extensive counseling with the patient, parents, guardians, and caregivers.

Clinical Vignette # 1

Early Adolescent

EM is an 11-year-old virginal female with ASD who presented with her mother for discussion of menstrual management. The patient is mostly nonverbal and uses an iPad and pictures to communicate. She is toilet trained during the day and dresses and toilets with direct supervision. She is able to feed herself and lives at home with her mother, father, sister, and brother. She is a very active young woman. She attends school and has a "private" teacher who accompanied the patient and her mother to the visit.

She underwent menarche at age 10.5 years and has had light bleeding for the first 6 months. Most recently, however, her menses have increased in flow and duration. According to her mother, the patient does not seem distressed by the bleeding, but she does not like to keep the pads on. She repetitively removes them soon after they are placed, which is causing significant difficulty with hygiene now that her menstrual flow is heavier. Neither the patient's mother nor teacher has noticed cyclic behavior changes nor do they feel she is experiencing physical discomfort during her menses. They report that her bowel function and appetite have remained stable as well.

Vital signs revealed a BMI of 22 with a normal blood pressure. Physical exam was deemed unnecessary at the visit due to the patient's age, the regularity with which she was menstruating, and the normal duration of her vaginal bleeding.

After discussion with the patient's mother and teacher, menstrual suppression with oral contraceptive pills was prescribed. The patient is able to take pills without issue per her mother's report. She had no family history of stroke or DVT. She was offered a low-dose combination contraceptive pill to be taken daily with no placebo pills.

She initially experienced persistent vaginal spotting with the low-dose OCPs she was given. The OCP was changed to increase the dose of the estrogen component, and the irregular bleeding has resolved.

Clinical Vignette # 2

Adolescent with a Seizure Disorder

SA is a 17-year-old young woman who developed a seizure disorder at age 11. Her seizures were well controlled on lamotrigine and ethosuximide until the onset of menarche right before her 14th birthday, after which she would have multiple generalized tonic-clonic seizures during her menstrual periods. Her medications were adjusted, but she continued to have one seizure per period. During her most recent period, she had a seizure while in the shower and fell and hit her head. Her periods would last 4–5 days and would occur every 30–40 days.

In addition to the seizure disorder, SA has diagnoses of attention-deficit/hyperactivity disorder, nonverbal learning disorder, and dysgenesis of the corpus callosum. Her medications include dexmethylphenidate ER 10 mg every morning, fluticasone nasal spray two sprays each nostril daily, and lamotrigine 400 mg twice a day.

She lives with her mother, father, brother, and maternal grandmother. She is in the 10th grade and is active in dance and gymnastics. She has never been sexually active and does not plan on becoming sexually active in the near future. She has no family history of stroke or DVT.

SA and her mother very much wanted to try a combined OCP to treat her catamenial seizures. Given that OCPs can increase the metabolism of lamotrisine, this was discussed with her neurologist, and a baseline lamotrigine level was checked the day of the office visit, with a follow-up level checked at the end of the 3rd week of active pills. Her seizure activity initially decreased, but after three OCP packs, she experienced another generalized tonic-clonic seizure, resulting in a fall, concussion, and fracture of her left scaphoid. Her lamotrigine level was on the low end of the normal range, so her dose was increased. She subsequently only experienced one seizure in the following 12 months.

Clinical Vignette # 3

Young Adult

MC is a 22-year-old G0 woman diagnosed at age 18 years with ASD who presented by herself to the office to discuss management of her persistent pelvic pain. She has attended college and currently is planning a trip abroad for 6 months with a not-for-profit organization.

Her medical history includes diagnoses of depression with a history of suicide attempt, anxiety, and a long-standing history of migraine headaches without aura.

She experienced menarche at age 13 years with menses every 25 days lasting up to 12 days of heavy bleeding. She was placed on combination OCPs, which successfully increased the interval between menses to 28 days and decreased her menstrual flow to light for 5–6 days. Endometriosis was diagnosed via laparoscopy at age 15, and, due to an increase in pelvic pain, she was switched to DepoLupron to suppress the pain she was experiencing with her menses despite OCPs. She was also treated with add-back therapy (Aygestin) to mitigate the hot flashes from the DepoLupron. Four years ago, she underwent an endometrial ablation for persistent bleeding.

MC denies bleeding following sexual intercourse and reports that she is active with both men and women. She reports using condoms with every episode of penile intercourse. She is not currently in a sexual relationship. She denies changes in her bowel or bladder habits, weight, appetite, or abdominal girth.

She reports significant and persistent hot flashes and thick, "funny" smelling vaginal discharge since receiving the DepoLupron and wishes to stop it for these reasons. She received her last dose 3 months to the date of this visit. She continues taking the Aygestin 5 mg per day but has not noticed a change in her pain or irregular bleeding symptoms. She recently had a physical exam with her primary care provider complete with normal Pap smear and negative sexually transmitted disease screening.

While the patient was open to changing her treatment from DepoLupron and Aygestin to a combination OCP, she states that adding a new medication to her daily routine would be particularly challenging for her. The decision was made to stop the DepoLupron due to its side effects and continue her on Aygestin but increase the dose to 10 mg every night. The nightly dose was offered because it was the time at which she currently took the medication. Should she continue to have irregular bleeding, she will be counseled to take the Aygestin twice daily.

Clinical Pearls

- Use the patient's preferred method of communication (e.g., verbal vs. pictorial), and use simple, straightforward language, including the words the patient uses to refer to different body parts.
- A "reproductive health visit" can be an important opportunity to review "rules" of appropriate touching, basic toileting and menstrual hygiene, contraception, and fertility.
- The ability of patients with ASD to consent to and comply with an office exam varies, and physical and emotional trauma can be minimized through multiple visits with the provider as well as extra time and support staff. Some patients may require a mild oral sedative or an exam under anesthesia in an operating room.
- Cervical cancer screening starts at age 21 years with a PAP test, regardless of the reported sexual activity of the patient.
- Adolescents with disabilities have concerns about sexuality similar to their peers without disabilities. The provider should discuss normal anatomy, sexuality, contraception, and sexually transmitted diseases with the patient and potentially with her caregivers depending on her degree of intellectual and developmental disability.
- Individuals with disabilities have rates of sexual assault ranging from 25% to 83%, so assessing for signs and symptoms of sexual abuse is vital to the health of women with ASD, particularly for those who may not be able to communicate the details of abuse. HPV immunization is recommended for the ASD population because of the high risk of sexual assault.
- Menstrual hygiene can be challenging for patients with ASD and their caregivers and should be discussed proactively to determine a management plan. This can include management of cyclic changes in mood or behavior, treatments for dysmenorrhea and/or menorrhagia, and menstrual suppression.
- Menstruation is not physiologically necessary. A wide array of both hormonal and nonhormonal methods is available for menstrual suppression. The provider must take

into account the treatment goals, side effects from various regimens, ease of administration, comorbid medical conditions, and interactions with other medications that the patient is taking.

- Endometrial ablation for adolescents with menorrhagia is not recommended. Hysterectomy is only indicated in extreme situations such as a cancer diagnosis. Surgical sterilization is used only for contraception and not for medical indications.
- Contraception methods should be selected based on effectiveness, convenience, reversibility, and cost.

References

1. American College of Obstetricians and Gynecologists. Adolescents and long-acting reversible contraception: implants and intrauterine devices. ACOG Committee Opinion No. 539. Obstet Gynecol. 2012;120:983–8.
2. American College of Obstetricians and Gynecologists. Guidelines for women's health care: a resource manual. 3rd ed. Washington DC: ACOG; 2007.
3. American College of Obstetricians and Gynecologists. Reproductive health care for adolescents with disabilities. Supplement to Guidelines for Adolescent Health Care. 2nd ed. Washington DC: American College of Obstetricians and Gynecologists; 2012.
4. Bergendal A, Persson I, Odeberg J, et al. Association of venous thromboembolism with hormonal contraception and thrombophilic genotypes. Obstet Gynecol. 2014;124:600.
5. American College of Obstetricians and Gynecologists. Breast cancer screening. ACOG Practice Bulletin No. 122. Obstet Gynecol. 2011;118:372–82.
6. Blum RW, Kelly A, Ireland M. Health-risk behaviors and protective factors among adolescents with mobility impairments and learning and emotional disabilities. J Adolesc Heath. 2001;28:481–90.
7. Centers for Disease Control and Prevention. Vaccine safety: human papilloma virus (HPV) vaccine. Available at: http://www.cdc.gov/vaccinesafety/vaccines/HPV/index.html.
8. American College of Obstetricians and Gynecologists. Cervical cytology screening. ACOG Practice Bulletin No. 109. Obstet Gynecol. 2009;114:1409–20.
9. Chumlea WC, Schubert CM, Roche AF, Kulin HE, Lee PA, Himes JH, et al. Age at menarche and racial comparisons in US girls. Pediatrics. 2003;111:110–3.
10. Copen CE, Chandra A, Martinez G. Prevalence and timing of oral sex with the opposite sex partners among female and males ages 15-25years; United States 2007-2010. Natl Health Stat Report. 2012;(56):1–14.
11. Darney P, Patel A, Rosen K, et al. Safety and efficacy of a single-rod etonogestrel implant (Implanon): results from 11 international clinical trials. Fertil Steril. 2009;91:1646.
12. Darney P, Etonogestrel contraceptive implant. UpToDate. Walters Kluwer Heath 6/24/2016.
13. American College of Obstetricians and Gynecologists. Depot medroxyprogesterone acetate and bone effects. ACOG Committee Opinion No. 415. Obstet Gynecol. 2008;112:727–30.
14. American College of Obstetricians and Gynecologists. Endometrial ablation ACOG Practice Bulletin No. 81. Obstet Gynecol. 2007;109:1233–48.
15. Fraser IS, Porte RJ, Kouides PA, Lukes AS. A benefit-risk review of systemic hemostatic agents: part 2: in excessive or heavy menstrual bleeding. Drug Saf. 2008;31:275–82.
16. Fritz MA, Speroff L. Long-acting methods of contraception. In: Clinical gynecology and infertility. 8th ed. Philadelphia: Walters Kluwer Heath; 2011. p. 1059–93.
17. Harden C, Leppik I. Optimizing therapy for seizures in women who use oral contraceptives. Neurology. 2006;67:S56–8.
18. American College of Obstetricians and Gynecologists. Human papilloma virus immunization. ACOG Committee Opinion No. 448. Obstet Gynecol. 2010;116:800–3.
19. Jentick J, Loane MA, Dolk H, Barisic I, Garne E, Morris JK, et al. Valproic acid monotherapy in pregnancy and major congenital Malformations. N Engl J Med. 2010;362:2185–93.
20. Kaunitz AM. Depot medroxyprogesterone acetate for contraception. UpToDate. Walters Kluwer Heath 1/26/2016.
21. Kaunitz AM. Hormonal contraception for suppression of menstruation. UpToDate. May 4, 2016.
22. Kirkham YA, Allen L, Kives S, Caccia N, Spitzer RF, Ornstein MP. Trends in menstrual concerns and suppression in adolescents with developmental disabilities. J Adolesc Health. 2013;53:407–12.
23. Kluft C, Meijer P, LaGuardia KD, Fisher AC. Comparison of a transdermal contraceptive patch vs. oral contraceptives on hemostasis variables. Contraception. 2008;77:77.
24. Knickmeyer RC, Wheelwright S, Hoekstra R, Baron-Cohen S. Age of Menarche in females with autisms spectrum conditions. Dev Med Child Neurol. 2006;48:1007–8.
25. Krauss GL, Brandt J, Campbell M, Plate C, Summerfield M. Antiepileptic medication and oral contraceptive interactions: a national survey of neurologists and obstetricians. Neurology. 1996;46:1534–9.
26. Lin K, Barnhart K. The clinical rational for menses-free contraception. J Woman's health (Larchmt). 2007; 16/1171.
27. Lopez LM, Edelman A, Chen M, et al. Progestin-only contraceptives: effects on weight. Cochrane Database Syst Rev. 2013:CD008815.

28. Lopez LM Grimes DA, Schulz KF, Curtis KM. Steroidal contraceptives: effect on bone fractures in women. Cochrane Database Syst Rev. 2011;(7).
29. Lukes AS, Moore KA, Muse KN, Gersten JK, Hecht BR, Edlund M, et al. Tranexamic acid treatment for heavy menstrual bleeding; a randomized controlled trial. Obstet Gynecol. 2010;116:865–75.
30. Mattson RH, Cramer JA, Darney PD, Naftolin F. Use of oral contraceptives by women with epilepsy. JAMA. 1986;256:238–40.
31. American College of Obstetricians and Gynecologists. Menstrual manipulation for adolescents with physical and developmental disabilities. ACOG Committee Opinion No. 668. Obstet Gynecol. 2016;128:e20–5.
32. American College of Obstetricians and Gynecologists. Menstruation in girls and adolescents: using menstrual cycle as a vital sign. ACOG Committee Opinion No. 651. Obstet Gynecol. 2015;126:e143–6.
33. Milsom I, Korver T. Ovulation incidence with oral contraceptives: a literature review. J Fam Plann Reprod Health Care. 2008;34:237.
34. American College of Obstetricians and Gynecologists. Options for prevention and management of heavy menstrual bleeding in adolescent patients undergoing cancer treatment. Committee Opinion No. 606. Obstet Gynecol. 2014;124:397.
35. Pearlman MD, Griffin IL. Benign breast disease. Obstet Gynecol. 2010;116:747–58.
36. American College of Obstetricians and Gynecologists. Premenstrual syndrome. ACOG Practice Bulletin No. 15. Washington DC; 2000.
37. Quint EH, Elkins TE, Sorg CA, Kope S. The treatment of cyclic behavior changes in women with mental disabilities. J Pediatr Adolesc Gynecol. 1999;12:139–42.
38. Quint EH. Menstrual and reproductive issues in adolescents with physical and developmental disabilities. Ann N Y Acad Sci. 2008;1135:230–6.
39. Quint EH. Adolescents with special needs:clinical challenges in reproductive health care. J Pediatr Adolesc Gynecol. 2016;29:2–6.
40. Reddy DS. Clinical pharmacokinetic interactions between antiepileptic drugs and hormonal contraceptives. Expert Rev Clin Pharmacol. 210(3):183–92.
41. Savelli SL, Kerlin BA, Springer MA, Monda KL, Thornton JD, Blanchong CA. Recommendations for screening for thrombophilic tendencies in teenage female prior to contraceptive initiation. J Pediatr Adolesc Gynecol. 2006;19:313–6.
42. US Prevention Services Task Force. Screening for breast cancer: US Prevention Services Task Force recommendations statement. Ann Intern Med. 2009;151:716–26.
43. Sobey D, Doe T. Patterns of sexual abuse and assault. Sex Disabil. 1991;9:243–59.
44. American College of Obstetricians and Gynecologists. Sterilization of women, including those with mental disabilities. ACOG Committee Opinion No. 371. Obstet Gynecol. 2007;110:217–20.
45. Stewart FH, Harper CC, Ellertson CE, Grimes DA, Sawaya GF, Trussell J. Clinical breast and pelvic examination requirements for hormonal contraception. Current practice vs. evidence. JAMA. 2001;285:2232–9.
46. Stoegerer-Hecher E, Kirchengast S, Huber JC, Hartmann B. Amenorrhea and BMI as independent determinants of patient satisfaction in LNG-IUD users: cross sectional study in a Central European district. Gynecol Endocrinol. 2012;28:119–24.
47. American College of Obstetricians and Gynecologists. The initial reproductive health visit. ACOG Committee Opinion No. 598. Obstet Gynecol. 2014;123:1143–7.
48. U.S. Department of Justice. Office of Victims of Crime. Working with victims of crime with disabilities. Washington DC; 1998.
49. U.S. medical eligibility criteria for contraceptive use, 2016 Centers for Disease Control and Prevention (CDC). MMWR Recomm Rep. 2016;65(3):1–104.
50. American College of Obstetricians and Gynecologists. Use of hormonal contraception in women with coexisting medical conditions. ACOG practice Bulletin # 73. Obstet Gynecol. 2006;107:1453–72.
51. American College of Obstetricians and Gynecologists. Well-woman visit. ACOG Committee Opinion No. 534. Obstet Gynecol. 2012;120:421–4.

Musculoskeletal Disorders

16

Gleeson Rebello

Introduction

Though neither essential for diagnosis nor pathognomonic of autism spectrum disorder (ASD), the condition is often accompanied by clinically important neuromuscular and musculoskeletal manifestations. Some of these manifestations have the potential to interfere with an individual's everyday function, self-esteem, and interactions with peers. In addition, musculoskeletal conditions common to all children, such as bone fractures, may require a different management approach in those with ASD. The specific neuromuscular and musculoskeletal manifestations commonly encountered in the management of a patient with ASD both in outpatient and inpatient settings are discussed in this chapter.

History and Physical Examination

The pertinent points to be considered in the orthopedic history of a patient with ASD would begin with the timing of the motor milestones and the gait pattern at the onset of ambulation. A detailed history and assessment would be directed at inquiries into pain at specific sites with loss of function leading to limitation of activity. Challenges in communication and eliciting an accurate history in a patient with ASD should make the examining healthcare provider even more vigilant and thorough. Classic symptoms associated with a condition may not be as clearly defined in a patient with ASD.

When taking the history of a patient with ASD, specific questions pertinent to orthopedics must be directed at the presence of pain, swelling, history of trauma if any, gait pattern (for instance, history of toe-walking), and the ability to perform activities of daily living. If the clinician is planning sophisticated imaging like magnetic resonance imaging (MRI), it is important to determine the patient's ability to lay still for protracted periods of time.

The physical examination must be directed at the presence of limp, gait pattern, areas of pain and tenderness in the body, and contractures of the joints. The heel cords could be tight especially if the patient has a long-standing history of toe-walking.

The classic orthopedic examination follows the "look, feel, move, and measure" approach and can be found in any basic orthopedic textbook of clinical examination and applied in the assessment of individuals with ASD [1]. When examining a patient with pain, it often helps to

G. Rebello
Department of Orthopedic Surgery, Massachusetts General Hospital, Boston, MA, USA
e-mail: grebello@mgh.harvard.edu

E. P. Hazen, C. J. McDougle (eds.), *The Massachusetts General Hospital Guide to Medical Care in Patients with Autism Spectrum Disorder*, Current Clinical Psychiatry,
https://doi.org/10.1007/978-3-319-94458-6_16

examine the most painful area last, or the examination might have to be aborted due to noncompliance.

Common Conditions

Abnormalities of Gross Motor Function

Motor Planning Abnormalities

The functions of anticipation, coordination, and adaptation enable us to carry out an action toward a goal that facilitates our integration into the environment. The optimal development of such functions is necessary for harmonious and efficient motor planning. The main deficits commonly observed in ASD are either poverty of interactions between the person with ASD and his environment or carrying out non-purposeful repetitive activity [2, 3].

Numerous studies in children with ASD have reported a deficit in the organization of action toward a goal [2, 3]. Study of movements involved in the major motor milestones in development indicates that disturbances of motion could be present in early infancy and may be considered one of the earliest signs of ASD. In the process of learning to perform a movement, the brain builds an association between motor commands and sensory feedback. These internal models allow the brain to predict the sensory consequences of self-generated motor commands and produce motor commands that maximize expected rewards at a minimum effort. Children with ASD exhibit impairments in motor control and imitation.

Clinical descriptions of children with ASD frequently mention "hypotonia" [4]. Hypotonia appears to be clinically more prevalent in children with ASD than in IQ-matched non-autistic peers and tends to decrease with age. Hypotonia with preserved muscle strength and normal tendon reflexes has multiple possible causes. It is unclear whether clinical descriptions of hypotonia in children with ASD are a reflection of ligamentous laxity, a subtle disorder of muscles, or dysfunction of central nervous system subcortical circuitry controlling muscle tone. All of these might contribute to a clinician's perception of hypotonia.

Gait Abnormalities

Toe-walking is the best documented gait abnormality in children with ASD [5–9]. Intermittent toe-walking is common in normally developing toddlers but usually disappears by age 3 years, although it can persist in an otherwise developmentally normal individual. Rates of toe-walking among children with ASD have been reported to be as high as 63%. It is not uncommon to encounter children ranging from 5 to 12 years of age with ASD displaying a toe-walking gait on presentation. At times, toe-walking can persist into adulthood. Clinical assessment of this finding involves ruling out an organic cause for the toe-walking. Treatment can consist of heel cord stretching by way of physical therapy with constant reinforcement at home, as well as the use of carbon fiber footplates in the shoes that prevent toe-walking by increasing the rigidity of the sole of the shoe. In some cases, ankle foot orthotics (AFOs) may be considered as an option (and see Chap. 18).

As long as the heel cords are supple to the point where the ankle can achieve neutral dorsiflexion and permit placement of a plantigrade foot on the ground, no active intervention is necessary. Development of an equinus contracture as a result of prolonged positioning can result in the inability to place a plantigrade foot on the ground. This can lead to concentration of pressure on the balls of the feet and formation of callosities on the soles of the feet. Interventions for this problem include serial casting, botulinum toxin injections into the gastrosoleus muscles with serial casting, and heel cord lengthening surgery followed by serial casting. Inability to follow up on interventions like botulinum toxin injections or heel cord lengthening surgery with serial casting and AFOs or carbon fiber foot plates can lead to recurrence of toe-walking and equinus contractures. Management of this condition in a child with ASD can be a challenge as it requires compliance with a physical therapy program. The need to wear orthotics, such as an AFO or carbon foot plates, to maintain correction or prevent worsening of deformity can also add to the challenge, as many children with ASD have sensory integration issues that may make them sensitive to these interventions. Anecdotal evidence also suggests that toe-walking in some of these individuals can resolve with antianxiety medication.

Dysmorphic Physical Features

Evidence is available that there is a positive association between musculoskeletal morphological abnormalities and ASD [10]. Clinically significant musculoskeletal morphological abnormalities in children with ASD have been shown to occur in the appendicular skeleton but not the axial skeleton. The fact that there is no increase in the risk for development of axial musculoskeletal morphological abnormalities, such as scoliosis, in individuals with ASD is important to remember for the following reasons. First, it provides indirect evidence that ASD is related to abnormal neuromuscular development at a later stage of nervous system development when the appendicular skeleton is also developing. In addition, it helps to differentiate ASD from Rett's disorder, which is strongly associated with axial musculoskeletal morphological abnormalities such as neuromuscular scoliosis.

Hypermobility of the joints is yet another dysmorphic feature associated with ASD. Shetreat-Klein et al. [11] measured the maximum passive range of mobility at the elbow, wrist, and metacarpophalangeal joint of the index finger and ankle joints in children with ASD and their non-autistic peers and found that children with ASD had significantly greater joint mobility. The clinical significance of hypermobility of joints in children with ASD is unknown. Future studies should look into the clinical consequences of hypermobility of joints in children with ASD, such as increased risks of subluxation/dislocation of the joint and arthritis. Regardless, joint hypermobility needs to be addressed with improving muscle strength and conditioning through physical and occupational therapy whenever possible.

Bone Pain with Rash and Growth Failure due to Vitamin C Deficiency (Scurvy)

Scurvy is the result of vitamin C (ascorbic acid) deficiency, and its manifestations are predominantly due to collagen structural and functional abnormalities. Due to lack of the enzyme gulonolactone oxidase, humans lack the ability to synthesize vitamin C from glucose. Hence, dietary vitamin C from fruits, vegetables, or multivitamin supplements is essential for survival. As vitamin C storage levels last only several weeks, deficiency symptoms can develop in as few as 30–40 days [12]. Compared to peers with typical development, children with ASD are more prone to vitamin C deficiency due to an unbalanced diet. Many children with ASD have significant nutritional deficiencies, often related to very restricted diets with limited dietary intake of energy, macronutrients, and micronutrients, which is why a daily complete multivitamin is generally recommended.

The typical musculoskeletal manifestation of scurvy in a child with ASD is pain in the hip joint or anterior thigh with decreased energy and refusal to walk [12, 13]. Associated findings include skin rash and gingival swelling. Musculoskeletal exam findings are disproportionately subtle compared to clinical symptoms [12, 13]. The typical hip exam is normal except for pain on terminal hip abduction and a wide-based gait. Skin examination may reveal a petechial rash which is typically raised/flat, punctuate, and erythematous around the hair follicles that is seen over the dorsum of the feet to the upper thighs and scattered on the arms. Oral exam may reveal gingival hypertrophy with deep purple discoloration.

Laboratory tests, including total and differential white blood cell counts, red blood cell studies, iron, and bone marrow studies, are typically normal. The two possible abnormal studies in scurvy are elevated C-reactive protein and erythrocyte sedimentation rate [12]. The serum vitamin C level is low in scurvy (normal range 0.2–1.90 mg/deciliter).

Radiological evaluation of scurvy must include plain films. Abnormal radiological findings on a plain film include white lines surrounding epiphysis due to osteoporosis (Wimberger's sign), metaphyseal irregularities with spurring (Pelkan's sign), and a sclerotic metaphyseal white line (Frankl) in the zone of provisional calcification with a lucent line immediately below this (Trummerfeld zone of scurvy line). Bone scans are not very informative. On MRI of the pelvis, striking lesions are seen around the pelvis and hip joint [13]. On fat suppressed T2-weighted sequence imaging with short tau inversion recovery (STIR), multifocal contrast-enhancing lesions are seen both in the cancellous bone and periosteum.

Treatment of scurvy involves supplementation of vitamin C, typically at a dose of 160 mg daily, along with a pediatric multivitamin. A dramatic response will be noted in 3–4 days with continued improvement in strength and motor function over a period of 2–3 months.

Bone Health and Fractures

There is evidence that bone mineral density (BMD) is lower in boys with ASD compared with age-matched neurotypical controls at the spine, femoral neck, and total hip [14, 15]. Data from these studies raised significant concerns regarding bone health in the ASD population and the question of whether peak bone mass acquisition is negatively affected in children with ASD. Theories about the cause of the diminution in BMD include higher prevalence of malabsorptive symptoms and lactose intolerance leading to decreased vitamin D intake and absorption in children with ASD. Additionally, reduced activity and time spent outdoors by individuals with ASD could adversely affect endogenous vitamin D synthesis. Given that adequate vitamin D serum levels are essential for optimal bone mineralization and pubertal bone accrual, the long-term bone health of these individuals is of concern, and therefore studies are necessary to determine whether vitamin D supplementation in boys with ASD is effective in improving bone health in this population.

Physical activity has a favorable effect on BMD, and boys with ASD are known to have lower activity levels than controls. If future studies indicate that a lower exercise level is an important determinant of bone density in boys with ASD, structured exercise programs may be necessary to optimize pubertal bone accrual in this condition. However, it is not clear whether lower BMD in children with ASD translates to an increased fracture rate either during childhood or in adult life. In an attempt to answer that question, a study querying a national database of emergency department visits reported a higher risk of hip fracture in children and adults with ASD than in those without ASD and a higher risk for forearm and spine fracture in women with ASD [16]. With the increasing prevalence of ASD and the reduced communication skills in these patients, the need to address this increase in fracture rate is important, particularly with regard to the morbidity of hip fractures in the elderly. Hence, the childhood years will be specifically important to target, as bone accrual during the childhood years is a critical determinant of future bone health.

The Child with ASD in a Body Cast: Challenges in Managing Behavior

Placing a child with behavioral problems related to ASD in a body cast, especially a hip spica, is quite often a management challenge for all involved [17, 18]. Hip spica casts extend from nipples to toes and can include one entire leg, one entire leg with the other thigh, or both legs. The purpose of a hip spica cast is to immobilize the joint after an osteotomy (cutting the bone) of the pelvis or proximal femur in conditions like hip dysplasia or a posttraumatic fracture of the femur. There are described non-medication and medication strategies that can be helpful in the management of a child with ASD who requires a hip spica cast.

Non-medication strategies of managing behavior challenges for a child with ASD in a hip spica cast are based on facilitating the child's communication and understanding of the procedure. Picture-based descriptions of what a child can expect when casted help improve understanding of the upcoming event of spica casting. Communication with the child can be facilitated by learning of specific signs or words to describe discomfort. See Chap. 4, for additional discussion of behavioral strategies to help patients with ASD tolerate procedures.

Medication strategies of managing behavioral challenges related to spica casting should focus on optimizing pain control and reducing hyperactivity. Post-procedural pain in a child with ASD is better controlled by either scheduled or PRN pain medication than continuous pain medication. The aim of scheduled and/or PRN pain medication is to reduce pain while minimizing the sedation that often accompanies continuous pain medication.

Controlling hyperactivity of a child with ASD in a hip spica cast is possible in two ways: altering the dosage of an existing medication based on its adverse effect profile or addition of a new drug(s). If a child with ASD has coexisting attention-deficit/hyperactivity disorder, working with the child's psychopharmacologist to optimize treatment of hyperactivity during the casting period is essential. Some children may need an increase in the dosage of current medications, and others may benefit from the addition of a medication, such as an alpha-2 agonist, which can reduce hyperactivity and impulsivity [19] to help them during a time when their mobility is limited and excessive activity can put them at risk of re-injury.

Clinical Vignette #1

John is a 9-year-old boy with a diagnosis of ASD who has been a toe-walker for as long as his parents can remember. When asked about his gait pattern at 3 years of age, his pediatrician noted that there was a possibility that his gait pattern would normalize on its own. When it still persisted at the age of 5 years, a pediatric orthopedic surgeon was consulted, and he recommended physical therapy aimed at keeping the heel cords stretched, coupled with use of carbon fiber foot plates in his shoes. Over the next couple of years, John and his parents became busy with school and therapies aimed at helping him integrate socially. In the meantime, John continued to toe-walk and began to complain of occasional calf pain. The pediatric orthopedic surgeon was consulted again, and he noted that John had tight heel cords and that his ankle, when passively dorsiflexed, stopped a couple of degrees short of neutral dorsiflexion, indicating that he was on the verge of developing a fixed plantar flexion contracture. He was also developing mild callosities under the balls of his feet. After discussion with parents, serial casting was recommended and initiated. Casts were changed every couple of weeks for a period of 6 weeks. In the interim John needed to come in for a couple of unscheduled visits because he got the cast wet at one time and was uncomfortable with pain in his heel the other time. At those visits, the casts were removed and reapplied. After 6 weeks of casting, it was noted that John's ankle dorsiflexion had improved to 5° of dorsiflexion, which meant he could now put his feet plantigrade if he wanted to do so. Though his gait demonstrated heel toe progression, he was a little weak and unsteady from his prolonged casting. He was provided carbon fiber foot plates and referred to physical therapy to relearn heel cord stretching. A home program was emphasized. He was asked to follow up every 3 months for the first year to make sure his heel cords remained stretched and a contracture did not develop.

Musculoskeletal Issues in Adults with ASD

There is not much literature on musculoskeletal issues in adults with ASD. A study utilizing a national database of emergency department visits found a higher risk of hip fracture in children and adults with ASD than in those without ASD and a higher risk for forearm and spine fracture in women with ASD [16]. The increasing prevalence of ASD (to above 1% of the population) combined with the known morbidity of hip fractures in the elderly could result in the average adult orthopedic surgeon treating more of these patients that have serious musculoskeletal problems complicated by altered communication skills. A better understanding of an adult with ASD would be an asset for the orthopedic surgeon or healthcare professional when treating this individual's musculoskeletal issues. Performing sophisticated imaging like an MRI on an individual with ASD may require sedation as many patients with ASD may not be able to lie still for the time required to obtain an MRI. The logistics of obtaining an MRI in an adult with ASD with a musculoskeletal problem makes a detailed clinical examination essential to pinpoint the locus of pathology prior to ordering the MRI. If the exact area is not pinpointed clinically, it might result in obtaining an MRI of the wrong area, for instance, doing an MRI of the foot instead of the ankle which would result in the need to perform an additional MRI on the ankle of the patient.

Understanding an orthopedic procedure preoperatively and postoperative compliance with instructions for mobilization and physical therapy can be challenging in many patients with ASD. Measures used in pediatric patients like video games, visual aids, and adult versions of "child life specialists" may have to be utilized to help this group of patients navigate an orthopedic condition that necessitates surgery.

Clinical Vignette #2

Bradley is a 19-year-old male patient with ASD with idiopathic scoliosis with a spinal curve that demonstrated progression after skeletal maturity necessitating posterior spinal instrumented fusion. Prior to undergoing surgery, he was evaluated by the psychiatry and physical and occupations therapy teams. He also was given a tour of the operating room prior to the procedure to help him get acclimated to the location of surgery and its surroundings. Postoperatively he was put on trazodone by the psychiatry team to help normalize his sleep pattern. Challenges in mobilizing him postsurgery included helping him differentiate between pain and discomfort, reestablishing a daily routine, observing postsurgical precautions to prevent hardware failure, and adjusting to new movement patterns. His spinal instrumentation was clinically and radiographically monitored with regular follow-up visits until bony fusion of his vertebral column took place.

Conclusion

ASD is often accompanied by clinically important neuromuscular and musculoskeletal manifestations that are neither essential for diagnosis nor pathognomonic of the condition. Some of these manifestations could potentially interfere with an individual's everyday function, self-esteem, and interactions with peers. Toe-walking is the best documented gait abnormality in children with ASD and can be treated with physical therapy and orthotics where the treatment is aimed at preventing the formation of fixed contractures. Application of body casts when indicated for children with ASD can be challenging and needs to be backed with appropriate psychopharmacological treatment. Compared to peers with typical development, children with ASD could be more prone to vitamin C deficiency due to imbalances in diet.

Clinical Pearls

- There is no pathognomonic sign or symptom that is consistently seen in the musculoskeletal examination of an individual with ASD.
- Idiopathic toe-walking is the most frequently documented gait abnormality in children with ASD.
- The cornerstone of treatment of idiopathic toe-walking in children with ASD is to preserve ankle dorsiflexion using a combination of physical therapy and orthotics.
- If a plantar flexion contracture develops, manipulations and serial casting could be attempted in order to preserve the ability of the foot to be placed plantigrade on the ground so as to prevent skin breakdown or callosity formation.
- Lower bone mineral density in children with ASD could translate to an increased fracture

rate either during childhood or in adult life and vigilance and counseling about appropriate dietary supplementation, and exercise to improve bone health should be strongly considered.

- Poor dietary habits in individuals with ASD could result in rare conditions like scurvy and present to a musculoskeletal physician as an inability to walk.
- Application of body casts when indicated for children with ASD can be challenging and needs to be backed with appropriate psychopharmacological treatment.
- Sophisticated imaging that requires prolonged periods of laying immobile, like an MRI, may need sedation.

References

1. McRae R. Clinical orthopaedic examination. 5th ed. Edinburgh: Churchill Livingstone; 2004.
2. Gowen E, Hamilton A. Motor abilities in autism: a review using a computational context. J Autism Dev Disord. 2013;43(2):323–44.
3. Haswell C, Izawa J, Dowell L, Mostofsky S, Shadmehr R. Representation of internal models of action in the autistic brain. Nat Neurosci. 2009;12(8):970–2.
4. Stoit AM, van Schie HT, Slaats-Willemse DI, Buitelaar JK. Grasping motor impairments in autism: not action planning but movement execution is deficient. J Autism Dev Disord. 2013;43(12):2793–806.
5. Schmitz C, Martineau J, Barthélémy C, Assaiante C. Motor control and children with autism: deficit of anticipatory function? Neurosci Lett. 2003;348(1):17–20.
6. Ming X, Brimacombe M, Wagner GC. Prevalence of motor impairment in autism spectrum disorders. Brain Dev. 2007;29(9):565–70.
7. Barrow WJ, Jaworski M, Accardo PJ. Persistent toe walking in autism. J Child Neurol. 2011;26(5):619–21.
8. Accardo PJ, Barrow W. Toe walking in autism: further observations. J Child Neurol. 2015;30(5):606–9.
9. Kindregan D, Gallagher L, Gormley J. Gait deviations in children with autism spectrum disorders: a review. Autism Res Treat. 2015;2015:74–48.
10. Ozgen H, Hellemann GS, Stellato RK, Lahuis B, van Daalen E, Staal WG, Rozendal M, Hennekam RC, Beemer FA, van Engeland H. Morphological features in children with autism spectrum disorders: a matched case-control study. J Autism Dev Disord. 2011;41(1):23–31.
11. Shetreat-Klein M, Shinnar S, Rapin I. Abnormalities of joint mobility and gait in children with autism spectrum disorders. Brain Dev. 2014;36(2):91–6.
12. Duggan CP, Westra SJ, Rosenberg AE. Case records of the Massachusetts General Hospital. Case 23-2007. A 9-year-old boy with bone pain, rash, and gingival hypertrophy. N Engl J Med. 2007;357(4):392–400.
13. Niwa T, Aida N, Tanaka Y, Tanaka M, Shiomi M, Machida J. Scurvy in a child with autism: magnetic resonance imaging and pathological findings. J Pediatr Hematol Oncol. 2012;34(6):484–7.
14. Furlano RI, Bloechliger M, Jick H, Meier CR. Bone fractures in children with autistic spectrum disorder. J Dev Behav Pediatr. 2014;35(6):353–9.
15. Roke Y, van Harten PN, Buitelaar JK, Tenback DE, Quekel LG, de Rijke YB, Boot AM. Bone mineral density in male adolescents with autism spectrum disorders and disruptive behavior disorder with or without antipsychotic treatment. Eur J Endocrinol. 2012;167(6):855–63.
16. Neumeyer AM, O'Rourke JA, Massa A, Lee H, Lawson EA, McDougle CJ, Misra M. Brief report: bone fractures in children and adults with autism spectrum disorders. J Autism Dev Disord. 2015;45(3):881–7.
17. Chambers H, Becker RE, Hoffman MT, Hartley-McAndrew M, Stein MT. Managing behavior for a child with autism in a body cast. J Dev Behav Pediatr. 2012;33(6):506–8.
18. Sakai C, Miller K, Brussa AK, MacPherson C, Augustyn M. Challenges of autism in the inpatient setting. J Dev Behav Pediatr. 2014;35(1):82–4.
19. Scahill L, McCracken JT, King BH, Rockhill C, Shah B, Politte L, Sanders R, Minjarez M, Cowen J, Mullett J, Page C, Ward D, Deng Y, Loo S, Dziura J, McDougle CJ. Extended-release guanfacine for hyperactivity in children with autism spectrum disorder. Res Units Pediatr Psychopharmacol Autism Netw. 2015;172(12):1197–206.

Dermatology

17

Anna Cristina Garza-Mayers
and Daniela Kroshinsky

Introduction

Dermatologic concerns can present a challenge in the medical care of individuals with autism spectrum disorder (ASD). Some genetic syndromes (see Table 17.1) manifest dermatologically and are associated with a greater frequency of ASD than in the general population [15]. A summary of these syndromes has recently been published [1]. More commonly, providers are likely to encounter general dermatologic issues that require evaluation and treatment tailored to the ASD population. Data from 5 years of National Health Interview Surveys showed that children with ASD have a higher prevalence of multiple health conditions, including eczema. Parents of children with ASD were also more likely to report "unmet health needs" [32], suggesting barriers to diagnosis and treatment of common skin disorders in the ASD population that may contribute to increased prevalence of dermatologic disease. In this chapter we will provide a general approach to the dermatologic examination and discuss a selection of common dermatologic diseases with particular attention to potential exacerbation in the care of patients with ASD.

A general dermatologic examination must take into account the sensory processing dysfunction often found in individuals with ASD. Patients may exhibit hyposensitivity or hypersensitivity to stimuli including touch [23]. Differences in sensory processing are in fact a consideration when making a diagnosis of ASD [6] and have been shown to present similar challenges in dental evaluation and care [21]. Deficits in communication, particularly in nonverbal patients, and difficulty accommodating changes in routine may present additional challenges.

Table 17.1 Genetic syndromes with dermatologic comorbidity and association with ASD

Syndrome	Dermatologic finding
Tuberous sclerosis complex	"Ash leaf" hypomelanotic macules, facial angiofibromas, ungual (nail fold) fibromas, shagreen patches (areas of thickened skin)
Angelman syndrome	Hypopigmentation
Neurofibromatosis type 1	Café-au-lait spots, axillary and/or inguinal freckling, neurofibromas of the skin
Hypomelanosis of Ito	Hypopigmentation in a blaschkoid distribution (following lines of neural crest cell migration)

A. C. Garza-Mayers
Harvard Combined Program in Dermatology, Massachusetts General Hospital, Boston, MA, USA

D. Kroshinsky (✉)
Department of Dermatology, Massachusetts General Hospital, Boston, MA, USA
e-mail: dkroshinsky@mgh.harvard.edu

E. P. Hazen, C. J. McDougle (eds.), *The Massachusetts General Hospital Guide to Medical Care in Patients with Autism Spectrum Disorder*, Current Clinical Psychiatry,
https://doi.org/10.1007/978-3-319-94458-6_17

Providers should consider the stimuli present in the examination setting, including lighting and background noise such as that from medical equipment. It is often preferable to schedule a patient with ASD during a less busy time, such as the first appointment of the day, to minimize time spent in a crowded waiting room and to allow for more time with the patient as needed [29]. The examination itself should be accompanied by direct and concrete verbal explanation with the use of touch that is minimal but firm [21] and a soothing tone of voice. When appropriate, communication with a caregiver prior to the exam can help determine whether particular distractors, such as a cell phone, may increase the comfort of the patient and if there are specific areas of the body that are distressing for the patient when touched.

As a final note, it is our experience that procedures can be stressful or painful for all patients and particularly difficult for pediatric patients and patients with ASD who experience difficulties in sensory processing and communication. Patients with ASD may react in unpredictable ways in times of stress; thus, sedation, such as with benzodiazepine or with the aid of an anesthesiologist, may be required to ensure the safety of both patient and provider. When possible, explaining the procedure and scheduling a subsequent visit may be helpful, especially if the use of pre-procedural agents such as numbing creams may help decrease procedure-associated pain and anxiety. With adult patients, it is important to confirm whether the patient consents for him- or herself or there is a legal guardian who should be contacted. In all instances and with all patients, we emphasize that patients with ASD present with a spectrum of unique needs to be considered on an individual basis.

A Pediatric Approach to Common Conditions

Self-Injurious Behavior and Related Dermatologic Concerns

Clinical Evaluation

History Stereotyped and repetitive movements and behaviors are a part of the diagnostic criteria for ASD and may include flicking fingers in front of the eyes, hand flapping, or whole-body rocking, among others. In individuals with sensory processing deficits, data suggests such behaviors may serve a self-stimulating purpose or may satisfy ritualistic or routine tendencies [7]. These behaviors may also be self-injurious to the patient. Self-injurious behavior (SIB) may be present in as many as half of patients with ASD and may begin as early as 2 years of age [7]. Relevant to dermatologic care, these behaviors may include biting oneself or skin picking that result in injury to the skin. Behaviors such as onychophagia (nail biting) or trichotillomania (hair pulling) may also be seen.

It is important to determine whether a dermatologic or systemic cause of discomfort is driving SIB, particularly in cases of new onset behaviors. A common complaint to consider is pruritus (itch), which may manifest as a strong need or desire to pick the skin. Pruritus has multiple etiologies (Table 17.2) for which a thorough history, including a complete review of systems, can help focus the differential [38]. For instance, a history of atopy, such as asthma or allergic rhinitis, may accompany atopic dermatitis (also known as eczema). Systemic disease such as liver or renal disease may cause pruritus without accompanying skin lesions, the origin of which is not fully understood, though this is less common in pediatric patients. Other affected

Table 17.2 Potential causes of pruritus

Xerosis
Inflammation (e.g., eczema, psoriasis)
Contact dermatitis
Hypersensitivity reaction
Insect bite
Scabies
Parasitic infection
Fungal infection of the skin
Chronic renal disease
Liver disease, such as cholestasis or primary biliary cholangitis
Hematopoietic disease, such as polycythemia vera or lymphoma
HIV infection
Hypo- or hyperthyroidism
Neuropathic causes such as postherpetic itch

family members or contacts may indicate an infectious etiology such as scabies. Information regarding new exposures such as to medications (discussed in further detail below) and contact irritants should be obtained.

Physical Examination Attention should be paid to the area of the body affected as well as to the distribution and morphology of evident lesions. It should also be noted whether lesions are primary (native) or secondary (reflecting manipulation, such as by scratching or rubbing). For instance, linear burrows are a pathognomonic primary lesion of scabies, particularly if found on the hands and feet. Atopic dermatitis may have diverse presentations. In older children, adolescents, and adults, it may present acutely as erythematous scaling with papules or plaques of the antecubital and popliteal fossae, with widespread xerosis (dry skin) [38]. Chronic lesions may appear as lichenified plaques (raised areas of increased skin markings and thickened skin).

Picking or excoriating (scratching) without a dermatologic cause is most likely to be identified as lesions of a variety of shapes and states of evolution, in a symmetric distribution that reflects areas easily accessible to the patient. For instance, such lesions are more likely to be found on the face and upper extremities but not along the thoracic spine. Post-inflammatory pigmentation changes may also be seen in and around older lesions. If untreated, excoriation can progress to prurigo nodularis, firm dome-shaped nodules that may be hyperpigmented or scaly. Similar to cases of chronic atopic dermatitis, lichen simplex chronicus may develop, identified as plaques with exaggerated skin lines secondary to habitual rubbing. Ulceration or secondary infection may also result.

Other types of SIB have a limited number of etiologies to consider. Onychophagia (nail biting) presents with characteristic uneven destruction of the nail plate. Trichotillomania (hair pulling) presents with alopecia, typically of a single area, with hairs of varying lengths. This is distinguishable from alopecia areata in which remaining hairs are of a uniform length and in which case hair-pulling behavior is likely not to be elicited in the patient's history.

Studies If history and physical examination indicate pruritus is driving SIB, there are many potential laboratory tests that may be of use in determining etiology, including a complete blood count (CBC) with differential, liver and renal function tests, thyroid hormone levels, HIV serologies, serum IgE levels, and, if indicated, allergen-specific blood or skin testing [38]. Careful selection guided by the patient's presentation should be employed. In cases where fungal or parasitic infection is suspected, a skin scraping is easily and quickly obtainable and may reveal causative organisms. If a primary dermatologic disorder, such as eczema or contact dermatitis, is suspected, skin biopsy may be informative. Its use should be judicious, for reasons described above. Though repetitive behaviors are part of a diagnosis of ASD, attributing skin lesions to behavior alone should be a diagnosis of exclusion, similar to the approach to psychogenic itch or neurotic excoriation in the general population [9].

Treatment

Cases in which an obvious etiology or systemic disease is identified may be treated accordingly, such as anti-parasitic treatment of scabies, complete work-up and management of liver disease, or identification and treatment of malignancy. Lesions concerning for infection should be swabbed for bacterial, fungal, or viral culture as clinically indicated to guide antimicrobial therapy. Lesions that appear eroded or ulcerated should be treated with antibiotic ointment or petrolatum and covered daily until fully healed.

In cases where pruritus is the driving force or dermatologic disease is suspected, it is important to note that symptomatic treatment may be implemented, if the patient and family desire, even in cases of unknown etiology. Topical medications are the mainstays of treatment in pruritus [10]. For xerosis (dry skin) with or without atopic dermatitis, moisturizers may help to prevent exacerbation. Ointments followed by creams generally have higher lipid content than lotions and are preferred. Ideally moisturizer is applied twice daily and immediately after bathing. Regarding prescription topical medications, topical corticosteroids are first-line therapy and are most effective when inflammation of the skin is apparent. These range in potency, with ointments generally more potent than creams and lotions, and should be applied twice daily for 1–3 weeks. In general higher-potency corticosteroids will take effect more quickly and should be used for shorter amounts of time. If a greater length of treatment is considered necessary, referral for dermatologic management is recommended. Long-term corticosteroid use is associated with local side effects such as atrophy, striae, and telangiectasia, particularly where the skin is thin such as on the face and dorsal hands. Clear discussion on proper use and duration of treatment with corticosteroids is critical.

Tactile processing in patients with ASD may also affect the use of topical therapeutics, the mainstay of dermatologic care. Based on frequent anecdotal parent reports of difficulties, Ellis and colleagues used graduated exposure, modeling product use, and social attention or praise to promote desensitization and tolerance of lotion and/or cream in two children with ASD. Progressing through a hierarchy of steps, from visualizing the product to the child applying it himself, both children achieved successful product use that continued after the study's conclusion (for one child, up to 3 years) [8]. This presents a promising approach when prescribing topical medications. It also serves as a reminder to focus on what the patient and his or her family most wishes to address, to simplify care regimens as much as possible, and to follow up regularly to assess progress. When encountering multiple issues requiring multiple prescriptions, adherence can be maximized by introducing only a few agents at each visit with a focus on the most distressing or pressing issues first and then building on the regimen with subsequent close follow-up visits. When possible, written instructions outlining the plan of therapy should be provided. If varying over time or in complexity, writing out instructions on a printed calendar can be helpful. Many individuals with ASD have strengths in visual processing. Utilizing pictures and diagrams may also be a successful approach.

Oral medications may also be useful in breaking the "itch-scratch" cycle. We recommend the non-sedating oral H1 antihistamine fexofenadine at off-label dosing for itch, 180 mg twice daily in adults. Hydroxyzine is often more effective but may cause sedation and is thus most often used before bedtime. Rarely, an idiosyncratic activating reaction can take place with hydroxyzine, so it is important to discuss and monitor for this possibility, particularly in individuals with ASD. Hydroxyzine is typically dosed up to every 6 h with a maximum dosage of 2 mg/kg/day recommended in pediatric patients. In most cases, a starting dosage ranges from 5 to 10 mg given 30 min before nap and/or before bed with up-titration based on response and tolerability. This can be particularly helpful as itch is often reported to be more severe at night and can interfere with sleep.

Particularly when the etiology driving a problematic behavior eludes identification, treatment may alternatively focus on behavior modification techniques, as supported by case reports and small observational studies [22]. These include differential reinforcement, either of time spent not engaging in the behavior or of another behavior. Redirection and the use of competing activities have also been shown to be effective, while limited data suggest that punishment, including verbal and physical overcorrection, is not effective. Consider referral to a behavioral specialist or a psychologist if behavioral therapy is desired. Some psychiatric medications, including atypical antipsychotics, have been shown to be helpful in reducing SIB or harmful repetitive behaviors resulting in skin injury or irritation. Comorbid anxiety may underlie these behaviors in many cases. Thus, referral to a psychiatrist may be indicated for some patients.

Finally, occlusion may also be used to break the "itch-scratch" cycle. Dressings or bandages may be applied to encourage healing of the lesions and also to discourage further excoriation or picking. For lesions on the extremities, an Unna boot may be utilized. Conventionally used for lesions resulting from venous stasis dermatitis, this consists of an impregnated gauze wrap followed by a dry gauze wrap with or without overlying ACE wrapping that promotes healing and can be left in place for several days [30]. Data suggest that occlusion may serve not only to physically prevent injury but may also affect tactile processing such that the behavior is no longer desired by the patient [27].

Drug Eruptions

Clinical Evaluation

History ASD is often treated with a combination of behavioral and pharmacologic therapies. Prescription medications may be used to target some symptoms associated with ASD, including hyperactive behavior, anxiety, depression, self-injurious, and aggressive behavior [24]. Individuals with ASD may also have associated medical conditions, such as a seizure disorder, that require pharmacologic treatment. As such, individuals with ASD may be exposed to a variety of medications, any of which may result in an adverse reaction (Table 17.3).

Anticonvulsant medications are frequently implicated in drug eruptions. Adverse cutaneous reactions to such medications have been reported in four small studies and case reports of individuals with ASD specifically, totaling 3 children and 1 adult affected out of a total of 34 children and 3 adults, treated with either topiramate for seizures [13], guanfacine for attention-deficit hyperactivity/disorder [31], or memantine or galantamine to promote language [11, 14]. As up to 56% of children with ASD have a prescription medication of any kind [24], and may be prescribed medications off-label, it is likely the incidence of such reactions is much higher than reported.

Table 17.3 Medications frequently associated with drug eruption

Antibiotics
Carbamazepine
Lamotrigine
Lithium
Phenytoin

A rash or cutaneous eruption is one of the most common adverse drug reactions. If an adverse cutaneous drug reaction is suspected, chronology is of the utmost importance. A history of all medications to which the patient has been exposed, including over-the-counter medications and all medications taken previously without incident in important, as reaction may occur even after years of exposure. Dates of administration, dosages, recent changes in dosage or formulation, and date and evolution of drug eruption (including after the drug is discontinued) should be compiled. Further history obtained should include potential exposure to sick contacts, as drug eruptions may often closely resemble viral exanthem. History of immunosuppression or immunodeficiency may be a risk factor for drug reaction. A full review of systems should be documented; systemic symptoms such as fever, skin pain, dysuria, dysphagia, photophobia, and abdominal pain may indicate a more severe adverse reaction, discussed in further detail below.

Physical Examination Drug-related rashes vary widely in their presentation and severity. They are most often self-limited, pruritic, exanthematous eruptions, also referred to as morbilliform or maculopapular rashes, presenting as symmetric, widespread discrete pink erythematous macules and papules that can become confluent (Fig. 17.1a). The eruption most often arises 4–21 days after drug administration and can progress even up to 7 days after the offending agent is withdrawn [35]. Blisters and pustules are rare and suggest more severe drug reaction subtypes warranting urgent evaluation.

Urticarial reactions are also common, with associated angioedema and anaphylaxis possible. Urticaria presents as "hives" or "wheals," transient erythematous and edematous papules, and plaques that are usually pruritic. Angioedema reflects edema of subcutaneous tissues beneath the epidermis and most often presents as acute swelling of the face, lips, and larynx. Anaphylaxis is a rare and potentially life-threatening rapid onset hypersensitivity reaction. Both angioedema and anaphylaxis may be accompanied by urti-

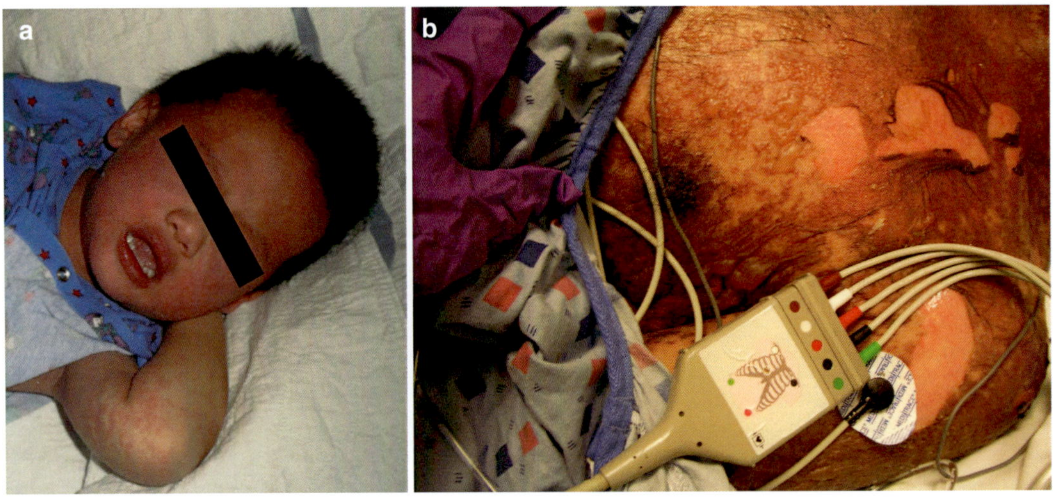

Fig. 17.1 Morbiliform drug eruption

caria and pruritus as well as signs of respiratory compromise (dyspnea, wheeze, or stridor).

Photosensitivity drug reactions are less common and are most often due to phototoxicity [12]. Phototoxicity occurs with certain drugs in combination with sufficient ultraviolet radiation exposure. A sunburn-like reaction occurs (generally in less time than would be expected for sunburn) in sun-exposed areas and may blister. This can occur with tetracyclines, nonsteroidal anti-inflammatory drugs (NSAIDs), and selective serotonin reuptake inhibitors (SSRIs), among others. Photoallergy describes the effect of light on a drug or its metabolite resulting in a hypersensitivity reaction, resulting in a dermatitis of sun-exposed areas that is more chronic in nature. Photoallergy has been associated with tricyclic antidepressants. Photosensitivity drug reactions have otherwise not been described in drugs commonly administered for ASD-related conditions.

More severe cutaneous adverse drug reactions include drug reaction with eosinophilia and systemic symptoms (DRESS) also known as drug hypersensitivity syndrome, Stevens-Johnson syndrome (SJS), and toxic epidermal necrolysis (TEN). A full skin examination is required to assess for mucosal involvement. History and physical should include vital signs as well as general assessment for lymphadenopathy and other systemic symptoms [36].

DRESS is most commonly attributed to anticonvulsant medications. It may initially resemble an exanthematous reaction but presents after a longer latent period, up to 6 weeks after drug exposure. It progresses to diffuse erythema with follicular accentuation, affecting greater than 50% body surface area (BSA). Facial edema, fever greater than 38 °C, lymphadenopathy, and symptoms related to visceral organ involvement (most frequently of the liver, kidney, and lung) may occur [19].

SJS and TEN are rare but life-threatening cutaneous reactions that consist of separation of the skin at the dermal-epidermal junction with mucosal involvement (Fig. 17.1b). SJS describes less than 10% BSA, while TEN describes greater than 30% BSA involvement. Fever greater than 39 °C, conjunctival pain or pruritus, and pain on swallowing may precede cutaneous lesions by 1–3 days. Lesions present as painful dusky erythematous or purpuric macules that spread and coalesce, progressing to the vesicles and bullae that break easily and slough to reveal the dermis. If skin detachment is suspected but not evident, a positive Nikolsky sign may be elicited (separation of the skin with exertion of tangential mechanical pressure on an erythematous area). Bullae and erosions may present on oral, ocular, or urogenital mucosa. Patients presenting with any of these features should be sent for immediate dermatologic or emergency department evaluation, while morbilliform eruptions can be monitored closely.

Studies If a severe drug reaction is suspected, laboratory studies should include a CBC with differential, a complete metabolic panel, and urinalysis. Urticaria, angioedema, and anaphylaxis are IgE-mediated, and serum IgE antibody levels may be assessed. Otherwise, diagnostic testing to identify the culprit drug in cases of drug eruption is generally not commercially available [35]. Patch testing (deliberate exposure to potential allergen in a defined location to assess reaction) is of limited value given low specificity and sensitivity and is thus not recommended [28]. Response to drug withdrawal may be informative, as clearance of the eruption would generally be expected. Conversely, rechallenge is not recommended as response is not predictable and a more severe reaction is possible. Skin biopsy is not likely to reveal distinguishing histopathological features.

Treatment

In cases of a suspected drug reaction, it is generally recommended that all nonessential medications be stopped. However, if the reaction is mild or easily managed, or the medication is not easily replaced by a similar acting medication without chemical and/or pharmacologic cross-reactivity, overall risks and benefits in patient management must be weighed [5]. Antihistamines and topical corticosteroids may be used for symptomatic relief of pruritus, as described in the preceding section.

In severe cases, such as reactions with systemic symptoms, concern for breathing, or suspected SJS/TEN, the patient should be admitted to the hospital for monitoring and supportive care, potentially in an intensive care or burn unit. Infection and sepsis are a risk. If ophthalmic or mucosal (such as urethral or vaginal) involvement is suspected, ophthalmologic, urologic, and gynecologic consultation should be sought as needed. There are no established guidelines regarding systemic treatment, which may include systemic corticosteroids, intravenous immune globulin (IVIG), and cyclosporine. Data on all therapies is limited and conflicting [33, 36].

Acne

Clinical Evaluation

History Acne vulgaris is the most common dermatologic condition affecting adolescents and can persist well into adulthood. While there is no data specific to the ASD population, acne can have profound psychosocial impact in all individuals, leading to anxiety and depression as well as physical scarring. Acne is often readily recognized clinically, and history may not be as informative as physical examination. Nevertheless, age of onset and lesion location should be noted, as these may indicate a less common dermatologic condition or an inciting factor. Additionally, a medication list should be obtained as well as a thorough past medical history. Glucocorticoids, androgens, phenytoin, and lithium may induce acne. In girls, hyperandrogenism of polycystic ovary syndrome (PCOS), which has been shown to be associated with valproic acid, may contribute to acne. Other information that may be useful when determining treatment includes the patient's motivation for treatment and current skin care regimen.

Physical Examination Acne is a disorder of the pilosebaceous unit and progresses through the formation of a comedo, which can accumulate keratin and sebum, expand, become colonized with *Propionibacterium acnes*, and rupture, ultimately producing inflammation [4]. It is thus typically found in areas of the body with well-developed sebaceous glands, including the face, neck, chest, and back.

The patient's skin type (oily or dry), skin color, lesion distribution, and overall degree of involvement should be noted. Typical lesions reflect the progression described. Closed comedones (or "whiteheads") are subtle small skin-colored papules. Open comedones (or "blackheads") are dark papules in which comedonal debris is exposed to air via a follicular opening and is thus oxidized. Both typically do not have associated erythema or inflammation. Inflammatory lesions consist of papules, pustules, nodules, or cysts that can be painful or tender. Resolved lesions may have post-inflammatory hyperpigmentation. Scarring is possible, particularly in severe cases or with lesions that have been manipulated or picked. This may be problematic in individuals with ASD, who may pick at acne lesions secondary to anxiety or pain, thereby causing further discomfort.

Studies Laboratory studies are generally not required or obtained. For lesions that appear superinfected, swabbing for bacterial Gram stain and culture may help guide antibiotic treatment directed at the infection prior to initiating long-term acne management. If hyperandrogenism in a female patient is suspected, referral for laboratory evaluation for PCOS or further endocrinology work-up may be helpful in establishing a diagnosis and treatment of an underlying condition.

Treatment

The treatment approach must take into consideration lesion type and severity of involvement (Table 17.4), as well as the patient's motivation level. Medications work to decrease follicular keratinization, decrease sebum production, target *P. acnes*, and decrease inflammation [37].

For comedonal acne, a topical retinoid such as tretinoin or adapalene is first-line. Retinoids may cause dryness and peeling; patients should be counseled to use only a pea-sized amount on the entire face every other night for 2 weeks before moving to nightly use and to moisturize as needed [20]. The agent should be held in cases of irritation and restarted more gradually. For mildly inflammatory acne, topical clindamycin or erythromycin may be added each morning. This can be in addition to retinoid cream in the evening or in addition to a 4–10% benzoyl peroxide wash with skin contact for 20–30 s.

For moderate to severe inflammatory acne, a topical retinoid may be used in combination with oral minocycline or doxycycline 100 mg twice daily with food. Topical or oral antibiotic monotherapy is not recommended due to the risk of antibiotic resistance [37]. Antibiotic therapy should be of limited duration, typically not longer than 3 months.

Oral isotretinoin is proven effective in recalcitrant nodular acne. It is also used in milder cases that have proven resistant to other treatment or have resulted in significant scarring. Concerns for increased risk of depression and suicide and isotretinoin therapy have not been borne out in large-scale analysis [18]. Though close monitoring of individuals with a history of mood disorder or suicide attempt is advised, it is not a contraindication to therapy, particularly given the psychological distress of acne itself. We recommend referral to a dermatologist for patient registration and monitoring of fasting triglyceride and cholesterol levels, liver function, complete blood count, as well as pregnancy status and plans for conception prior to and during medication use.

In general, a management plan should be designed to optimize adherence. For instance, a particular patient may be more inclined to take an oral medication than to apply a topical cream; in such a case, one topical and one oral medication may be preferable to two topical medications. Additionally, there are combina-

Table 17.4 First-line treatment of acne vulgaris

Acne severity	Mild		Moderate	
Lesion type	Comedonal	Papular/pustular	Papular/pustular	Nodular
	Topical retinoid or topical salicylic acid 2% wash (open comedones only)	Topical retinoid + topical antimicrobial	Oral antibiotic + topical retinoid +/– benzoyl peroxide	Oral isotretinoin

tion prescription products, such as clindamycin and benzoyl peroxide together. To date there is no evidence to suggest that combination products are more effective, but it is possible they may improve adherence, provided that they are not cost prohibitive. Patients and their caregivers should be cautioned as dryness may occur. Finally, oral isotretinoin may be of use in cases of moderately severe acne in individuals who are more psychologically affected by acne lesions or are more prone to induce scarring.

Pigmentation and scarring secondary to acne may fade over time but may require months to years for resolution, underscoring the need for prompt treatment of inflammatory disease. Scarring may be permanent and is generally not responsive to topical treatment. Laser treatment of scarring is possible; while the details are outside the scope of this chapter, treatment usually consists of multiple sessions and can be painful; thus the goals and tolerance of the patient should be considered prior to referral to a laser specialist.

Dermatologic Manifestation of Nutritional Deficiency

Clinical Evaluation

History Concern for nutritional deficiency in the ASD population stems from a multitude of factors. While children generally may be described as "picky eaters," review of the literature demonstrates food selectivity in children with ASD may arise secondary to sensory processing deficits, leading to intolerance of certain smells or textures, as well as due to ritualistic tendencies leading to food refusal [2]. Additionally, children with ASD may adhere to a restricted diet as part of an alternative or complementary approach to treatment. Though current data does not support its use [25], a gluten-free, casein-free diet is commonly used in an effort to reduce symptoms of ASD. This and other restrictive diets carry the risks of calcium, vitamin D, and other nutrient deficiencies.

Data to suggest nutritional deficiency is more prevalent in the ASD population compared to the general population is mixed. One study found that children with ASD are more likely to consume less of some nutrients, particularly vitamins A and C, but all children, both with ASD and control individuals, are at risk for some nutritional deficiencies, including vitamin D deficiency [16]. There are nevertheless case reports of children with ASD presenting with nutritional deficiency, two with scurvy (vitamin C deficiency) secondary to an extremely restricted diet [3, 26], and one reported case of eruptive xanthomas, yellow papules associated with hyperlipidemia, described in a boy in the setting of ASD, restricted diet, and accompanying hyperphagia of tolerated foods [34].

If dermatologic concerns arise, history obtained should include the patient's diet, which may be assessed by a food diary of 1–3 days. A parent or caregiver may provide insight into particular foods that are liked or disliked by the patient, any particular mealtime routines, or other dietary restrictions. Any changes in diet with an accompanying timeline may also be helpful.

Physical Examination We focus here on dermatologic findings of vitamin A and C deficiencies, respectively, as these have been suggested and/or reported in the literature and have prominent mucocutaneous findings, whereas vitamin D deficiency does not. Skin and hair findings of vitamin A deficiency include dry skin, sebaceous gland atrophy, hair fragility, and phrynoderma, follicular hyperkeratosis that manifests as follicular-based papules with a central hyperkeratotic plug [17]. Extradermatologic findings are largely ophthalmic and are in fact more prominent and concerning. Dryness of the cornea and conjunctiva as well as night blindness should prompt ophthalmic evaluation.

Findings concerning for vitamin C deficiency include bleeding or eroded gingivae, petechiae, ecchymoses, and follicular hyperkeratosis. "Corkscrew" hairs with perifollicular erythema are a classic finding. Outside of the skin, effects can be numerous and profound, including poor growth and joint pain secondary to osteopenia, anemia, and hemorrhage.

Studies Clinical diagnosis is often sufficient. Laboratory studies to confirm can include serum levels; less than 20 μg/dL retinol is consistent with vitamin A deficiency. Less than 0.2 mg/dL ascorbic acid is consistent with vitamin C deficiency [17]. In both cases, serum measurements may be impacted by recent dietary intake, overall nutrition status, and presence of infection.

Treatment

Deficiencies can be corrected with changes to diet or supplementation. Vitamin A is found in green leafy vegetables, liver, kidney, egg yolk, and animal fat. Supplementation with vitamin A should be in collaboration with a nutrition specialist, as excess is possible given its fat solubility. While skin and hair findings will resolve, ophthalmic deficits may be permanent.

Vitamin C is found in fresh fruits and vegetables, particularly citrus fruits. Supplementation in children is 100 mg three times per day for 1 week and then 100 mg once daily until symptoms resolve [17]. Adults are treated with 300–1000 mg per day for 1 month.

While vitamin A is available as a capsule or by intramuscular injection, ascorbic acid is available as a capsule, powder, or liquid for oral intake or by subcutaneous injection. Dietary modifications may be achieved through a behavioral approach through work with a behavioral therapist, a speech/language pathologist, and/or a nutritionist. Supplementation should likewise adapt to the modality best tolerated by the patient.

Clinical Vignette # 1

A 10-year-old boy with ASD and his mother present with a concern for eczema. His mother notes that he incessantly scratches at his skin, particularly at the antecubital fossae. She is concerned that his skin in the affected areas is "whiter." The boy is otherwise well and has no known allergies or recent contact with irritants.

On exam the boy has erythematous papules and excoriations of the antecubital and popliteal fossae consistent with eczema, with post-inflammatory hypopigmentation. His mother notes that she has difficulty applying lotions or creams. While in the office, you try applying an ointment steroid, while the boy plays with a favorite toy. When this is successful, you instruct his mother to apply the ointment immediately after baths, to bathe in lukewarm water for short periods of time, and to bath him every other day if possible. You schedule a short-term follow-up to assess adherence and effect.

An Adult Approach to Common Conditions

Dermatologic concerns in patients with ASD are similar in both pediatric and adult patients. There is no data to suggest that SIB and nutritional deficiencies should not remain a concern for adult providers. Regarding pruritus and drug eruption, there is likewise no evidence to suggest distinctions in prevalence between pediatric and adult populations, though it should be noted that adults are more likely to have complex medical histories that are likely to impact both general health and the number of medications prescribed. In the general population, acne is more prevalent in the adolescent age group. It is nevertheless present in adults, and we would argue that patients who experience any barriers to care, including psychosocial such as may affect individuals with ASD, are more likely to experience acne into adulthood.

Finally, as is the case in all aspects of medical care of individuals with ASD, adulthood does not necessarily correspond with independence in medical decision-making. Patients may present for care with a parent or a guardian, and while the patient's wishes should always be considered first and foremost, attention should be paid to who has decision-making capacity.

Clinical Vignette # 2

A woman in her 20s presents with concern for moderately severe acne. She reports that she has been diagnosed with Asperger's disorder in the past. The decision is made to initiate isotretinoin. The patient reads and signs all necessary paperwork and completes bloodwork before receiving the prescription. You receive a phone call the following week from the woman's parents. They are in fact her legal guardians and must consent for all procedures, including signing the paperwork to initiate isotretinoin. You schedule the patient to return to the office with her parents, to explain the medication and obtain appropriate consent.

Clinical Pearls

- Repetitive or stereotypical behavior in patients with ASD may include self-injurious behavior such as skin picking.
- It is important to rule out primary causes of disease before attributing dermatologic complaints to clinical features of ASD, such as characteristic repetitive behavior.
- Adverse cutaneous drug reactions are common, particularly to antiepileptic and antibiotic medications.
- Most drug eruptions are self-limited and mild. Mucosal involvement, systemic symptoms including fever, and laboratory abnormalities should raise concern for a severe reaction.
- Acne is the most common dermatologic disorder of adolescence. Treatment in individuals with ASD should take into account both current treatment guidelines and the individual's motivation for and ability to adhere to treatment.
- Individuals with ASD may present with nutritional deficiency, such as vitamin A or C deficiency, secondary to restrictive diets.
- Both pediatric and adult patients with ASD may present with common dermatologic diseases that require an approach tailored to their unique situations.
- Adults with ASD may or may not have medical decision-making capacity required for procedures including biopsy as well as certain prescription medications.

References

1. Accordino RE, Lucarelli J, Yan AC. Cutaneous disease in autism spectrum disorder: a review. Pediatr Dermatol. 2015;32(4):455–60. PubMed PMID: 25824343.
2. Cermak SA, Curtin C, Bandini LG. Food selectivity and sensory sensitivity in children with autism spectrum disorders. J Am Diet Assoc. 2010;110(2):238–46. PubMed PMID: 20102851. Pubmed Central PMCID: 3601920.
3. Cole JA, Warthan MM, Hirano SA, Gowen CW Jr, Williams JV. Scurvy in a 10-year-old boy. Pediatr Dermatol. 2011;28(4):444–6. PubMed PMID: 20561240.
4. Das S, Reynolds RV. Recent advances in acne pathogenesis: implications for therapy. Am J Clin Dermatol. 2014;15(6):479–88. PubMed PMID: 25388823.
5. Drake LA, Dinehart SM, Farmer ER, Goltz RW, Graham GF, Hordinsky MK, et al. Guidelines of care for cutaneous adverse drug reactions. American Academy of Dermatology. J Am Acad Dermatol. 1996;35(3 Pt 1):458–61. PubMed PMID: 8784285.
6. DSM-5. Autism spectrum disorder. Diagnostic and statistical manual of mental disorders. 5th ed. Arlington: American Psychiatric Association; 2013.
7. Duerden EG, Oatley HK, Mak-Fan KM, McGrath PA, Taylor MJ, Szatmari P, et al. Risk factors associated with self-injurious behaviors in children and adolescents with autism spectrum disorders. J Autism Dev Disord. 2012;42(11):2460–70. PubMed PMID: 22422338.
8. Ellis EM, Ala'i-Rosales SS, Glenn SS, Rosales-Ruiz J, Greenspoon J. The effects of graduated exposure, modeling, and contingent social attention on tolerance to skin care products with two children with autism. Res Dev Disabil. 2006;27(6):585–98. PubMed PMID: 16242911.
9. Elmariah SB. Careful considerations concerning psychogenic itch. JAMA Intern Med. 2015;175(11):1861. PubMed PMID: 26524738.
10. Elmariah SB, Lerner EA. Topical therapies for pruritus. Semin Cutan Med Surg. 2011;30(2):118–26. PubMed PMID: 21767774. Pubmed Central PMCID: 3139917.
11. Erickson CA, Posey DJ, Stigler KA, Mullett J, Katschke AR, McDougle CJ. A retrospective study of memantine in children and adolescents with pervasive developmental disorders. Psychopharmacology. 2007;191(1):141–7. PubMed PMID: 17016714.
12. Ferguson J. Photosensitivity due to drugs. Photodermatol Photoimmunol Photomed. 2002;18(5):262–9. PubMed PMID: 12390668.
13. Hardan AY, Jou RJ, Handen BL. A retrospective assessment of topiramate in children and adolescents with pervasive developmental disorders. J Child Adolesc Psychopharmacol. 2004;14(3):426–32. PubMed PMID: 15650499.
14. Hertzman M. Galantamine in the treatment of adult autism: a report of three clinical cases. Int J Psychiatry Med. 2003;33(4):395–8. PubMed PMID: 15152789.
15. Hunt A, Shepherd C. A prevalence study of autism in tuberous sclerosis. J Autism Dev Disord. 1993;23(2):323–39. PubMed PMID: 8331050.
16. Hyman SL, Stewart PA, Schmidt B, Cain U, Lemcke N, Foley JT, et al. Nutrient intake from food in children with autism. Pediatrics. 2012;130(Suppl 2):S145–53. PubMed PMID: 23118245. Pubmed Central PMCID: 4536585.

17. Jen M, Yan AC. Syndromes associated with nutritional deficiency and excess. Clin Dermatol. 2010;28(6):669–85. PubMed PMID: 21034991.
18. Jick SS, Kremers HM, Vasilakis-Scaramozza C. Isotretinoin use and risk of depression, psychotic symptoms, suicide, and attempted suicide. Arch Dermatol. 2000;136(10):1231–6. PubMed PMID: 11030769.
19. Kardaun SH, Sekula P, Valeyrie-Allanore L, Liss Y, Chu CY, Creamer D, et al. Drug reaction with eosinophilia and systemic symptoms (DRESS): an original multisystem adverse drug reaction. Results from the prospective RegiSCAR study. Br J Dermatol. 2013;169(5):1071–80. PubMed PMID: 23855313.
20. Kroshinsky D. Adolescent dermatology. In: Goldstein MA, editor. The MassGeneral Hospital for children adolescent medicine handbook. New York: Springer; 2011. p. 43–9.
21. Kuhaneck HM, Chisholm EC. Improving dental visits for individuals with autism spectrum disorders through an understanding of sensory processing. Spec Care Dentist. 2012;32(6):229–33. PubMed PMID: 23095065.
22. Lang R, Didden R, Machalicek W, Rispoli M, Sigafoos J, Lancioni G, et al. Behavioral treatment of chronic skin-picking in individuals with developmental disabilities: a systematic review. Res Dev Disabil. 2010;31(2):304–15. PubMed PMID: 19963341.
23. Leekam SR, Nieto C, Libby SJ, Wing L, Gould J. Describing the sensory abnormalities of children and adults with autism. J Autism Dev Disord. 2007;37(5):894–910. PubMed PMID: 17016677.
24. Logan SL, Nicholas JS, Carpenter LA, King LB, Garrett-Mayer E, Charles JM. High prescription drug use and associated costs among Medicaid-eligible children with autism spectrum disorders identified by a population-based surveillance network. Ann Epidemiol. 2012;22(1):1–8. PubMed PMID: 22153288. Pubmed Central PMCID: 3240812.
25. Millward C, Ferriter M, Calver S, Connell-Jones G. Gluten- and casein-free diets for autistic spectrum disorder. Cochrane Database Syst Rev. 2008;(2):CD003498. PubMed PMID: 18425890. Pubmed Central PMCID: 4164915.
26. Monks G, Juracek L, Weigand D, Magro C, Cornelison R, Crowson AN. A case of scurvy in an autistic boy. J Drugs Dermatol JDD. 2002;1(1):67–9. PubMed PMID: 12847759.
27. Moore JW, Fisher WW, Pennington A. Systematic application and removal of protective equipment in the assessment of multiple topographies of self-injury. J Appl Behav Anal. 2004;37(1):73–7. PubMed PMID: 15154217. Pubmed Central PMCID: 1284479.
28. Ohtoshi S, Kitami Y, Sueki H, Nakada T. Utility of patch testing for patients with drug eruption. Clin Exp Dermatol. 2014;39(3):279–83. PubMed PMID: 24635061.
29. Oza VS, Marco E, Frieden IJ. Improving the dermatologic care of individuals with autism: a review of relevant issues and a perspective. Pediatr Dermatol. 2015;32(4):447–54. PubMed PMID: 25779667.
30. Paley K, Prevost N, English JC 3rd. Unna sleeve for neurotic excoriations. Cutis. 2010;85(3):149–52. PubMed PMID: 20408514.
31. Romanelli M, Rhodes A. Guanfacine-induced lichenoid drug eruption in a child with autism and attention deficit hyperactivity disorder. Pediatr Dermatol. 2014;31(5):614–5. PubMed PMID: 23869619.
32. Schieve LA, Gonzalez V, Boulet SL, Visser SN, Rice CE, Van Naarden Braun K, et al. Concurrent medical conditions and health care use and needs among children with learning and behavioral developmental disabilities, National Health Interview Survey, 2006–2010. Res Dev Disabil. 2012;33(2):467–76. PubMed PMID: 22119694.
33. Schneck J, Fagot JP, Sekula P, Sassolas B, Roujeau JC, Mockenhaupt M. Effects of treatments on the mortality of Stevens-Johnson syndrome and toxic epidermal necrolysis: a retrospective study on patients included in the prospective EuroSCAR Study. J Am Acad Dermatol. 2008;58(1):33–40. PubMed PMID: 17919775.
34. Sorrell J, Salvaggio H, Garg A, Guo L, Duck SC, Paller AS. Eruptive xanthomas masquerading as molluscum contagiosum. Pediatrics. 2014;134(1):e257–60. PubMed PMID: 24918225.
35. Stern RS. Clinical practice. Exanthematous drug eruptions. N Engl J Med. 2012;366(26):2492–501. PubMed PMID: 22738099.
36. Swanson L, Colven RM. Approach to the patient with a suspected cutaneous adverse drug reaction. Med Clin North Am. 2015;99(6):1337–48. PubMed PMID: 26476256.
37. Thiboutot D, Gollnick H, Bettoli V, Dreno B, Kang S, Leyden JJ, et al. New insights into the management of acne: an update from the global alliance to improve outcomes in acne group. J Am Acad Dermatol. 2009;60(5 Suppl):S1–50. PubMed PMID: 19376456.
38. Yosipovitch G, Bernhard JD. Clinical practice. Chronic pruritus. N Engl J Med. 2013;368(17):1625–34. PubMed PMID: 23614588.

Podiatry

18

Stuart E. Kigner, Archibald J. Loch, and Joseph H. Bahn

Introduction

Autism spectrum disorder (ASD) and other developmental disorders can present with a wide array of clinical findings that can be both diagnostic and sequelae of the disorder. Patients with ASD may present with several findings in the lower extremity and specifically in the foot and ankle that should be addressed by the treating provider.

Podiatrists may encounter several conditions or symptoms in patients with ASD, which include but are not limited to toe walking, hypotonia, pes planus, and cutaneous/nail lesions. By recognizing these conditions, providers can help ASD patients receive more prompt and appropriate treatment, leading to improved patient outcomes.

S. E. Kigner (✉)
Department of Orthopaedic Surgery, Massachusetts General Hospital, Boston, MA, USA
e-mail: SKIGNER@mgh.harvard.edu

A. J. Loch
Mercyhealth Hospital and Medical Center-Walworth, Lake Geneva, WI, USA

J. H. Bahn
Kaiser Permanente Northern California, Sacramento, CA, USA

Foot and Ankle Examination

History

The history for a patient with ASD presenting with foot and ankle concerns should begin with a focus on the patient and/or parents' chief concerns as well as their beliefs and attitudes toward the problem. Important areas to explore in the history include:

- Developmental milestones.
- Previous treatment and patient and/or parents' attitudes toward bracing if orthoses have been tried previously.
- Family history of foot disorders.
- Patient's physical activities including likes and dislikes regarding the activities and whether the foot disorder may be a barrier to physical activity.
- The shoe gear currently worn in the house and outside the house.
- How consistently the patient has been wearing the foot orthoses and performing prescribed exercises such as stretches for tight heel cords.
- The presence of pain or fatigue (which may occur in the absence of pain) in the feet, recognizing that pain under the arch and medial aspect of the foot may be the result of flatfeet.

E. P. Hazen, C. J. McDougle (eds.), *The Massachusetts General Hospital Guide to Medical Care in Patients with Autism Spectrum Disorder*, Current Clinical Psychiatry,
https://doi.org/10.1007/978-3-319-94458-6_18

- Children around the age of 10 years should be assessed for heel pain, which may be the result of calcaneal apophysitis.

Physical Examination

During the physical examination, the patient should be observed walking barefoot and wearing shoes, while the clinician looks for signs of toe walking, limping, or excessive foot pronation. The patient may also be observed walking at a faster than usual speed to see whether toe walking appears. While standing, the patient may be evaluated for a flexible or rigid flatfoot. This may be evaluated by externally rotating the leg or dorsiflexing the hallux (great toe) and then observing whether the arch appears higher.

Other important elements of the physical examination include evaluation of the following:

- Signs of hallux valgus (great toe points toward the second toe) or contracted or curling toes
- Toenails for signs of periungual fibromas, which are small soft growths around the nails (see Fig. 18.1)
- Areas of tenderness on palpation
- Tenderness and guarding when the joints are taken through their range of motion

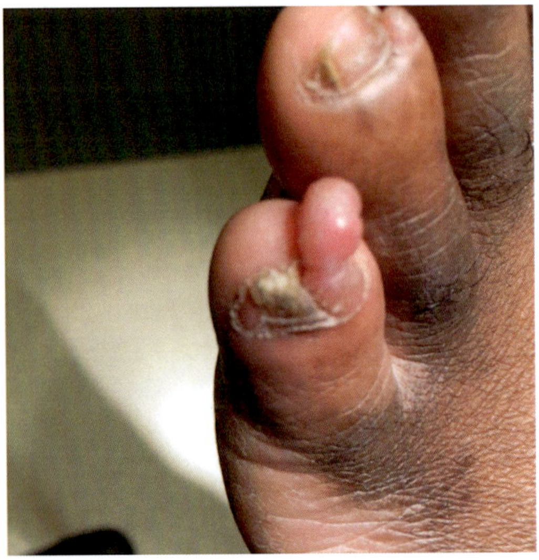

Fig. 18.1 Ungual fibromas

- Range of motion at the hip, knee, ankle, subtalar, midtarsal, and metatarsal phalangeal (MTP) joints
- Ankle dorsiflexion range of motion including the range of motion with the subtalar joint in neutral position with the knee flexed and extended to determine whether restricted dorsiflexion at the ankle is the result of a tight gastrocnemius
- Balance, posture, muscle strength and tone, and deep tendon reflexes
- Overall ligamentous laxity and for the presence of hypomobility
- Leg length discrepancy and scoliosis
- Cutaneous sensation and vascular status of feet
- Radiological (standing x-rays of the foot and ankle) and laboratory tests, as clinically indicated

Gait Evaluation

Evaluation of gait is a complex science that involves analyzing many moving segments in the body in real time. An in-depth study often involves a gait lab with high-speed cameras, sensors, and force plates. In-office examination should focus on findings easily appreciated by the naked eye. The body should be observed in the following segments: head, shoulders, upper extremities, back, hips, knees, ankles, and finally feet [54].

Many kinematic and kinetic studies of gait have been conducted on the pediatric ASD population in an effort to better classify and describe these clinical findings. The most common finding noted by most clinicians is toe walking, which will be addressed later in this section. It is important that adequate time is put into the evaluation since motor deficits and abnormalities may lead to a decrease in social interactions in individuals with ASD [10].

Kinematics

Kinematic evaluation often includes measurements of stride length and width, cadence, and velocity. A number of studies have shown that individuals with ASD have a greater likelihood of abnormal gait kinematics, which may affect their mobility. At least four studies have found increased step width in individuals with ASD [2, 31, 48, 62], and stride length has been noted to be reduced or have greater variability in the ASD population [2, 53, 58, 62]. The majority of studies that have evaluated cadence and velocity found no significant difference between typically developing and ASD populations. Asymmetry in hip, knee, and ankle positions throughout the gait cycle was noted by Eggleston and colleagues, who postulated that if this continues to adulthood, one extremity would compensate for the other resulting in a gait-related injury [63].

In one pediatric study, 21 children with ASD with a mean age of 6.1 years were filmed using high-speed cameras. The children with ASD had shorter strides, longer stance phase, increased hip flexion at toe off, and decreased knee extension at heel contact. The children with ASD also plantarflexed their ankles to a greater extent when the foot initially contacted the ground [53].

In another study, the kinematics of older teenagers and young adults ages 16–22 years with severe ASD were measured and compared to those of university undergraduates. The subjects with ASD demonstrated shorter step length, shorter stride length, shorter cadence, shorter gait cycle time, longer step time, longer stance phase, longer double support time, and greater percent of gait cycle in stance phase compared to the controls. In summary, the older teenagers and young adults with severe ASD took shorter steps, walked slower, and were in stance phase longer [58]. However, the findings of the studies have not always been consistent [6, 24].

As a matter of reassurance to parents, a study of a small group of adults with ASD found no differences in kinetic and kinematic measures including gait velocity, step length, cadence, step width, stance time, and vertical ground-reactive forces except that the ASD group had a decrease in ankle range of motion [14].

In summary, the results of the kinematic studies have not been consistent due to in part to differences in the ASD study populations, but it is felt that the gait abnormalities may reflect strategies to increase stability while participating in activities such as walking and running [24]. Eggleston et al. (2017) support the premise that evaluation of motor development and movement patterns should be considered in the process of diagnosing ASD [63].

Kinetics

Kinetics, which refers to the effect of forces on motion, has not been extensively studied in ambulation of those with ASD, but several studies have reported reduced lever arm moment in ankle joint dorsiflexion and plantar flexion [5]. The decreased moments were accompanied by decreased peak hip flexor and extensor moments [5]. The cumulative effect of these findings can increase vertical ground-reactive forces, which may increase the risk of injuries as a result of abnormal gait [2]. After evaluating three-dimensional ground reaction forces during gait in children with ASD compared with typically developing children, it was noted that children with ASD had reduced second peak vertical ground reaction forces (105%) compared with the typically developing children (110%). The children with ASD also had higher maximum breaking force, earlier maximum breaking force, and lower relative time to zero force during midstance. It was postulated that the earlier time to maximum breaking may reflect a lack of control during the breaking phase. These findings may be signs of gait instability in children with ASD and difficulties supporting their body weight during terminal stance [61].

Toe Walking

The major neurologic manifestation seen in the foot and ankle in individuals with ASD is toe walking. Toe walking was first described in the literature in 1943, and at one point it was thought to occur in upward of 80% of individuals with ASD [23]. With refinements in the diagnostic criteria for ASD over the last several decades, it is currently thought that the incidence of toe walking in this population is closer to 20% [3, 46]. Toe walking may be present in the early screening of the patient with ASD, though toe walking may be observed in some children with other developmental disorders as well those with otherwise normal development. Toe walking gait pattern may be disturbing to the parents of children with ASD, though many may find reassurance in the fact that toe walking generally resolves without treatment before adulthood.

Toe walking can be defined as the absence of heel strike during the contact phase of gait and the absence of full foot contact during the stance phase of gait [52]. Prolonged toe walking can result in a fixed deformity of the lower extremity, most commonly as a shortened Achilles tendon that limits the dorsiflexion of the ankle joint [3]. In a developmental pediatrics clinic, persistent toe walking was noted in 20.1% and tight heel cords in 12.0% of the children diagnosed with ASD with a mean age of 5.6 years. Persistent toe walking and tight heel cords have been shown to be more common in children with a DSM-IV diagnosis of autistic disorder than in those with a diagnosis of Asperger's disorder [3].

Several treatment options for toe walking have been described in the literature with acceptable results [44]. Some of the common treatments include stretching, physical therapy, casting, botulinum toxin injection, and surgical interventions. In one study, Stricker and colleagues found the outcome of Achilles tendon lengthening was superior to cast and brace treatment [49]. They also observed little improvement with cast and brace treatment compared to the non-treatment group and found recurrence after all three treatments.

Enstrom (2013) conducted a randomized controlled trial comparing the effectiveness of botulinum toxin A as an adjunct to casting treatment [11]. He found improvements in the dorsiflexion of the ankle joint in both groups but found no significant difference between the cast group and the cast with botulinum injection group.

Ruzbarsky et al. (2016) recommended observing the child under 5 years that is able to dorsiflex the ankle past 90°. If the child is 5 years or older and can dorsiflex the ankle greater than 10°, then observation would be an option, or the ankle could be placed in a cast in maximum dorsiflexion for 6 weeks. If the child is 5 years of age or older and cannot dorsiflex the ankle 10°, then serial casts can be applied every 1–2 weeks increasing dorsiflexion during each cast change until no additional correction is needed or adequate dorsiflexion is achieved. These investigators noted that serial casting may not be effective in children older than 7 years. Surgical lengthening of the gastrocsoleus muscle or Achilles tendon would be considered when casting or dorsiflexion of the ankle to 90° is not successful [44].

Morozova and colleagues (2017) have noted that it is not known whether toe walking children progress to a normal heel-toe gait or develop a fixed contracture of the heel cord and question whether toe walking may have a negative psychosocial impact on the child and family [66]. For additional information on toe walking see Chap. 16.

Orthoses

In a study involving 154 children with ASD, Ming et al. [35] identified a prevalence of hypotonia of 63% in children ages 2–6 years and 38% in children ages 7–18 years of age. In a smaller study, Calhoun et al. identified hypotonia in 33% of children with ASD ages 5–9 years old [5]. The most commonly agreed-upon characteristics of hypotonia in a survey of pediatric physical therapists and occupational therapists were hypermobile joints, increased flexibility/muscle extensibility, and decreased strength [33, 34]. Weber et al. noted that hypotonia and ligamentous laxity may result in inadequate stability affecting postural control, lower extremity malalignment, and orthopedic disorders more proximal on the kinetic chain which may include disorders of the knee, hip, or back [56]. Ozgen et al. evaluated morphological features in 224 children ages 3–18 years with ASD in the Netherlands with controls from the local area noting that the children with ASD had a higher prevalence of hypermobile/hyperlax joints and pes planus compared to a control group of children from the general population in the Netherlands [38].

The hypotonia observed in children with ASD may be addressed through the use of physical therapy [20], which may involve orthoses. A survey of Canadian physical therapists indicated that the most commonly identified condition indicated for foot orthoses was hypotonia (91% of respondents) and the most commonly cited indications for foot orthoses were abnormal lower extremity alignment and the appearance of excessive subtalar joint pronation and calcaneovalgus [22]. Weber et al. reported in 2014 that it is the current standard of care to treat hypotonia with foot orthoses and supra-malleolar orthoses (SMO) to promote stability and functional mobility [56].

Several studies have demonstrated a positive effect of orthoses on flatfeet. Children age 18 months to 5 years with hypotonia and flatfeet with developmental delays (including ASD and tuberous sclerosis) participating in gross motor therapy developed a higher arch index (arch width/heel width while barefoot) after wearing custom foot orthoses for 6 months compared to the children that did not wear the foot orthoses [43]. The use of flexible SMO resulted in improvement after 3 weeks and 7 weeks in the Standing and Walking, Running, and Jumping dimension of the Gross Motor Function Measure in children with a mean age of 5 years 10 months with Down syndrome, indicative of improvement in postural stability [32]. "Growing pain" frequency and degree of pain decreased when children wore foot orthoses for 1 month and 3 months. Despite the absence of a control group, the authors reported a decrease in pain compared to the baseline frequency of pain [25].

University of California Biomechanics Laboratory (UCBL) foot orthoses reduced eversion of the calcaneus indicative of a decrease in foot pronation during the stance phase of gait in children with flatfeet seen in a pediatric orthopedic clinic between the ages of 4 and 11 years [26]. Children with Down syndrome wearing SMO demonstrated a significant increase in the Gross Motor Function Measure in the Standing and Walking, Running, and Jumping dimensions compared to a control group wearing shoes only. It was concluded that a flexible SMO increased postural stability in children with Down syndrome [32]. The center of gravity sway velocity while balancing on one foot was reduced in children with flatfeet, especially with the eyes closed in children that wore the foot orthoses. It was felt that wearing the foot orthoses may have enhanced proprioception or tactile sense from the sole [25]. The orthoses should stabilize and enhance alignment of osseous and soft tissue structures, allowing the foot to function as a more rigid lever before heel off [47]. Enhancing the child's stability through the use of the orthoses may facilitate development of more complex motor tasks. This may in turn facilitate the child's ability to explore the environment and enhance social integration.

However, it has been noted that many of the studies investigating the efficacy of nonsurgical interventions to address the pediatric flexible flatfoot did not include a control group and therefore it is difficult to determine whether radiographic and postural changes were the result of natural maturation of the arch [30]. A randomized controlled trial involving children between the ages of 7 and 11 years provided with custom-made and ready-made foot orthoses to treat flexible hyperpronation of the feet found after 3 and 12 months, there was no improvement in motor skills, exercise efficiency, self-perception, and pain [59]. A Cochrane review in 2012 indicated that there was no evidence from randomized trials supporting any nonsurgical treatment, including the use of foot orthoses, to treat asymptomatic flatfeet in children [42]. Looper et al. indicated that the SMO may limit the ability to problem solve and acquire motor skills necessary for crawling and kneeling [27] in children with Down syndrome and that the SMO may limit motion in the foot and ankle diminishing this learning experience while learning to walk [27]. They recommended postponing the use of SMO until the child is able to walk independently [27].

There is no strong evidence supporting the use of a therapeutic shoe to address flexible flatfeet. Gould et al. provided children ages 11–14 months with straight last shoes (control group), straight last shoes with pads under the arch, orthopedic shoes, and shoes with a longitudinal arch support. At age 5 years, there was no difference between the groups with flatfeet, though it should be noted that the study had a high dropout rate of 58% [13]. In a study of children that had been independent walkers for 0–5 months, plantar pressures wearing the most flexible shoe (highest torsional flexibility) in the study were similar to those walking barefoot, which may enhance proprioception for children learning to walk [18]. Epidemiological studies have indicated that children that wear shoes have a greater prevalence of flatfeet [40, 45].

Parents frequently present to a physician's office concerned with their child's flatfeet. However, Pfeiffer and colleagues found that the prevalence of flatfeet was 54% at age 3 years and 24% at age 6 years [39]. It therefore may be difficult to determine whether the flatfoot is physiological or pathological. Pfeiffer classified weight-bearing heel valgus between 5° and 20° physiological and greater than or equal to 20° a pathological flatfoot. He recommended treatment for children with symptomatic or pathological flatfeet and concluded that 90% of the orthoses worn by children in the study were unnecessary [39]. In a review article on the effect of children's shoes on gait, Wegener et al. postulated that shoes may reduce proprioception feedback [57]. Buckland et al. also questioned whether the sole of the shoe may act as mechanical filter reducing proprioceptive feedback compared to barefoot walking [4].

It has been proposed that children wear orthoses to maintain the proper alignment of the lower extremity, while osseous and soft tissue structures are developing [19]. Some researchers have suggested that there may be a window of opportunity for early intervention, while the bones and soft tissue structures in the foot are developing [8], while others have recommended considering treatment of some flexible flatfeet by maintaining the foot in better alignment, while the bones are developing during the endochondral ossification process [15]. However, Dare et al. indicated that while orthoses may be an option in the treatment of a symptomatic child with flatfeet, there is no evidence that the orthoses can change the natural history of arch development [9]. It is also noted that it has not been possible to determine which children with flatfeet will be symptomatic when they are adults [9, 15].

Given the conflicting views discussed above, it may be reasonable to recommend the use of orthoses for children with ASD who are symptomatic or exhibit signs of an antalgic gait. Consideration may be given to also recommending the use of orthoses for children with a moderately severe valgus rear foot who are not very physically active or who have a strong family history of foot disorders given the high prevalence of obesity in children with ASD and low participation in physical activity [7, 12, 29, 60]. Physically inactive children with mild to moderate deformities may try orthoses on a trial basis. Consideration may be given to the use of a prefabricated device for these children. Active children with mild to moderate deformities may be monitored for symptoms or a change in activity level.

The selection of the type of orthotic required will depend on the level and extent of the deformity. If the child has a flatfoot with mild valgus orientation of the rear foot, then a foot orthotic may be sufficient. Jay and Schoenhaus have suggested that controlling the forefoot and rear foot may require not just controlling the frontal plane (inversion/eversion of the foot) but also the transverse (adduction/abduction) and sagittal planes (plantarflexion/dorsiflexion) [19].

If there is a more severe valgus deformity, then a UCBL, SMO, or ankle foot orthotic (AFO) may be necessary to provide medial-lateral stability. Frequent follow-up visits are necessary to reassess the effectiveness of the orthotic. During the visit the child and parent should be asked whether there have been any changes in physical activities and how often the orthotic is worn. The fit of the orthotic should be assessed, and skin should be inspected for signs of pressure such as redness, blisters, or callus. Children with ASD should be encouraged to wear a long seamless tube sock that can wick perspiration away from the skin. Velcro closure or a tie shoe with extra depth and a removable insole is preferable. A wider shoe such as a skateboard shoe may be helpful depending on the type of orthotic. Tamminga noted that the Surestep SMO is composed of a thin flexible plastic and has a trim line medially proximal to the first metatarsal head and laterally distal to the fifth metatarsal head, while the Cascade DAFO#4 is fabricated from custom impressions of the child's feet and has a full length footplate. Tamminga felt that this did not allow for as much mobility within the orthotic [50]. The role of the Sensory Dynamic Orthosis in the treatment of children with ASD has not been established.

Dermatological Manifestations of the Foot

Dermatological manifestations of the foot in those with ASD are most commonly observed in individuals with tuberous sclerosis. The 2012 International Tuberous Sclerosis Complex Consensus Conference designated ungual fibromas (≥2) a major feature in the clinical diagnostic criteria [64]. Annual skin examinations of children with tuberous sclerosis were recommended [64]. The incidence of ASD in individuals with tuberous sclerosis was noted to be about 25% (60). Ungual fibromas appear in individuals with tuberous sclerosis with an incidence of 23% in children age 5–14 years, 68% in adolescents age 15–29 years, and 88% in adults ≥ age 30 years) [55]. Jozwiak did not note any periungual fibromas in children under the age of 2 years [21]. Ungual fibromas are among the last skin lesions to appear [1]. They may appear as late as the fifth decade [55].

Multiple ungual fibromas were present in 75% of individuals with tuberous sclerosis [55]. The mean number of fibromas present was 3.6 [1]. Ungual fibromas are more common in toenails than fingernails [1]. Ungual fibromas appear as pink papules resembling garlic cloves, globoid, fusiform, or vermiform [1]. They originate under the proximal or lateral nail fold [1]. A groove may be present in the underlying nail plate approximately the width of the fibroma [1, 52]. Ungual fibromas appear as pink papules originating under the nail plate [1]. Other dermatological features observed on the toes of individuals with tuberous sclerosis include splinter hemorrhages, longitudinal leukonychia, and red comets [1].

Treatment of a symptomatic ungual fibroma may involve removal of the nail followed by excision or punch biopsy [41]. The 2012 International Tuberous Sclerosis Complex Consensus Conference indicated that ablative laser or surgical excision may be considered if the lesions are symptomatic or larger than 3 mm [65].

Coffin-Siris syndrome has been associated with ASD. A clinical characteristic is a hypoplastic/absent toenail on the fifth toe [17]. It is also associated with hypotonia, microcephaly, feeding difficulties, and coarse facial features.

Musculoskeletal Manifestations of ASD

Foot Morphology

One large study of children with ASD showed a higher incidence of the following foot deformities compared to age-matched controls [38].

Syndactyly toes[a]
Hallux valgus[a]
Widely spaced toes
2nd toe longer than first
Pes planus[a]
Sandal gap (between digits 1 and 2)[a]
Hypermobile/hyperlax joints[a]

[a]Denotes found to be more common in male ASD patients

Coffin-Siris syndrome: Hypoplastic middle and distal phalanges are noted particularly on the fifth toe [17, 28].

XXYY syndrome: In a series of 95 males with a mean age of 14.9 years, common physical features included clinodactyly (present in 80% of children under age 10 years), pes planus, and hypotonia [51]. Clinodactyly is the bending of the finger or toe toward the adjacent digit. Most commonly the fifth digit will point toward the fourth.

Osseous

Although there is conflicting data, an increased risk of several bone abnormalities has been noted in the ASD population. Bone mineral density (BMD) has been shown to be decreased in boys with ASD at the femoral neck and hip, even after controlling for maturity, BMI, decreased vitamin D intake, decreased exercise, and increased sedentary behavior [37]. Evaluation of cortical thickness of femoral heads of boys with ASD revealed a 25–30% decrease in cortical thickness compared to controls [16].

The Danish National Hospital Register indicated that over the course of 30 years, 11.9% of individuals with ASD had fractures compared with 24.7% in the comparison group. In the ASD group, 1.7% had a foot fracture compared to 4.2% in the control group. The reason for the lower rate of fractures among those with ASD shown in this study is not known, but it is noted that individuals with ASD may be more likely to live in institutions and less likely to drive or participate in sports and they may use fewer tools and have lower consumption of alcohol [36].

In another study, both male and female subjects with ASD across a broad age range had a higher odds ratio for hip fractures, and adult females had a higher risk of forearm and spine fractures compared to individuals without ASD. It was felt that this may be the result of reduced physical activity and vitamin D intake and the use of particular medications. However, boys had a lower risk of forearm fractures, which are usually the result of trauma associated with participation in sports. This may be the result of decreased participation in sports by children with ASD [37]. Young adults with ASD and a history of trauma resulting in a painful foot or limping should be evaluated to rule out a fracture.

Clinical Vignette # 1

A 10-year-old boy with ASD and global developmental delay presented to clinic for evaluation of bilateral foot pain in the setting of recent surgical intervention for pes planus deformity. He underwent calcaneal lengthening osteotomy (Evans) with posterior tibial tendon transfer on the left foot at another local hospital. The patient continued to complain of foot pain and difficulty with walking.

On examination, he displayed bilateral flexible flatfeet with normal subtalar range of motion and tight heel cords bilaterally and multiple healed surgical scars on the left foot. Gait evaluation revealed externally rotated feet with a higher arch on the left. Plain film radiographs revealed the presence of bone allograft at the anterior aspect of the calcaneus on the left foot and collapse of the arch on the right foot.

Wearing sturdy shoes was recommended, and he was prescribed bilateral UCBL orthotics to provide him with better arch support and relief of foot pain. The patient was followed every 6 months for adjustment and modification of the UCBL. He tolerated the orthotics well without significant complaints. He was able to fully participate in gym class and other activities without pain.

At age 15, he returned to clinic with the complaint of intermittent right foot pain. His symptoms were being managed with modifications to the UCBL and seemed to improve with aggressive physical therapy and rest. He continued to have foot pain and subsequently developed knee pain as well. An MRI was obtained and lab work was ordered to rule out a rheumatologic etiology. Lab findings were negative with the exception of a vitamin D deficiency.

Two years later at a follow-up visit, the patient had discontinued the use of his UCBL due to discomfort and no improvement of his pain. The pain prevented him from participating in activities at school and home. After careful evaluation, surgical intervention was recommended on the right foot. Plain film radiographs revealed complete closure of his physeal plates. Surgical intervention involved right medial calcaneal slide osteotomy and medial cuneiform osteotomy with opening wedge and heel cord lengthening. Postoperatively, the patient was placed into a short-leg cast and was non-weight bearing for 6 weeks. He recovered well from the operation, and at his final postoperative visit, he was able to bear full weight on his right foot without pain. Final follow-up radiographs showed improvement of the medial arch and healing of the osteotomy sites.

Clinical Pearls

- Ungual fibromas often present in the second decade of life in individuals with ASD and comorbid tuberous sclerosis complex.
- Hypotonia is found in approximately 63% of children ages 2–6 years and 38% of children 7–18 years with ASD [35].
- Gait evaluation is an important aspect of the exam in the pediatric patient with ASD. Gait abnormalities may be considered in the diagnostic process and should be addressed in the treatment recommendations.
- Gait abnormalities are common in individuals with ASD, with toe walking being the most common. The majority of children with toe walking will have resolution of this symptom by adulthood.
- Symptomatic flatfoot should be treated with orthotic/bracing and physical therapy.
- There is little evidence to support the use of orthoses to treat asymptomatic flatfeet.
- The optimal age to initiate the use of orthoses has not been established and will vary for each child.
- More flexible shoes may aid in proprioception in early walkers.
- There are no studies demonstrating that the use of orthoses in children can prevent foot disorders in adults.

References

1. Aldrich S. Acral lesions in tuberous sclerosis complex: insights into pathogenesis. J Am Acad Dermatol. 2010;63:244–51.
2. Ambrosini D. Motion analysis of patients with infantile autism. Gait Posture. 1998;7:188.
3. Barrow W, Jaworski M, Accardo P. Persistent toe walking in autism. J Child Neurol. 2011;26(5):619–21.
4. Buckland M, Slevin C, Hafer J, Choate C, Krazeski A. The effect of torsional shoe flexibility on gait and stability in children learning to walk. Pediatr Phys Ther. 2014;26:411–7.
5. Calhoun M, Longworth M, Chester V. Gait patterns in children with autism. Clin Biomech. 2011;26:200–6.
6. Chester V, Calhoun M. Gait symmetry in children with autism. Autism Res Treat. 2012;2012:1–6.
7. Curtin C, Anderson S, Must A, Bandini L. The prevalence of obesity in children with autism: a secondary data analysis using nationally representative data from the National Survey of Children's health. BMC Pediatr. 2010;10:11.
8. D'Amico J. The flat-footed child- to treat or not to treat. J Am Podiatr Med Assoc. 2009;99(3):267.
9. Dare D, Dodwell E. Pediatric flatfoot: cause epidemiology, assessment, and treatment. Curr Open Pediatr. 2014;26(1):93–100.
10. Downey R, Rapport M. Motor activity in children with autism: a review of current literature. Pediatr Phys Ther. 2012;24:2–20.
11. Enstrom P. Botulinum toxin A does not improve the results of cast treatment for idiopathic toe-walking. JBJS. 2013;95:400–7.
12. Evans A. The flat-footed child-to treat or not to treat. J Am Podiatr Med Assoc. 2008;98(5):386–93.
13. Gould N, Morelan M, Alvarez R, Trevino S, Fenwick J. Development of the child's arch. Foot Ankle. 1989;9(5):241–5.
14. Hallett M, Lebiedowska M, Thomas S, Stanhope S, Denckla M, Rumsey J. Locomotion of autistic adults. Arch Neurol. 1993;50:1304–8.
15. Harris E. The natural history and pathophysiology of flexible flatfoot. Clin Podiatr Med Surg. 2010;27:1–23.
16. Hediger M, Englan L. Reduced cortical thickness in boys with autism or autism spectrum disorder. J Autism Dev Disord. 2008;38:848–56.
17. Hersh J. Childhood autism in a female with coffin Siris syndrome. Dev Behav Pediatr. 1982;3(4):249–52.
18. Hillstrom H. Effect of shoe flexibility on plantar loading in children learning to walk. J Am Podiatr Med Assoc. 2013;103(4):297–305.
19. Jay R, Schoenhaus H. The dynamic stabilizing innersole system (DSIS): the management of hyperpronation in children. JFAS. 1995;34(2):124–31.
20. Jeste S. The neurology of autism spectrum disorders. Curr Opin Neurol. 2011;24:132–9.
21. Jozwiak S, Schwartz R, Janniger C, Michalowicz R, Chmielek J. Skin lesions in children with tuberous sclerosis complex: their prevalence, natural course, and diagnostic significance. Int J Dermatol. 1998;37:911–7.
22. Kane K. Foot orthoses for pediatric flexible flatfoot: evidence and current practices among Canadian physical therapists. Pediatr Phys Ther. 2015:53–9.
23. Kanner L. Autistic disturbances of affective contact. Acta Paedopsychiatr. 1968;40(4):100–36.
24. Kindregan D, Gallagher L, Gormlet J. Gait deviations in children with autism spectrum disorders: a review. Autism Res Treat. 2015;2015:1–8.
25. Lee H. Effect of custom molded foot orthoses on foot pain and balance in children with symptomatic flexible flat feet. Ann Rehabil Med. 2015;39(6):905–13.

26. Leung A, Mak A, Evans J. Biomechanical gait evaluation of the immediate effect of orthotic treatment for flexible flat foot. Prosthet Orthot Int. 1998;22: 25–34.
27. Looper J, Ulrich D. Effect of treadmill training and supramalleolar orthosis use on motor skill development in infants with Down syndrome: a randomized controlled trial. Phys Ther. 2010;90(3):382–90.
28. Lucaya J, Garcia-Conesa A, Bosch-Banyeras J, Pons-Peradejordi G. The Coffin-Siris syndrome. Pediatr Radiol. 1981;11:35–8.
29. MacDonald M, Esposito P, Ulrich D. The physical activity patterns of children with autism. BMC Res Notes. 2011;4:442.
30. MacKenzie A, Rome K, Evans A. The efficacy of non-surgical interventions for pediatric flexible flat foot: a critical review. J Pediatr Orthop. 2012;32:830–4.
31. Manning J, Callow P. Finger and toe ratios in humans and mice: implications for the aetiology of diseases influenced by HOX genes. Med Hypotheses. 2003;60(3):340–3.
32. Martin K. Effects of supramalleolar orthoses on postural stability in children with Down syndrome. Dev Med Child Neurol. 2004;46:406–11.
33. Martin K, Kaltenmark T, Lewallem A, Smith C, Yoshida A. Clinical characteristics of hypotonia: a survey of pediatric physical and occupational therapists. Pediatr Phys Ther. 2007;19:217–26.
34. Martin K, McCoy S, Wrotniak B. Diagnosis dialog for pediatric physical therapists: hypotonia, developmental coordination disorder, and pediatric obesity as examples. Pediatr Phys Ther. 2013;25:431–43.
35. Ming X, Brimacombe M, Wagner G. Prevalence of motor impairment in autism spectrum disorders. Brain Dev. 2007;29:565–70.
36. Mouridsen S, Rich B, Isager T. Fractures in individuals with and without a history of infantile autism. A Danish register study based on hospital discharge diagnosis. J Autism Dev Disord. 2012;42:619–24.
37. Neumeyer A, Gates A, Ferrone C, Lee H, Misra M. Bone density in peripubertal boys with autism spectrum disorders. J Autism Dev Disord. 2013;43(7):1623–9.
38. Ozgen H, Hellmenan G, et al. Morphologic features in children with autism spectrum disorders: a matched case control study. J Autism Dev Disord. 2011;41:23–31.
39. Pfieffer M, Kotz R, Ledl T. Prevalence of flatfoot in preschool aged children. Paediatrics. 2006;118:634–9.
40. Rao U. The influence of footwear on the prevalence of flat foot. JBJS [Br]. 1992;74–B:525–7.
41. Rich P. Nail surgery. In: Bolognia J, Jorizzo J, Rapini R, editors. Dermatology. 2nd ed. London: Elsevier Health Sciences; 2008. p. 2435–44.
42. Rome K, Ashford RL, Evans A. Non-surgical interventions for paediatric pes planus (review). Cochrane Collab. 2012;(11):1–31.
43. Ross C, Shore S. The effect of gross motor therapy and orthotic intervention in children with hypotonia and flexible flatfeet. J Prosthet Orthop. 2011;23(3):149–56.
44. Ruzbarsky J, Scher D, Dodwell E. Toe walking: causes, epidemiology, assessment and treatment. Curr Opin Pediatr. 2016;28:40–6.
45. Sachithanandam V. The influence of footwear on the prevalence of flat foot. JBJS [Br]. 1995;77 B:254–7.
46. Schattuck P. The contribution of diagnostic substitution to the growing administrative prevalence of autism in US special education. Paediatrics. 2006;117:1028–37.
47. Scherer P. Pediatric flexible flatfoot and functional orthoses. Recent advances in orthotic therapy. 1st ed. Albany: Lower Extremity Review; 2011. p. 69–87.
48. Shetreat-Klein M, et al. Abnormalities of joint mobility and gait in children with autism spectrum disorders. Brain Dev. 2014;36:91–6.
49. Stricker S, Angulo J. Idiopathic toe walking: a comparison of treatment methods. J Pediatr Orthop. 1998;18:293–8.
50. Tamminga J, Martin K, Miller E. Single-subject design study of 2 types of supramalleolar orthoses for young children with Down syndrome. Pediatr Phys Ther. 2012;24:278–84.
51. Tartaglia N, et al. A new look at XXYY syndrome: medical and psychological features. Am J Med Genet. 2008;146A:1509–22.
52. Van Kuijk A, Kosters R, Vugts M, Gerurts A. Treatment for idiopathic toe walking: a systematic review of the literature. J Rehabil Med. 2014;46:945–57.
53. Vilensky J. Gait disturbances in patients with autistic behavior. Arch Neurol. 1981;38:646–9.
54. Warnock A, Raducanu R, Deheer P. Lower extremity pediatric history and physical examination. Clin Podiatr Med Surg. 30:461–73.
55. Webb D, Clarke A, Fryer A, Osborne J. The cutaneous features of tuberous sclerosis: a population study. Br J Dermatol. 1996;135:1–5.
56. Weber A, Martin K. Efficacy of orthoses for children with hypotonia: a systematic review. Pediatr Phys Ther. 2014;26:38–47.
57. Wegener C, Hunt A, Vanwanseele B, Burns J, Smith R. Effect of children's shoes on gait: a systematic review and meta-analysis. J Foot Ankle Res. 2011;4:3.
58. Weiss M, Moran M, Parker M, Foley J. Gait analysis of teenagers and young adults diagnosed with autism and severe verbal communication disorders. Front Integr Neurosci. 2013;7(33):1–10.
59. Whitford D, Esterman A. A randomized controlled trial of two types of in-shoe orthoses in children with flexible excess pronation of the feet. Foot Ankle Int. 2007;28(6):715–23.
60. Yeagerman S, Cross M, Positano R, Doyle S. Evaluation and treatment of symptomatic pes planus. Curr Opin Pediatr. 23:60–7.
61. Hasas C, Jailani R, Tahir N. The analysis of three-dimensional ground reaction forces during gait in children with autism spectrum disorders. Res Dev Disabil. 2017;66:55–63.

62. Lim B, O'Sullivan D, Choi B, Kim M. Comparative gait analysis between children with autism and age-matched controls: analysis with temporal-spatial and foot pressure variables. J Phys Ther Sci. 2016;28:286–92.
63. Eggleston J, Harry J, Hickman R, Dufek J. Analysis of gait symmetry during over-ground walking in children with autism spectrum disorder. Gait Posture. 2017;55:162–6.
64. Northrup H, Krueger D. Tuberous sclerosis complex diagnostic criteria update: recommendations of the 2012 international tuberous sclerosis complex consensus conference. Pediatr Neurol. 2013;49:243–54.
65. Teng J, Cowen E, Wataya-Kaneda M. Dermatologic and dental aspects of the 2012 international tuberous sclerosis complex consensus statements. JAMA Dermatol. 2014;150(10):1095–101.
66. Morozova O, Chang T, Brown M. Toe walking: when do we need to worry. Curr Probl Adolesc Health Care. 2017;47(7):156–60.

Index

E. P. Hazen, C. J. McDougle (eds.), *The Massachusetts General Hospital Guide to Medical Care in Patients with Autism Spectrum Disorder*, Current Clinical Psychiatry,
https://doi.org/10.1007/978-3-319-94458-6

P